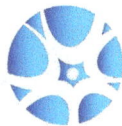

FNNR
Foundation for Neurofeedback
& Neuromodulation Research

Also by Helena Bester

Help, My Kind Makeer Iets

Help, my Child is Causing Chaos: Hyperactive or creative?

How to cope with ADHD

New Hope for ADHD in Children and Adults: A Practical Guide

Neurofeedback. The non-invasive alternative: An Intervention for
ADHD, anxiety, depression, dyslexia, epilepsy, fibromyalgia, PTSD and
other causes of discomfort

neurofeedback

the non-invasive alternative

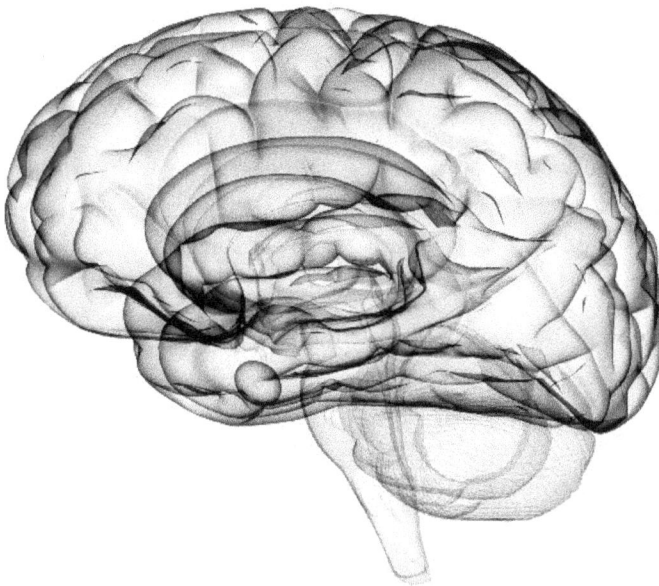

2nd edition

An intervention for ADHD, anxiety, depression, dyslexia, epilepsy, fibromyalgia, PTSD and other causes of discomfort.

Helena Bester, BCN

Foreword by Sebern F. Fisher

FNNR Publications

Longo, R. E., & Soutar, R. (2020). *Becoming certified in neurofeedback: A guide to the neurofeedback mentoring process for mentors and mentees.* Foundation for Neurofeedback and Neuromodulation Research.

Sokhadze, E., & Casanova, M. F. (Eds.). (2019). *Autism spectrum disorder: Neuromodulation, neurofeedback, and sensory integration approaches to research and treatment.* Foundation for Neurofeedback and Neuromodulation Research.

Martins-Mourao, A., & Kerson, C. (Eds.). (2017). *Alpha-theta neurofeedback in the 21st century: A handbook for clinicians and researchers* (2nd ed.). Foundation for Neurofeedback and Neuromodulation Research.

Soutar, R., & Longo, R. E. (2011). *Doing neurofeedback: An introduction.* The ISNR Research Foundation.

Hammond, D. C., & Gunkelman, J. (2011). *The art of artifacting.* The ISNR Research Foundation.

Carmichael, J. (2011). *Multi-component treatment for post-traumatic stress disorder, including strategies from clinical psycho-physiology and applied neuroscience.* The ISNR Research Foundation.

Donaldson, S. (2012). *The other side of the desk.* The ISNR Research Foundation.

Thompson, M., Thompson, J., & Wenqing, W. (2009). *ADD center Brodmann areas booklet.* The ISNR Research Foundation.

Neurofeedback
The Non-Invasive Alternative

An intervention for ADHD, anxiety, depression, epilepsy, insomnia,
dyslexia, fibromyalgia, PTSD and other causes of discomfort

2nd Edition

Helena Bester, BCN
Foreword by Sebern F. Fisher

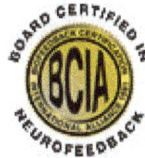

Publisher:

The FNNR

The Foundation for Neurofeedback & Neuromodulation
Research 2131 Woodruff Rd, Ste 2100 #121 Greenville,
SC 29607 http://www.theFNNR.org

Correspondence: admin@theFNNR.org

Publisher:
The FNNR
The Foundation for Neurofeedback & Neuromodulation Research 2131 Woodruff Rd, Ste 2100 #121 Greenville, SC 29607 http://www.theFNNR.org. Correspondence: Admin@theFNNR.org
Layout Design: Megan Stevens
Correspondence: Publishing@theFNNR.org

Neurofeedback: The Non-Invasive Alternative
An intervention for ADHD, anxiety, depression, epilepsy, insomnia, dyslexia, fibromyalgia, PTSD, and other causes of discomfort
Second sedition, first impression 2020 ISBN: 978-0-9978194-6-5 (print)
Cover concept: Isabel Viseu Cover design: Alesha Otto

Exclusive distribution by: BMED Press, LLC

Knowing
others is wisdom
Knowing yourself is
enlightenment

– Lao Tzu

Contents

Chapter 3
Brain Basics and Neuro-Anatomical Structures

Chapter 4
Neurophysiological Basis of the EEG; the Role of Neurotransmitters; Instrumentation; Electronics

Part Two

We have knowledge
Beyond the scope of words
Once we turn inward
And reach beyond the mind

For you who have gentled the black horse
And brought me white horse longing

Foreword

It is time to think differently about the treatment of emotional suffering and mental illness. We need only look at the statistics. The World Health Organization estimates that by 2020 there will be a death by suicide every 20 seconds. In the last 20 years, the suicide rate in the United States has gone up over 28%. Suicide is the fourth leading cause of death for young people in South Africa. 90% of suicides relate to mental illness.

Suicide is the leading statistical indicator used by Thomas Insel, former director of the National Institute of Mental Health to show that we are failing in our treatment of mental illness and to suggest that we have to think of mental disorders and behavioral disorders first and foremost as brain disorders. He goes further. The subtitle of his article Faulty Circuits published in Scientific American (April, 2010) reads "Neuroscience is revealing the malfunctioning connections underlying psychological disorders and forcing psychiatrists to rethink the causes of mental illness" It is true that neuroscience, particularly in the field of PTSD, is revealing malfunctioning brain circuitries, but it is less true that these discoveries are propelling widespread changes in the way psychiatrists or psychotherapists think about causes and about treatments.

As you are about to discover when you read the book in your hands, this is a tragic hesitation in the face of the paradigm shift. Psychotherapists need to understand how the brain works, how its circuitry errors give rise to problems in behavior and mental states and how we can encourage it to function better regardless of its particular malaise. We can help people address the very disorders that so often lead to suicide by holding a gentle mirror up to the brain so that it can observe and change its own functioning. This mirror is called neurofeedback or biofeedback to the brain. In this comprehensive book, Helena Bester will take you through how this all works, so I'll just tempt you to keep reading with a vignette from my own practice in neurofeedback. I was first trained in 1996 (almost 30 years after neurofeedback was discovered!).

The week I returned from the training with my computer I set the system up in my office with the sole intent of using it with my friends and family. My own experience that led me to train in the first place served as a caution to take this learning curve slowly. Then Ann arrived for her session crying. Although she had a lifelong history of unipolar depression, I had never seen her cry. "I can't meet my classes – I can hardly get out of bed. I can't sleep or eat. I am falling into this depression so fast it's terrifying me". We'd been engaged in understanding her depression for almost a year, but her mood did not yield to her insight. Her younger sister, diagnosed with bipolar illness, had committed suicide seven years before. We both acknowledged that Ann suffered from a "chemical" depression; but she had researched anti-depressants and could not bring herself to take them. This idea of chemical depression is still very much accepted – it is the basis of a billion-dollar industry – but as I was about to learn and as you will see, her brain chemistry was not the issue.

Ann knew I'd been away for this training in neurofeedback and saw the system set up in my waiting room. She wanted me to use it for her. I reminded her that I was brand new to this and was hesitant for her, in these desperate straits, to be my first patient. "I'm scared I'm dying, Sebern. We have to try it.' There was literally nothing else to do. We trained her brain for depression as I had been instructed to do, with a sensor on the left hemisphere and rewarding her brain to make beta waves (15–18 Hz). Ann played a video game just with her brain that gave her points when she made these wave forms. This is what happened. Almost immediately as she oriented to the training, she stopped crying, she straightened out of her slump and her color returned. Neither of us could believe what we were seeing. At the end of 30 minutes she declared, "Sebern, I am out of this! I could meet my class today. I feel like I will sleep tonight." Both were accurate readings of her change in state. Ann had fully recovered. We trained 23 sessions to allow her brain to learn and over-learn its new capacity.

I had reason to check in with Ann twelve years later before a speaking engagement in Australia. She said, "Let your audience know that I've never had another episode of depression. I can wake up blue sometimes, but it's nothing that meditation or a cup of coffee doesn't handle.' It is important to say that it is unusual for neurofeedback to provide this level of relief so quickly. Ann's case in that sense may be rare but it also provides a proof of principle. Brains respond to learning about themselves and given time and feedback, can learn how to rewire themselves, how to correct their faulty circuits.

Circuitry underwrites plasticity in the brain. Ann had gained access to her brain's capacity to change itself. Once the brain learns its path toward self-regulation, when it optimizes its own neural plasticity, it will practice its new level of function. As a colleague once said, "The brain is devoted to its own regulation. It has to be."

The DSM has led us to think that there are many discreet types of mental illness. In her subtitle, Bester says that neurofeedback is "an intervention for ADHD, anxiety, depression, epilepsy, insomnia, dyslexia, fibromyalgia, PTSD and other causes of discomfort." Some readers might be discouraged right here, thinking that she is making an exaggerated claim that one intervention could help in so many disorders. The problem however is not in the claim that neurofeedback helps, it is in the belief that the brain parcels out its "discomforts" in so many packages. Even the NIMH isn't thinking this way anymore. The same year that the DSM 5 was published, NIMH began to refuse funding for research on discreet disorders. They turned their attention toward a search for the common factors that give rise to mental illness. Although there is yet to be consensus on these common factors, the two that have been identified are fear circuits and working memory. Cases abound that show that neurofeedback addresses these common factors and in so addresses the conditions they give rise to.

Bester rises to the challenge presented by this rapidly evolving field of study and the many technologies and ideologies it has given rise to. She does so with articulate compassion both for those suffering and for those trying to understand neurofeedback's many pathways to ease if not end it. She discusses waveforms, and she takes us through the brain and its structures. She provides a deep and clear understanding of stress and its many tolls. Every chapter is relevant to neurofeedback practice, but the chapter on stress may be the most so. The USFDA has granted its approval to some neurofeedback systems. The approval is for addressing stress. Stress is of course a common factor in all mental illness either as a cause or as an effect or both. Training a brain to become stress resilient will change the life of its owner. She ends with case studies of her own and of other practitioners in South Africa which demonstrate exactly this.

This book is an invaluable resource for neurofeedback practitioners, whether you are new to the practice or have been, like me, practicing for decades as well as to those who are considering neurofeedback for themselves as patients, as therapists, or as researchers.

On her first page, Bester quotes Lao Tzu— 'Knowing others is wisdom— Knowing yourself, is enlightenment" The greater blessing may be the ability to change what we know to be our self. This is the promise of neurofeedback.

The night after her first session Ann had a dream. It was entirely auditory. The dream voice said one thing: "The path to the enigma is now clear". As Bester so thoroughly explores, neurofeedback is the path. The enigma has yet to yield.

-Sebern F. Fisher, M.A., BCN

Acknowledgments

Collaboration is teamwork taken to a higher level. Despite the fact that I often pursue goals on my own, my journey with neurofeedback has taught me the importance of teamwork. Since I joined the Biofeedback Association of South Africa (BFSA) I have witnessed the achievement of many goals that cannot even be perceived of alone. When I was elected vice-president of the BFSA I was very nervous and hesitant at first. That did not last long, because Louise van der Westhuyzen (previous president of the BFSA) and the other Board Members soon proved to me the power of "flying in formation" (Louise's favorite phrase). Thank you to all the BFSA Board Members for the selfless and tireless contributions to placing Bio-/Neurofeedback in South Africa on a firm footing. Thank you for the bridges that especially you Louise, McGill, Justine and Karlien built to interact with the international Bio-/Neurofeedback fraternity.

Thank you for the contributions of case studies by the following clinicians and colleagues: Mitzi Hollander, Rika Scribante, Louise van der Westhuyzen, McGill Scott and Justine Loewenthal. It is so valuable to other clinicians to read about different approaches and witness how different skill sets are incorporated into neurotherapy. The bigger purpose that you have contributed to is the purpose of demonstrating to the world—the healthcare professionals as well as to those individuals seeking alternative approaches to addressing their discomfort-that neurofeedback is a viable treatment option.

I feel so privileged to be able to work with the clients I work with. Thank you to each and every one of you that was willing to share your story for the greater good. Your stories bring hope and shine light.

Sebern, when I met you in March 2016 at a workshop in Cape Town, I felt blessed. I remember saying to a colleague on our way back at the end of the first day that the workshop with you was the most meaningful educational experience I have ever had. It felt as if my own thoughts were voiced and then there was so much more. I was amazed at the insight you conveyed and felt the need to go on a retreat to be able to integrate the richness of your knowledge and understanding into my own processes. And when you agreed to write the foreword to this book, I felt privileged and so grateful. Thank you for your precious time and the compassion with which you approached this task and the communication with me throughout. It is an inspiring and invaluable contribution to this book.

To Elize, my dear friend, thank you for your unwavering support and meticulous editing. Thank you for your willingness to abandon your convictions and follow to where the elephant could become a part of the book!

Thank you to our hosts at Shametu River Lodge in the Kavango Region in Namibia where the bulk of this book was written. Amori and Louis, you have also become friends while hosting us on the banks of the Kavango River where the sunsets bleed into the river and life rises from it every morning. Thank you for sharing your piece of paradise with us so graciously.

Isabel, we are so different and yet so alike. You add the detail and polish the products of my endeavors to where they shine. I am amazed at your talent of beautifying and trust that you will soon put many of your own creations out there for the world to bask in. Thank you for making it possible for me to have the practice, the ambiance with all that goes with it, exactly as is necessary for me to be the hollow bamboo I wish to be when I work.

Thank you to Dr Roger DeBeus for the suggestion to communicate with Professor Tato Sokhadze, the president of the FNNR (The Foundation for Neurofeedback and Neuromodulation Research) which resulted not only in assistance with the marketing of the first edition, but sprouted into the concept of the second edition of this book. Tato, your openness and enthusiasm pertaining to the support of the field of neurofeedback is very encouraging. Thank you for your support.

Thank you to Megan Stevens, the publishing coordinator of the FNNR. Megan your friendliness, efficiency and professionalism made this journey involving all the processes of going to press, pleasant.

The final thank you is to you, the reader. By choosing this book amongst millions of books by acclaimed authors, you are contributing to change— much needed and sought-after transformation. We can no longer judge that which we are not familiar with because of fear. We ought to embrace different vantage points if we are to truly contribute to a holistic approach to relieving suffering and discomfort which we claim we have achieved a long time ago. Neurofeedback is no longer an experimental treatment and yet prejudice still exists but doesn't prevail. Pythagoras also met with prejudice

. . . So, all is at it should be. We are all part of the process of growth and change.

Introduction

Do you also sometimes wonder what it feels like inside someone else's head– inside someone else's life? I'm not referring here to the external circumstances and the drama that we all manage to create, but to the inner perception. It is after all the perception that creates the experience. Should there be clinical evidence that you ought to have a really severe toothache and you did not have the ability to experience pain, the toothache would not exist. Your experience is what is relevant.

People who feel depressed or anxious, or people who are volatile, seemingly unreasonable, aggressive, self-centered, or who present with any symptoms that cause discomfort, are often judged. They are considered to be ungrateful or to be in a lower league by which ever prejudiced criteria we apply to weigh them or evaluate them. They ought to be grateful for all the privileges they were born into and get their act together – we say or at least think. They should compare their lives to those who have "real" problems like the millions of people in South Africa who are unemployed or those who have been traumatized by violent crime. Truth be told, the seemingly privileged individual with the high-end job, the apparent ideal partner and the sought after address, may be struggling much more with life than the person from a crime ridden area earning minimum wage and raising three children without a life partner.

What is it then that creates our experience of life if it is not external circumstances? Why do the perceptions of life of two people with very similar circumstances often differ so drastically?

There is a beautiful Buddhist teaching that tells the story of a person that unknowingly meets a master. He has just relocated and meets the master whom he considers to be an inhabitant of the area. He asks the master what the people of the area are like. The master responds with a question about the nature of the people in the area where the man used to live. He describes

xxiii

his previous neighbors and other people from the area where he relocated from as being unkind, unreliable, and generally unpleasant. The master responds and says that the man will find the people in the new suburb he has moved to, to be exactly the same. And so, it is: Were we go, there we are but only until it changes. And it can change. Our experience of life can change. In essence, that is what this book is about – what neurofeedback or neurotherapy is about. When we embark on a journey with neurofeedback, transformations are potentially possible and often occur.

Another title that I considered for this book is "Neurofeedback the Alternative to Discomfort" This is how strongly I feel about the potential of neurofeedback. You are not interested in what I feel, and you needn't be so I will provide the research outcomes as well as anecdotal evidence of the efficacy of neurofeedback in this book.

To get back to the question posed earlier: What determines our experience or perception? Of course there are genetic factors, personality factors (those determined mainly by genetics as well as those shaped by events and circumstances), diet (what we ingest apparently has a significant influence on energy levels and mood, hormone levels and neurochemistry) and who knows what else may be in the mix of factors that influence our experience of life. Different disciplines and modalities view problems through different lenses and from different perspectives and notice different determinants of mood and perception. The fact remains that many people, possibly most people, experience a lot of discomfort. We need not necessarily understand exactly what is causing the discomfort in order for the symptoms of the discomfort to be addressed in neurofeedback. The more information the neurotherapist can access about the causes of the discomfort, the more puzzle pieces there are to work with, but mostly, due to the neuroplasticity of the brain, the electrical communication patterns in the brain get altered with neurofeedback that results in – of course only when the trained and experienced neurotherapist uses the correct protocol - a diminishing or removal of the discomfort irrespective of whether we have a complete understanding of the determining factors or not. Sebern Fisher, clinical psychologist and renowned neurotherapist recently acknowledged by ISNR for her contribution to neurofeedback (2014), states it that "the brain has a natural bias toward self-regulation". That fact is one of the core reasons why neurofeedback can bring so much relief. In neurofeedback the brain is reminded of its ability to regulate.

The depressed person does not want to be depressed – if she has a choice to not be depressed, she will exercise that choice. She cannot just "get her act together". The volatile person wishes that he would not overreact when his child accidently drops a glass. He does not want to see his wife and children walk as if on eggshells when in close proximity to him. The wife with impulse control issues wishes that she won't offend a friend again by speaking without considering the effect her words may have. The business executive does not want to be imprisoned by the fear that he'll break out in a cold sweat at the next presentation. I have witnessed people with the above-mentioned symptoms and a myriad of other symptoms, become transformed people who are no longer plagued by symptoms causing them to be unpleasant to be around. Often people become very desperate and despondent after years of psychotherapy that does not bring about a desired outcome or bring lasting relief. I am definitely not implying that the talk therapies have become redundant, by no means so, but often the client or the patient benefits far more from psychotherapy, occupational therapy, speech therapy, remedial therapy or frankly any other therapy when the balance in the brain has been restored or when the regulation of the brain has improved through neurofeedback.

When I was introduced to neurotherapy, the person with whom I did my initial didactic training, Mitzi Hollander, said that the neurotherapy fraternity often jokingly say that whereas the motto of talk therapy is that one will feel better when you talk about it, the motto of neurotherapy is that you will feel better and then you'll want to talk about it.

In the decades of working with people I have truly come to know that inside the lives and minds of other people, life often seems unbearable. Some people truly are imprisoned by their minds. (The difference between mind and brain is another debate that will be referred to later). I have always wanted to almost desperately, help them and assist them in making a shift, liberating them from toxic thought patterns and self-damaging behavior patterns. My good intentions alone were mostly not enough.

Since I have added neurotherapy to my practice fifteen years ago, that has changed. I now have the privilege of witnessing changes in the lives of people that are truly transformational. Things that were perceived to be burdens dissipate. Those who did not have the energy to perform daily tasks begin to participate in life eagerly and engage meaningfully with their loved ones; underachieving children that have become withdrawn and painfully alone, start soaring academically, gain confidence and find friends. There are case studies in this book that bear testimony to such and many more positive changes that occur due to neurotherapy. Neurotherapy does not only have the potential to relieve emotional discomfort but is also often used in rehabilitation of those that have suffered traumatic brain injury or to remedy an array of physical symptoms. Research shows us different efficacy levels of neurofeedback for different disorders and symptoms. Some of the significant research studies that highlight the efficacy levels will be discussed. Generally speaking, and more often than not, the perceptions of people who engage in a neurofeedback training program change. Their experience of life changes – they become lighter, happier, more content and liberated.

The second edition includes a chapter entitled Neurofeedback for PTSD and Developmental Trauma. This addition is relevant, significant and urgent. The incidence of those suffering in the aftermath of trauma probably surpasses the alarming statistics pertaining to those diagnosed with depressive and anxiety disorders. The viability of neurofeedback as an intervention for this population that often don't respond well to medication and talk therapy, is evident.

When one embarks on a journey of writing a book, one has a specific audience in mind. A book is almost like a letter in a way. It is a means of communication. One also has certain goals in mind. I am writing this to you, the individual suffering discomfort for whatever reason and searching for an intervention that may bring relief. I am also writing to all the neurofeedback practitioners, more and less experienced that have chosen to include this therapy in their practices. Neurotherapist are per definition, open minded, brave individuals who were willing to break away from mainstream approaches despite initial resistance and criticism from the medical fraternity. Neurotherapists are always eager to learn and investigate the perspectives of others.

This book is also intended to enlighten all medical and other healthcare practitioners on the principles and validity of neurofeedback. This modality of applied neuroscience can no longer be ignored or brushed off as an experimental treatment. The booming interest shown by mainstream medical specialists indicates the necessity of a condensed source made available to all professional healthcare practitioners who either wish to consider adding the modality of neurofeedback to their practice, make referrals to neurotherapists or keep themselves responsibly abreast of available therapies in the modern arena.

One goal that is of paramount importance to me personally is the wish to be able to contribute in paving the way for the future generations of neurotherapists in South Africa and all countries that are possibly less in touch with the latest developments in applied neuroscience and where neurotherapy is still perceived by most as an alternative therapy. Ignorance breeds skepticism, criticism, and fear. Those of us who initiated neurotherapy into our mainstream practices after we had been introduced to this modality by a few courageous individuals, who had ventured far beyond the boundaries of comfort, were chastised by the mainstream medical professionals. The medical specialists that were welcoming of alternative solutions to the treatment of both complicated and straight forward diagnoses and disorders were few and far between. It was often suggested that our professional conduct was questionable, and insinuations were made to shared clients and patients that there was no clear research evidence that proved the efficacy of neurofeedback. We lacked the numbers of trained neurotherapists that could stand united in our efforts to enlighten the medical fraternity about the validity of the modality. We had to simply keep our heads down and continue working until the anecdotal evidence started changing perceptions.

The story of neurotherapy gaining ground is the same throughout the world, but there is strength in numbers. In South Africa there were only sixteen board certified neuro- and/or biofeedback practitioners in 2019 and fortunately many more that are in the process of becoming Board Certified. I wish this book to be an aid that can encourage all neurotherapists to walk with their heads high in the knowledge that they have braved and are in the good company of some of the most forward thinking minds in the world. May each one of you know that you will, through the responsible application of this modality, make transformations in people's lives possible that will be paid forward for eternity. May this book serve as a barrier between you and unfounded and unfair judgement born of ignorance! The world of interventions is changing. I think of the development of neurofeedback as resulting from a natural and spontaneous action and reaction – like the swinging of a pendulum. When a pendulum starts moving in one direction, it then necessarily moves through the still point in the opposite direction. If we consider the origin of science as the still point, we could consider the general perception at the time to be one in which the views of the educated few would be accepted and not challenged. The general practitioner would make undisputed diagnoses, the minister or priest would pass uncontested judgements and the teachers' knowledge would be regarded irrefutable. This arrangement did not work well for very long for enquiring minds. So a few brave hearts lifted the pendulum to the left away from mainstream belief systems and started experimenting with the healing properties of plants, spiritual practices outside of dogmatic teachings which then lead to movement of the pendulum to the opposite side. Mainstream approaches started developing more sophisticated methods of evaluation for more accurate diagnoses like for instance the electrocardiograph and the electroencephalograph. The more advanced the techniques deployed by mainstream approaches became, the bigger the trajectory of the pendulum moving to the left, representing the alternative therapies and approaches became. The advances in mainstream healthcare and research are developing at a staggering rate and include possibilities such as gene editing, stem cell treatments, growing replacement organs production, PET and SPECT scans and other sophisticated examinations involving radioactive materials such as isotopes. Radioactive materials are used to test new drugs and conduct medical research. On the alternative side of things, sophisticated applications of sound technology, vision therapy, craniosacral therapy and many other therapies and approaches developed. Neurofeedback incorporates aspects of both sides of the spectrum: it uses highly sophisticated software applying latest findings from neuroscience; protocol decisions are often based on quantified electroencephalograms; event related potentials are incorporated in treatment plans and exact measurements of amplitudes and frequencies of the electrical activity in the brain are used. From the alternative pole it incorporates individualized treatment plans, considers the effects of meditation, and supports the concept of improved self-awareness.

Another factor that has probably impacted significantly on the growing interest in neurofeedback worldwide is the withdrawal of the funding by the NIMH (The National Institute of Mental Health) from the DSM – based diagnoses and the financial support invested in brain based therapies. The NIMH is the largest scientific organization in the world dedicated to research focused on the understanding, prevention and treatment of mental disorders. The organization is also dedicated to transforming the understanding and treatment of mental health. In psychology as in other disciplines alike, a holistic approach to physical and mental health has been advocated and endorsed for decades. Neurofeedback may be the best example of a truly holistic approach to date. The era has perhaps dawned in which the trajectory of the pendulum will complete the circle and all vantage points and specialties will be considered equal, significant, and important.

Chapter 1

Historical Overview and Relevant Learning Paradigms

1.1 Historical Overview of the Origin of the EEG and Neurofeedback

The main purpose of this section is to provide the reader with a brief historical overview of the field of neurofeedback and offer key names and concepts for further research, should it be required.

The first introduction of the terms "neuron" and "synapse" was done by Sir Charles Scott Sherrington (1857–1952). He received the Nobel Prize in Physiology or Medicine with Edgar Adrian for their work on the functions of neurons.

In 1875 Richard Caton discovered fluctuations in brainwave activity related to mental activity. These noted changes in the electrical activity of the brain in accordance with the tasks the brain engages in, is one of the cornerstones of neurofeedback.

Most regard Hans Berger's work as the origin of Neurofeedback as we know it today. He was a German psychiatrist who observed the alpha rhythm in humans. Ten hertz is known as the Berger Rhythm. He also observed patterns of smaller and de-synchronous waves which we know as beta waves. In addition, Berger noticed that alpha waves were more prominent when the brain was in a resting state. His findings were published in 1929 (Berger, 1929). He called the patterns of recorded brain wave activity the electroencephalogram, abbreviated EEG. Hans Berger believed that abnormalities in the EEG reflected clinical disorders.

In the 1930s Edgar Adrian and B. C. H. Matthews replicated Berger's measurement of brain waves and studied the entrainment of brain waves with photic stimulation (Adrian & Matthews, 1934). They also designed the differential amplifier and proved that brainwave patterns could be modified by using specific frequencies of flickering lights. This process however is not a biofeedback process because there is no feedback to the client. Brainwave entrainment can however also cause neuronal change and growth.

Fisher and Lowenbach recorded epileptiform spikes in 1934 which could later be included in software for easy detection during EEG recordings (Fischer & Lowenbach, 1934).

In 1935 Adrian and Matthews did a demonstration of an EEG recording at a Physiological Society meeting in England. This was very well received and lead to widespread application for diagnostic purposes.

Nathaniel Kleitman (1895–1999) made major contributions to our modern understanding of sleep cycles. He was a professor Emeritus in Physiology at the University of Chicago. He is widely recognized as the father of sleep research in America. He has done remarkable research on circadian rhythms, regulation of sleep-wake cycles and sleep patterns of different age groups. He has also studied the effects of sleep deprivation extensively (Kleitman, 1987).

Edward C. Beck, from the University of Utah was the first to document alpha blocking which is a phenomenon widely assessed in neurofeedback and which offers valuable information. The brain is supposed to produce lower amplitudes of alpha activity when the eyes are opened after a relaxing state with the eyes closed (Beck et al., 1958).

In 1964, Grey Walter and colleagues were the first to name delta and theta brain waves and the contingent negative variation. They reported on a steady, negative shift in the EEG in the interval between a warming signal and a second stimulus that required a response (Walter et al., 1964). This slow potential was the contingent negative variation (CNV).

Another significant role player was Joe Kamiya, a lecturer at the University of Chicago. He ascertained that individuals could identify when they were in an alpha dominant state (8–12 Hz) although they could not at will generate more alpha waves (Kamiya, 1962, 1969). This concept of being attuned to one's mental state in terms of the frequency of the dominant electrical activity is of course very relevant to neurofeedback. Extended research on the relation between EEG and states of consciousness ensued. Recording of the EEGs of meditating Buddhist monks was done by James Hardt who is to this day doing research in San Francisco on states of consciousness (Hardt, 1993). Many modern day neurotherapists include meditation techniques in their treatment programs. The influence of meditation on brain regulation will be discussed at length later in this book.

In the 1960s Neal Miller's research proved that ANS (autonomic nervous system) functions can be altered through operant conditioning (Miller, 1969).

There are others who regard Barry Sterman, a physiological psychologist, as the true father of neurofeedback. In the 1960s he proved that cats could be trained to increase brain wave activity in the 12–19 Hz range through a process of operant conditioning in his research work at the University of California in Los Angeles (Sterman, 1996; Sterman & Wyrwicka, 1967; Sterman et al., 1969, 1970). There was now proof that brain waves could be influenced through operant conditioning. Dr Sterman coined the phrase SMR (sensory motor rhythm) which he indicated as being brain wave activity in the frequency range of 12–15 Hz. It became clear that cats with increased amplitudes of SMR activity became more resistant to seizures when exposed to the toxic chemical hydrazine in rocket fuel. The same operant conditioning process was applied to humans with epilepsy and it was found that the duration as well as the frequency and the severity of the seizure activity had been reduced. In some cases, the seizures stopped completely. The same effects were achieved in duplicated studies. Sterman published an article on the findings in the January 2000 edition of Clinical Electroencephalography (Sterman, 2000).

In 1963, John Basmajan studied cells in the brain's motor cortex. He determined that subjects could control the firing of a single motor unit in the brain that governed a particular muscle. He thus illustrated the mind-body connection. Surface electromyography (SEMG) was born (Basmajian, 1963, 1989).

Prof. Joel Lubar, a physiological psychologist, had also been working with EEGs at the University of Tennessee at the time Dr Sterman was working on the effects of SMR training. He went to the University of California in Los Angeles on a grant to work with Dr Sterman. It had been noted that many patients with epilepsy also suffered ADHD symptoms and had become significantly calmer with the increased amplitudes of 12–15 Hz activity due to the SMR training. Prof. Lubar was the supervisor of a doctoral student who aimed her research at studying the effects of SMR training on hyperactive. It became clear from the outcome measures that a significant number of hyperactivity children benefited from SMR training. A paper was published in this regard by Lubar and Shouse (1976).

Another very significant finding by Lubar is the importance of the theta/

beta ratio in the ADHD population. Joel Lubar and his wife Judith continued with research and made major contributions to the field of neurofeedback (Lubar, 1991; Lubar & Lubar, 1984; Lubar et al., 1995ab). The theta/beta ratio was being considered as a key marker in distinguishing between ADHD and normal clients. Until very recently they offered many workshops and seminars in which they presented their findings and experience as educational opportunities to neurofeedback practitioners throughout the world. Sadly, Judith Lubar passed away in 2018.

The initial neurofeedback protocols were all based on amplitude or power training. In this type of training, more often than not, work is done with a single channel. The initial software also made provision for two channel training or for bipolar hook- ups. In amplitude training, a specific frequency band is usually rewarded while two frequency bands are being inhibited or discouraged. It is also possible to reward two different frequency bands or to down train all or specific frequency bands. The amplitudes of particular frequencies get influenced in power training. Power training is definitely still being used with great success and is often where the neurofeedback practitioner begins training or treatment before possibly moving on to using more channels or to training the brain of the individual against a normative data base. The different approaches will be addressed later in this book.

Contributions in terms of research and standardizing certain protocols for training the brains of individuals with different symptoms or disorders were made by many dedicated individuals. Information was shared and assistance offered on different forums, affiliate lines, clinical interchange conferences, workshops, and webinars. Mentoring and supervision programs were put in place as the neurofeedback fraternity went from strength to strength.

In 1965 Richard Sutton and colleague first reported on the P300 slow cortical potential (Sutton et al., 1965).

The clinical EEG was inaugurated by Gibbs, Davis, and Lennox through identifying abnormal EEG rhythms associated with epilepsy (Gibbs et al., 1935). In 1993, Elmar Green presented a paper at a symposium in Montreal Canada titled "Alpha- Theta Brainwave Training: Instrumental Vipassana" (Green, 1993). In this paper Dr Green addressed the similarities between alpha-theta brainwave feedback and vipassana meditation. He emphasized the usefulness of these practices in stimulating intuitive answers from the unconscious that are often valuable in relation to solving problems. His research findings became a core component of the alpha-theta protocol of Peniston and Kulkosky at the Menninger Foundation for the treatment of alcoholism (Peniston & Kulkosky, 1989, 1990, 1991).

Niels Birbaumer, professor of Medical Psychology and Behavioral Neurobiology from the University of Tübingen in Germany, received the Albert Einstein World Award of Science in 2001. He has been studying brain-computer interfaces for 40 years. His work on the efficacy of slow cortical potential biofeedback in the treatment of ADHD, epilepsy and schizophrenia, is groundbreaking (Birbaumer, 1999; Birbaumer et al., 1990).

Peter Rosenfeld, a professor at Northwestern University in Chicago's work on operant conditioning of cortically evoked responses is relevant to the field of neurofeedback (Rosenfeld, 1977).

Barbara Brown studied the relationship between reported subjective experience and brain rhythms in the 1970s based on feedback experiments using the three EEG frequency ranges of theta, alpha and beta to operate lights of three different colors (Brown, 1977).

The work of Margaret Ayers on the treatment of coma patients with open head injury for seizure control is well known in the neurofeedback fraternity and her protocols are still widely used. Ayers treated thirty-two level two coma patients who were comatose for more than two months. Twenty-five of these patients emerged from their coma after one to six neurofeedback treatments. This study was published in Biofeedback & Self-Regulation Journal (Ayers, 1995) and is probably the best known and most quoted study. Ayers published many other articles on neurofeedback as a treatment for closed and open head trauma.

The Neurofeedback Book—An Introduction to Basic Concepts in Applied Neurophysiology by Dr Michael Thompson and his wife, Dr Lynda Thompson, was first published in 2003 by the Association for Applied Psychophysiology and Biofeedback (Thompson & Thompson, 2003). The book has been updated and republished many times and has served as a neurofeedback textbook for many years. The book contains most of the information specified as the blueprint of knowledge by the Biofeedback Certification International Alliance (BCIA) for certification purposes. The second edition was published in 2015 and contains an update on the latest developments in the field (Thompson & Thompson, 2015).

In my opinion, Mike Cohen has made a huge contribution to neurofeedback both indirectly through the important role of the International Society for Neurofeedback & Research, in his previous capacity as the director of EEG Spectrum International, as well as in his private capacity as excellent and patient mentor and teacher. Leslie Sherlin, the previous president of the ISNR as well as Roger DeBeus, the newly elected president of the ISNR, have both made significant contributions to the field of neurofeedback. Dr DeBeus expanded the skills and knowledge of the South African neurofeedback practitioners when he presented a training course on an integrative introduction to the Quantitative Electroencephalogram for neurotherapy in South Africa in 2006.

John N. Demos is commended for the major contribution he made to the field of neurofeedback with his book *Getting Started with Neurofeedback* in 2005 when there was no other clear comprehensive guide to clinicians who chose to add neurotherapy to their practice (Demos, 2005). He furthermore contributed greatly with subsequent teachings and writings. The second edition of *Getting Started with Neurofeedback* was published recently (Demos, 2019).

Dr Hamlin, a noted expert in the field of neuroscience is a major role player in the development of neurofeedback programs. He also makes significant contributions in terms of training of neurofeedback practitioners internationally. Dr Hamlin is the lead instructor for EEG Education and Research and is on the faculty for Evidence- Based Neurotherapy of the Society for the Advancement of Brain Analysis.

Sebern Fisher is a psychotherapist and very experienced neurofeedback practitioner who specializes in trauma work and other attachment issues. She has been commended for her contribution to the field of neurofeedback by the ISNR. We as neurotherapists are privileged to have access to her insights and experience through her book, *Neurofeedback in the Treatment of Developmental Trauma: Calming the Fear-Driven Brain* (2014) and through her workshops and online teachings.

The work of Dr Bessel van der Kolk as teacher and researcher in the area of posttraumatic stress has influenced the mind-set of many biofeedback and neurofeedback practitioners in their approach to working with stress related problems. His book, *The Body Keeps the Score: Brain, Mind and Body in the Treatment of Trauma* is a New York Times Science bestseller (Van der Kolk, 2014).

The research analysis of neurofeedback protocols for PTSD and alcoholism by Peniston and Kulkosky offered further significant insight into the potential of neurofeedback (Peniston & Kulkosky, 1989, 1990, 1991).

Les Fehmi and his wife Judith have made and are still making significant contributions to newly trained and experienced neurofeedback practitioners through their teachings and writing (Fehmi & Robbins, 2008, 2010). Les Fehmi has received numerous awards amongst which is an award by the

ISNR for his book, *The Open Focus Brain-Harnessing the Power of Attention to Heal Mind and Body* (co- authored by Jim Robbins) which has brought valuable insight into the importance of alpha brain wave activity to the field of neurofeedback. The concept of "Open Focus", coined by Dr Fehmi, brings relief to many who access his books and online meditation and other exercises. He has authored or co-authored fifty-two papers to date on various aspects of neurofeedback including specific protocols for Open Focus™, aspects of autism, integrating neurofeedback with psychotherapy and overcoming chronic pain. I believe that all neurofeedback practitioners concur that the access that we have to Thomas Collura's books and teachings not only in his capacity as the president of Brain Master Technologies Incorporated, but also as past president of the ISNR and director of the Brain Enrichment Centre has taken neurofeedback as a viable intervention in all our private practices and globally, to the next level. As an educator and teacher, Tom is held in high esteem in the neurofeedback fraternity.

Jon A. Frederick serves on the editorial board of Neuro-regulation and board of directors for the Foundation for Neurofeedback and Neuromodulation Research. His ongoing work as well as his contribution to a cornerstone source entitled *Handbook of Clinical QEEG and Neurotherapy* plays a major role in the development and validation of neurofeedback in the modern-day arena (Collura & Frederick, 2017).

Many current neurofeedback practitioners know Mark Smith as a teacher of the methods, rationale, and benefits of Infra Slow Fluctuation Training. Mark Smith worked with bioengineers in the field for fifteen years to develop Infra Slow Fluctuation and is the owner and founder of Neurofeedback Services in New York (Smith, 2018; Smith et al., 2017).

Daniel Amen is an excellent teacher and presenter and as a psychiatrist offers an additional perspective to neurofeedback which he now publicly embraces (Amen, 1998, 2001, 2012, 2018). His presentations and teachings are generally informative and enjoyable. He has a large database of SPECT scans (single photon emission computed tomography) which he advocates for diagnostic purposes.

Of course, there are hundreds of other significant role players that ought to be mentioned. The recognition given to only a few is a result of the personal experience and exposure of the author. Many of the individuals that are currently doing wonderful work have not yet published articles and are known only for their contributions through workshops and personal interactions with practitioners. It is thus difficult to research their work. I trust that individuals worthy of recognition for their contribution to the field, who have not been mentioned here, will not be offended. Kindly accept the gratitude of many that have benefited from your work.

Recognition to the South African role players is mentioned under the acknowledgements section, due to their direct influence on and contributions to this book.

1.2 Learning Theories – Operant and Classical Conditioning

During neurofeedback intervention, training or treatment, changes occur in the electrical activity in the brain based on learning that happens during the feedback process. It is therefore important to understand what the underlying learning paradigms are and the rationale of the process.

The main underlying learning paradigm relevant to why and how the brain learns to make the required changes as suggested and rewarded by the specific training protocol, is operant conditioning. In the chosen protocol, in power training or amplitude training specifically, the amplitudes of specific frequencies are encouraged to increase and the amplitudes of other frequencies are inhibited or encouraged to decrease in specific areas of the brain determined by the placement areas of electrodes on the scalp. Although the processes involved in other types of neurofeedback, such as live Z-score and sLORETA training, which will be discussed later in this book, are different in some respects, the underlying principles remain the same. The brain is trained or taught to change through conditioning.

Operant conditioning or instrumental learning is a basic learning paradigm that underlies most of our learning. It is based on the law of effect and implies that the likelihood of behavior recurring is higher when that behavior is rewarded. This principle of learning was first established by Edward Thorndike in 1911 (Thorndike, 1911). Cats in puzzle boxes figured out how to reach food placed within sight outside the boxes. The efforts like mewing and scratching that did not lead to success were not repeated whereas the responses that lead to the success of finding the food were. Thorndike called this phenomenon the *law of effect*.

In 1938, Burrhus F. Skinner (1904–1990) a behaviorist and Edgar Pierce Professor at Harvard University from 1958 until 1974, further developed this principal of the instrumental learning paradigm which implies the law of effect and introduced the concept of *operant classes* or responses (Skinner, 1938, 1958).

In operant conditioning, an individual makes an association between a particular behavior and an outcome or result. Skinner's work stemmed from

36

a conviction that classical conditioning was far too simplistic an explanation for human behavior. Skinner considered human action dependent on consequences of previous actions. He studied human behavior by focusing on the causes of an action and its consequences. He established that reinforced behavior tends to be repeated whereas behavior that is not reinforced tends to be weakened or die out. He identified three types of responses or operants by studying the behavior of animals in puzzle boxes much like Thorndike's puzzle boxes. *Neutral operants* or responses from the environment are those that do not elicit either a greater or lesser probability of behavior being repeated. *Reinforcers* are responses from the environment that increase the probability of behavior being repeated in either a positive or a negative sense. *Punishers* are responses from the environment that decrease the likelihood of the behavior being repeated. Positive reinforcement thus strengthens a behavior by providing a consequence that an individual finds rewarding at some level.

Punishment that weakens or eliminates behavior occurs by either punishing the behavior directly by applying an unpleasant stimulus after a particular behavior or by removing a potentially rewarding response. An example of removing a potentially rewarding response is, not taking the child to a movie that would have been a positive response or operant to a good school report.

Aversive punishment is when the frequency of an operant behavior is reduced and results in a negative outcome. An example of aversive punishment would be if someone reduced his daily exercise due to muscle cramps.

Punishment and negative reinforcement are often confused. Punishment is an aversive event that follows behavior designed to eliminate or weaken a response. Negative reinforcement is removal of an unpleasant reinforcer that strengthens behavior. Negative reinforcement strengthens behavior because it removes the unpleasant experience. An example of negative reinforcement would be if a dyslexic child complains of stomach ache whenever she has to read. She has repeatedly been permitted to be excused from the activity when she experiences stomach pain. The unpleasant experience (reading) gets removed and negatively reinforces the stomach pain complaints.

Ferster and Skinner ascertained in 1957 that the ways in which reinforcement were delivered affected the response rate and the extinction rate of behavior (Ferster & Skinner, 1957). The reinforcement rate that had the quickest rate of extinction was continuous reinforcement. This is an important fact to consider in neurofeedback in terms of making threshold decisions that affect the frequency of the feedback stimuli. Equally important is the finding that fixed ratio reinforcement results in a fast response rate with a medium extinction rate. Fixed interval reinforcement results in medium response rate and medium extinction rate. Variable ratio reinforcement results in a fast response rate and slow extinction rate. Variable interval reinforcement also results in a fast response rate and slow extinction rate.

Another important component of operant conditioning relevant to neurotherapy is that of the different types of reinforcers. Primary reinforcement is when a reward strengthens behavior by itself. Secondary reinforcement is when something reinforces behavior because it leads to a primary reinforcer. The encouragement or the recognition provided by a therapist as well as little educational prizes or stickers offered to children can serve as secondary reinforcement in the neurofeedback environment.

The understanding of behavior shaping is another important contribution made by Skinner which is relevant to neurofeedback. In order for behavior to be shaped, the conditions required to receive the reward should keep on shifting. Generally speaking, operant conditioning or instrumental learning can be used for learning responses that can be controlled voluntarily. Operant conditioning can be used to explain a wide variety of behaviors and is one of the underlying principles of the efficacy of neurofeedback. A voluntary response is followed by a reinforcing stimulus.

Classical conditioning differs from operant conditioning. When the behavior that has been reinforced is voluntary, it is operant conditioning. Classical conditioning involves involuntary behavior. It involves a reflex response and is basically restricted to autonomic nervous system responses. Pavlov studied the reflex involved when dogs salivate when they perceive food. When the ringing of a bell was paired with the presentation of food, the dog "learned" to salivate at the ringing of a bell. The food was the unconditioned stimulus that produced the unconditioned response of salivation. The bell was the conditioned stimulus that caused a similar conditioned response, salivation. Second order conditioning then followed where a light went on just before the bell and the light then too, caused the same response as the bell. In classical conditioning, motivation is mostly irrelevant.

Emotional conditioning is classical conditioning. Emotional conditioning occurs when a reaction like anxiety or fear is paired with a neutral stimulus. A person that loved travelling by car for instance (an example from an actual case) needed to use the bathroom urgently while travelling with friends to a very remote destination where there was no bathroom anywhere near. He became very anxious and felt very vulnerable and embarrassed. He consequently became anxious (increased autonomic arousal) at any prospect of any outing that would take him out of reach of immediate access to a bathroom. He was not conscious of the pairing of the events. The anxiety was generalized to other situations as in the case of the often-quoted experiment of the white rat done by the behaviorist John B. Watson in 1920 (Watson & Rayner, 1920). "Little Albert" (his real name was Douglas Merritte) an eleven-month-old boy, was conditioned to fear white rats. Each time the child reached out to touch the rat; a loud noise was made. Albert then became fearful of touching all white furry objects including Watson's white hair and Santa's beard.

Both operant and classical conditioning are learning paradigms relevant to neurofeedback. Operant conditioning occurs in neurofeedback when the client is rewarded (through visual and auditory feedback fed back from the measuring instrument) for shifting to a desired state of consciousness or alertness that is in accordance with the thresholds specified in the training protocol. A secondary reward in the form of praise, recognition or a tangible object may or may not be present. The brain has the ability to learn about its own functioning when provided with information about its success. The information about the success is the reward that reinforces the behavior, being the desired state of arousal or regulation. With power training or amplitude training, it appears that the brain manages to achieve the desired state in which the symptoms associated dissipate with less complicated diagnoses, after approximately forty training sessions. The desired state of regulation needs to be transferred to beyond the training environment. Classical conditioning can possibly be involved in the second step of pairing the stimulus to the outcome. Reading or other relevant tasks may be incorporated during the training program. The desired mental state of focus for instance, is then paired with a reading task. The trainee will then first be allowed to find the ideal mental state by rewarding a particular brain wave pattern and then the desired state of focus (in the presence of ADHD) is paired with an academic task that requires focus. Should the auditory feedback become less, the client is then instructed to return her focus to the screen for the visual focus as well until the desired state of increased fast wave activity and a lower amplitude of slow brain wave activity is reached. When a person is trained to become more relaxed and faster frequencies are down- trained or alpha amplitudes are enhanced, the task with which the desired state of improved relaxation ought to be paired will be totally different. The chosen tasks will depend on the expertise and experience of the therapist. Metacognitive skills (to be discussed later in this book) ought to also be taught during the neurofeedback training should the therapists' original training, expertise and experience allow this.

Chapter 2

What is Neurofeedback? Definitions, Evidence-Based Research, Waveforms and Frequencies

2.1 Definitions of Neurofeedback

The electrical activity of the brain is measured from the scalp by means of sensors or electrodes that are placed in certain predetermined positions according to the international 10/20 placement system based on 20 placement areas on the scalp. (The 10/10 placement system is being used more frequently of late). The placement areas of the sensors are determined by the therapist after an evaluation. Evaluations may differ from therapist to therapist based on the therapist's original training, the presenting discomfort and the goals of the patient or client. Aids to assist with protocol decisions are referred to throughout the book.

The feedback the individual receives is based on the electrical activity in the brain during the training. The electrical activity is digitized by the use of computerized equipment including an amplifier and displayed in the form of brain waves of different frequencies. The nature, origin and description of the brain wave activity are discussed in the following section of this chapter. When certain goals are met in terms of changes in the amplitudes of particular frequencies of the measured brain wave activity as specified in the training protocol, the client receives positive visual and auditory feedback. The desired brain wave activity is rewarded and reinforced by the success the person experiences although it may not be registered consciously. Based on the principles of operant and classical conditioning (refer to chapter 1) the brain learns to change and reach a desired state of consciousness, arousal, or focus, depending on the training protocol.

Neurofeedback has a very strong and sound scientific foundation and has been going from strength to strength over the past six decades. Many leading neurofeedback practitioners have attempted to compile succinct definitions in attempts to be able to convey the essence of the process of neurofeedback in a nutshell. Due to the fast expanding research findings in neuroscience in what can be described as an proliferation in knowledge and findings that is continually integrated into neurofeedback methods and software, definitions keep changing and falling short in their capability to reflect the magnitude of the process.

Despite the sound scientifically based foundations of neurofeedback and the fact that it is in essence applied neuroscience and applied neurophysiology, there is a core almost hidden component to neurofeedback that makes it not only a science, but an art as well. Despite all the truly mind-boggling detail we can measure about the functioning of the brain from the recordings from the scalp, there are always more factors involved in any aspect of human behavior than what we can measure.

Sometimes a particular protocol that is clearly indicated from sophisticated quantified data obtained from an artefact free EEG recording in conjunction with psychometric evaluations, questionnaires and collateral information gathered from an intake procedure and significant others, does not have the anticipated outcome. In the words of Sebern Fisher (2014), "experience trumps measurement". It is of paramount importance that the therapist will remain ever mindful of the client's experience. Sometimes it is essential, and here I need to add, "-in my opinion-", that the therapist will move beyond science and access the sources of experience, inner wisdom and intuition, to adapt a protocol indicated by science, to one that results in relief from plaguing symptoms. I trust that this opinion will encourage therapists to turn within and consider the insights that often stem from an open and honest intent to heal. Should we wish to discard the field of limitless potential, as I assume Deepak Chopra would refer to this source of wisdom that I am attempting to describe (see Chopra, 1994) that we can access when we reflect mindfully on a process of an individual that is not responding to the neurofeedback training in a predictable manner, we would be doing the field of neurofeedback a disservice. There will be a protocol that will relieve the client of at least some of the debilitating symptoms. Finding the ideal protocol may in some cases just require the therapist to go to the silence between thoughts to access resources beyond our rational capabilities. I fully understand that this may be a scary prospect to some very analytically biased therapists who feel comfortable and secure with protocol recommendations based on sound scientific principles. It is furthermore important that we present the research and prove the scientific base of neurofeedback to all and especially to the mainstream medical fraternity that are not at all comfortable with intuitive approaches. And yes, as responsible and well trained, knowledgeable and experienced neurotherapists we need to do all of that. However, we need to also remember that the individual that approaches us for assistance is what it is all about. That person is not a research subject to serve science. Science and all the external as well as the internal resources that can be accessed, ought to be applied in service to the individual.

I have chosen to write this section here under the heading of definitions of neurofeedback to emphasize my conviction that neurofeedback is more than what can be defined by science alone. It is founded in viable and reliable scientific principles but ought to be integrated with all the other skills the therapist can bring to the training program. Opinions such as these have been voiced in some published articles by psychotherapists as well as by other therapists from different backgrounds that have mastered the art of integrating the science of the modality with therapeutic skills. Sebern Fisher (2014), Daniel Amen (2001, 2012, 2018), and others, have done valuable work in this regard. One aspect that is being emphasized here that is perhaps not discussed or referred to often in fear that it may dilute or harm the image of neurofeedback, is the aspect of the other sources we often unknowingly access. Often it is true that that which we regard as being an intuitive feeling or a gut feeling or inspired thought, is really an amalgamation of knowledge and experience, mingled together masterfully somewhere in the recesses of our minds and jumps to the fore as a suggested solution. I don't think that we can always ascertain what all the ingredients so to speak of an inspired thought are. Sometimes we may just accidently or purposefully access a knowledge bank of sorts beyond science. We as therapists ought not to discard these thoughts, feelings or insights as nonsense, and here again I need to add, in my humble opinion, but ought to develop a way in which to skillfully and responsibly balance science and knowledge with the particular skill set of the individual therapist. Should we choose to focus only on the science and wonderfully advanced technology we have access to, we will still have a very high success rate in our treatment and training of many individuals. However, we will then be functioning solely as technicians never achieving excellence because of our fear.

Many great minds, as mentioned earlier, have attempted to define neurofeedback concisely and aptly: Sterman described EEG biofeedback or neurofeedback as being "learned normalization of EEG patterns" (Sterman & Egner, 2006). (As a matter of interest, Sterman obtained good clinical outcomes in epilepsy even when the EEG patterns were not normalized). The normalization of EEG patterns occurs while changes in neuronal behavior are being rewarded. Significant and sustained physiological changes can be produced. Evidence of these changes have been well documented since the 1970s and are still been documented in a growing body of evidence-based research outcomes.

In his book, *Getting Started with Neurofeedback*, John N. Demos compared neurofeedback to an exercise program that strengthens neural pathways while "increasing mental endurance and flexibility" (Demos, 2005, 2019).

Because of the capability of the advanced available software, the individual that has felt shamed by impulsive decision making that results in adverse effects and consequences to his loved ones, or the individual that has feelings of guilt based on his inability to engage in life and experience joy, can now see logical explanations for their discomfort. The ADHD individual can be shown the high amplitude of slow brain wave activity in the left frontal lobe that could be the reason for the poor impulse control and resulting bad choices he has made. The individual can see a measurable explanation in the asymmetry of the alpha activity in the frontal lobes that has caused the depression-like symptoms and need no longer feel guilty or ashamed. This non-invasive therapy can potentially improve self-esteem and overall quality of life.

The non-invasive component of neurofeedback is important to mention to all prospective clients or patients that wish to embark on a neurofeedback treatment program. No signal is sent into the brain through the sensors. The process merely involves taking a reading of the neuronal activity in the brain and guiding the brain in terms of enhancing desired and discouraging undesired activity through the process of visual and auditory feedback. The activity that is being discouraged is also not done by punishing unwanted activity in any way – the activity is rather inhibited by ignoring it through the absence of positive feedback from the system being used.

A relevant factor in comparing neurofeedback to other interventions, is that it is often more difficult to set objective goals in other therapies. In neurofeedback many of the goals are easily quantifiable as for instance the necessity of improving the coherence between two particular relevant regions. The potential negative side effects of medication are also absent. It is however important that neurofeedback practitioners proceed cautiously in the face of many and complicated medications that have been prescribed. It is of paramount importance that we remain within our scope of practice and that any weaning off or phasing out of medication ought to be done by the prescribing practitioners.

In her book, *Neurofeedback in the Treatment of Developmental Trauma: Calming the Fear-Driven Brain,* Sebern Fisher (2014) describes the following as "core assumptions", about neurofeedback:

"Neurofeedback changes our attention from the mind to the brain; the brain organizes itself rhythmically in the frequency domain, and it is there that brain plasticity resides; we can access these rhythms through a type of computerized biofeedback to the brain, called neurofeedback."

Sebern Fisher's book is about neurofeedback as an intervention for development trauma and she chose the quoted assumptions accordingly, but these principles are relevant in a wider sense as well. Most people we see in our private practices on a daily basis are victims of their mindset and despite rationalizations and many therapies they have embarked on, find it difficult or impossible to shift negative thinking patterns that keep them stuck in the negative web of a narrative they have created. Wayne Dyer, previously a professor of psychology and spiritual teacher, mentioned in one of his many teachings or books that attempting to get beyond the mind with the mind, can be likened to attempting to stand on your own shoulders. It also reminds me of what one of my mentors, Mitzi Hollander, said during a training session mentioned above in the introduction that in neurofeedback one has a top down approach during which the training causes the person to feel better whereafter the other talk therapies can take effect. As the regulation in the brain improves, it becomes so much easier to identify and shift negative thought and behavior patterns. Very often the process happens automatically without added interventions.

One of my clients, a fifty-year-old female, recently asked me how it was possible that her experience of life has changed completely without her circumstances having changed at all. She was convinced that she would have to find the courage to get divorced so that her circumstances could change to enable her to have a better quality of life. She now has so much insight into the changes she needs to make within herself and does not find the presence and habits of her husband draining or overwhelming at all.

Brain plasticity which is one of the cornerstones of neurofeedback has been the talk of the town for at least the last decade. Neural plasticity is the ability of the brain to change throughout one's life. The implications of the plasticity of the brain impacts on most areas of our lives and also on the prognosis of so many brain-based diagnoses. It used to be common practice to terminate all therapies and interventions two years after a CVA (cerebrovascular accident) known as a stroke, which causes the sudden death of brain cells due to lack of oxygen to the brain caused either by the blockage or rupture of an artery to or in the brain. The general approach to all brain injuries, whether open head or closed head injuries, used to be the same. The general consensus was that that which could not be remedied or changed within two years after the incident, was not likely to improve. Many neurologists are still of the opinion that interventions for stroke patients longer than two years after the event are a waste of resources. I have had the privilege of witnessing significant progress with CVA patients after what was previously regarded as a limited window of opportunity as a result of neurofeedback in at least four cases that I have worked with and have often heard success stories in this regard from colleagues. There is a case study of a CVA patient further on in this book. Fortunately, we need not rely on anecdotal evidence in this regard alone. Valid research results on the efficacy of neurofeedback in the treatment of traumatic brain injury is available.

Neuroplasticity does not only imply that brain activity associated with a given function can be transferred to a different location, it also implies potential changes at neuronal level. Damaged or diseased neurons can actually be replaced or repaired. Changes occur in neural pathways and synapses according to Donaldson et al. in a chapter published in *Handbook of Clinical QEEG and Neurotherapy* (Collura & Frederick, 2017) as a result of various factors including neural processes influenced by neurofeedback.

Thomas F. Collura (2014) offers the following concise and encompassing definition of neurofeedback in his book – *Technical Foundations of Neurofeedback:* "At its core, neurofeedback embodies a process of neuronal self- regulation and re-education, leading the brain to find new and beneficial states and ways of processing information and feelings . However, it is by no means a weak intervention, and can be as efficacious as medication in many cases, and with fewer or no negative side effects."

2.2 Neurofeedback – A Summary of Evidence-Based Research Outcomes and a Practical Description of the Neurofeedback Process

This section is written mainly for the clients or patients that are considering neurofeedback as an intervention for themselves or for their children. The sections that follow after this section may be too technical for some and you may as a layperson, wish to skip those. Those sections are aimed at providing neurofeedback practitioners with relevant information accessible in one source as well as at healthcare practitioners that consider adding neurofeedback as a modality to their practice. Existing medical practitioners that want to ascertain whether neurofeedback is relevant and viable for referrals will also find valuable information from the more technical sections.

2.2.1 A Summary of Evidence-Based Research Outcomes

The information that follows is based on the *Evidence-Based Practice in Biofeedback and Neurofeedback* compiled by Tan et al. and published by The Association for Applied Psychophysiology and Biofeedback (Tan et al., 2016). This book is considered the most comprehensive review of research in the field of neurofeedback and biofeedback available to clinicians. More recent research information and results are woven into this book and specific recent studies are discussed in more detail later. This section serves as a summarized guide to indicate the efficacy of the intervention for the needs of the individual reader, be that to consider the therapy for themselves or for reference purposes.

Reference is made to biofeedback which is the broader modality and enables an individual to learn how to control physiological activity to improve health and performance (Moss & Shaffer, 2006). Neurofeedback, the focus of this book, is a specialty field within biofeedback that trains people to gain control over electro- physiological processes in the human brain.

(Refer to an elaboration of definitions of neurofeedback in section 2.1)

Neurofeedback is an intervention that involves a brain-computer interface process. There is ample research evidence of various levels of success of neurofeedback in the treatment of an array of disorders, symptoms, and discomfort. The levels of efficacy are statistical measures that indicate the strength of the available research data in support of the intervention as being relevant and viable. An important and very valuable aspect of *Evidence-Based Practice in Biofeedback & Neurofeedback* (Tan et al., 2016) is this ranking of the studies for each disorder based on the methodological quality of the research. The information provided in the guide is evidence-based and supported by neuroscience. The efficacy levels range from level 1 to level 5. A short description of efficacy levels follows:

Level 1: Not Empirically Supported

This rating pertains to findings which are supported only by anecdotal evidence from individual therapists without peer-reviewed publications.

Level 2: Possibly Efficacious

At least one study with sufficient statistical evidence with well-defined outcome measures exists but randomized assignment to a control condition is absent.

Level 3: Probably Efficacious

Multiple observational studies exist. There are also clinical studies, wait-list controlled studies and replication studies (within – subject and intra – subject) which demonstrate efficacy.

Level 4: Efficacious

The treatment is shown to be statistically significantly superior to the control condition or equal to another treatment with established efficacy.

The studies have been conducted with a population with a specific problem for which inclusion criteria have been delineated in a reliable manner.

The study has used valid and clearly defined outcome measures. The data has been subjected to appropriate data analyses.

Replication of the study by independent researchers is possible owing to diagnostic and treatment variables that have been specified clearly and are easily controlled.

The superiority or equivalence to other efficacious interventions has been proven in at least two independent studies.

Level 5: Efficacious and Specific

All the criteria of level 4 efficacy have been met plus the intervention has been proven to be superior to credible sham therapy, pill, or alternative bona fide treatment in at least two independent settings.

Below is a list of conditions for which Bio- and/or Neurofeedback have been used with specified efficacy levels according to *Evidence-Based Practice in Biofeedback & Neurofeedback* (Tan et al., 2016).

Attention Deficit Hyperactivity Disorder (ADHD)	Level 5
Alcoholism/Substance Use Disorder	Level 3
Anxiety and Anxiety Disorders	Level 4
Arthritis	Level 3
Asthma	Level 3
Autism	Level 3
Cerebral Palsy	Level 2
Chemobrain	Level 3
Chronic pain (excluding fibromyalgia, headache, Irritable bowel syndrome, Raymond's disease)	Level 4

Muscle related orofacial pain, non-cardiac chest pain, posture related pain	Level 4
Muscle related low-back pain, phantom limb pain, pelvic floor pain	Level 3
Subluxation of the patella and patellofemoral pain, cancer pain	Level 3
Pain from carpal tunnel, myofascial pain syndrome, PMS and dysmenorrhea	Level 2
Pain and spasticity due to not taking micro-breaks, reflex sympathetic dystrophy, trigeminal neuralgia	Level 1
Constipation	Level 4
Chronic Obstructive Pulmonary Disease	Level 2
Coronary Artery Disease	Level 2
Depressive Disorders	Level 4
Diabetes Mellitus	Level 4
Glycaemic Control	Level 4
Intermittent Claudication	Level 2
Diabetic Ulcers	Level 3
Epilepsy	Level 4
Erectile Dysfunction	Level 4
Facial Palsy	Level 3
Faecal Incontinence	Level 4
Fibromyalgia	Level 3
Functional/Recurrent Abdominal Pain	Level 2
Hyperhidrosis	Level 2
Hypertension	Level 4
Immune Function	Level 2
Insomnia	Level 3
Irritable Bowel Syndrome	Level 4
Motion Sickness	Level 3
Performance Enhancement	Level 3
Preeclampsia	Level 4
Post-Traumatic Stress Disorder	Level 3
Raynaud's Disease	Level 4
Stroke (Cardiovascular Accident)	Level 2
Syncope (Neuro-cardiogenic)	Level 1

Temporomandibular Muscle and Joint Disorder (TMJD) Pain	Level 4
Tinnitus (Level 3 for Biofeedback, Level 2 for NFB)	Level 3 & 2
Traumatic Brain Injury (TBI) and Posttraumatic Stress Disorder (PTSD)	Level 3
Urinary Incontinence in Males	Level 3
Urinary Incontinence in Children	Level 3
Urinary incontinence in Woman	Level 3
Vasovagal Syncope	Level 2

More recent research findings are available on some of the conditions mentioned above and has resulted in a change in efficacy levels. Some of the latest studies pertaining to particular disorders will be discussed further on in this book. The indicated efficacy levels on the above-mentioned official document, serves as an indication and as a quick reference. In many cases where efficacy levels 1 and 2 have been indicated, it is merely because of a lack of sufficient research. There have been many changes in rankings of the efficacy of bio- and neurofeedback pertaining to certain disorders since the second edition of *Evidence-Based Practice in Biofeedback & Neurofeedback* published in 2008 (Yucha & Montgomery, 2008) to the third edition published in 2016 (Tan et al., 2016). These changes and proof of higher levels of efficacy are due to a number of factors. More sophisticated measurements and protocols have been developed and there is more funding available for research. The body of clinicians that added neurofeedback as an intervention to their practices has grown phenomenally during the past decade which contributes to the expertise available from a variety of disciplines which inevitably advances the field in various ways.

2.2.2 A Description of the Neurofeedback Process

When one approaches a neurofeedback practitioner with the intention of embarking on a neurofeedback treatment/training program, the practitioner will usually have an intake consultation with the client or patient. (The terms client and patient will be used interchangeably). Background information relevant to the discomfort of the individual will be gathered in different ways by different therapists. Some request an interview prior to questionnaires and others will already provide certain intake questionnaires when the appointment is made.

During the intake procedure, the practitioner will explain the process and expected outcomes based on research findings. Reading material and a variety of reference sources ought to be suggested by the therapist after the he/she has acquired a very clear understanding of the client's needs.

The next step will normally be that the therapist will do a recording of the client's EEG. This will imply the placement of 19 electrodes or less in the case of a mini QEEG recording on the scalp on certain specific placement areas based on the 10/20 international placement system. Another electrode is placed elsewhere on the scalp to serve as a ground and two electrodes are placed on the mastoids behind the ears. In his recent work, Robert Coben encourages the use of 32 channel QEEG recordings (Coben et al., 2014). (The EEG and QEEG are discussed and explained in the following section in more detail). A recording of the electrical activity from the cortex produced mainly by the glial cells is made in two different states of consciousness or brain states. A recording is made of the electrical activity from the scalp of the client while her eyes are closed and another recording is made of the brain wave activity while the client's eyes are open. Some therapists also include ERP's or evoked related potentials in their recordings. In these instances, the activity in the brain will be recorded while the client is performing specific tasks. The recorded information is then either sent to a person or institution that removes the artefact from the recording with special software and thereafter the information is compared with a large normative data base or in some cases, a few data bases. Technically involved and very comprehensive reports are then compiled that involves the quantification of the digitized information. Some therapists are qualified to do the recording and analysis of the information and other therapists will make use of the services of others in this regard. On one of the reports that is an outcome of the quantified EEG recording of the client, the strength of the scientific support in terms of research evidence of the success of treatment for the particular condition or complaints, is indicated.

Some therapists do not suggest the acquisition of QEEG reports and follow a stronger symptom-based approach. This approach is more common in amplitude or power training, whereas more recent and more advanced types of neurofeedback that involve working with many channels and placements simultaneously and making use of live normative databases, usually necessitate the QEEG reports.

There are many protocols that were developed for the treatment of a number of conditions before the easy access that neurotherapists have to advanced technology and QEEG's currently. Many of those protocols are still very much in use and are a valuable part of neurofeedback.

Irrespective of whether the neurofeedback practitioner makes use of a

QEEG or not, it is of paramount importance that the symptoms of the client be understood and considered carefully. All the relevant information needs to be integrated in protocol decision-making.

In this regard, the importance of the art of neurofeedback emphasized in chapter 2, is relevant. All of us are infinitely more than thousands of quantified measures and should we simply have needed to train all brains towards the normative databases in terms of thousands of markers, we would just be able to hook everybody up to computers according to a standardized protocol. All measures that are deviant from the mean scores are not causes of negative symptoms. This fact cannot be emphasized enough.

The following step that the client embarking on a neurofeedback training program can expect, is that the therapist will either explain the QEEG reports with all the informative illustrations and conclusions and resulting protocol recommendations and decisions if such a report is available, or that the therapist will discuss and explain to the client how she/he has inferred a protocol decision from the questionnaires and other assessment measures that have been considered.

The number of sessions suggested used to be roughly forty for rather straight forward complaints such as attention problems or anxiety. Treatments for autism, traumatic brain injury and other more complicated conditions would last longer. It does appear that treatment goals are being reached sooner with more advanced software used in live Z-score training for instance and with sLORETA training which will be discussed in detail further on in this book. However, these treatments are not indicated for all individuals.

During a session, sensors are placed on the client's scalp after preparation of the placement areas with an abrasive gel and a conductive paste. Electrodes are connected to an amplifier that converts the signals from the scalp according to the Fast Fourier-Transform algorithm into brain waves displayed on the therapist's computer screen. Real time electrical activity measured from the scalp is displayed as brain waves of particular frequency bands with particular amplitudes. In the case of adults, the therapist would often show and explain the displayed EEG to the client. With children, the neurofeedback practitioners have a game of sorts or a video displayed on the screen that the child focuses on. The display on the feedback screen in front of the client, whether it displays the brain wave activity or a video game or video, responds to what is happening in the brain of the client in terms of certain goals that have been set. A straightforward and classical example of power training would for instance involve three goals set for three different bandwidths. The ADHD child with mainly inattentive symptoms would present with high amplitudes of slow brain wave activity and low amplitudes of fast brain wave activity. One would then typically set up a protocol on the computer that involves an inhibit of 4–7 Hz (slow brain wave activity), an enhance of 15–18 Hz (fast brain wave activity) and an inhibit of 22–36 Hz activity because high amplitudes of this frequency band usually causes anxiety. Thresholds are set for each frequency that are weighted according to importance of the change in amplitude for each of the bandwidths. The brain is then encouraged, through visual and auditory feedback, to meet the predetermined goals. The goals are to change the amplitudes of the selected frequency bands.

When the brain produces a lower amplitude of the two frequency bands that have been set as inhibits and produces a higher amplitude of the bandwidth set as an enhance, there is auditory feedback from the system in terms of beep sounds or continuous sound and visual feedback in the form of the continuous play of the video or success in the displayed graphics of the selected game. The brain then learns, based on the principles of operant and classical conditioning, to maintain a focused and alert state of focus associated with reduction in the slow brain wave activity and an increase in the fast brain wave activity within a particular frequency bandwidth. The principles of the learning paradigms involved and the characteristics of the different brain wave frequencies are explained elsewhere in this book.

There has to be at least one electrode on the scalp that is the active electrode, one electrode elsewhere (on the scalp or the mastoid or the earlobe) that serves as a reference and another electrode elsewhere that serves as a ground (on the scalp or the mastoid or the earlobe). There can however be many electrodes on different placement areas depending on the protocol decision and type of training. The area where the electrodes are placed is based on the protocol decision.

The international 10–20 system is a worldwide standardized system according to which placement areas on the scalp are named. The numbers "10" and "20" refer to the distances between the placement areas. The measurements are done from the nasion which is the little indentation above your nose and below your forehead, and the inion which is the ridge at the base of your skull and above your neck. A typical distance between these two points is 36 cm. Ten percent of the distance takes you to FPz and a further 20% of the total distance takes you to Fz. All of the other measurements as illustrated in the figure below, are either ten percent or 20% of the total distance apart from one another. (In the 10–10 system all the distances are measured in 10% increments). A measure across the head from ear to ear and more specifically from the indentation right at the front of the ear canal

− (called the pre-auricular notch) − to the other pre- auricular notch, is another relevant measurement for the placements referred to as T3, C3, Cz, C4 and T4. The letters refer to the relevant lobes of the brain. "T" is for the temporal lobes, "P" for the parietal lobes, "C" indicates the central area and "F" indicates the frontal lobe. The uneven numbers indicate areas on the left and the even numbers denote placement positions on the right. The letter "Z" indicates any placement along the midline between the nasion and the inion.

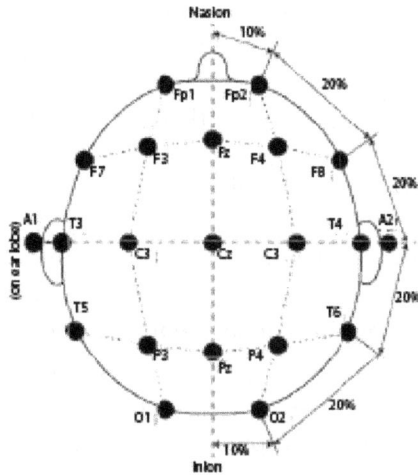

Figure 2.1: Positions on the scalp corresponding with the 10/20 International placement system. Reprinted from: Davidson, R. J., Putnam, K. M., & Larson, C. L. (2000). Dysfunction in the neural circuitry of emotion regulation--a possible prelude to violence. Science, 289(5479), 91-594. doi:10.1126/science.289.5479.591

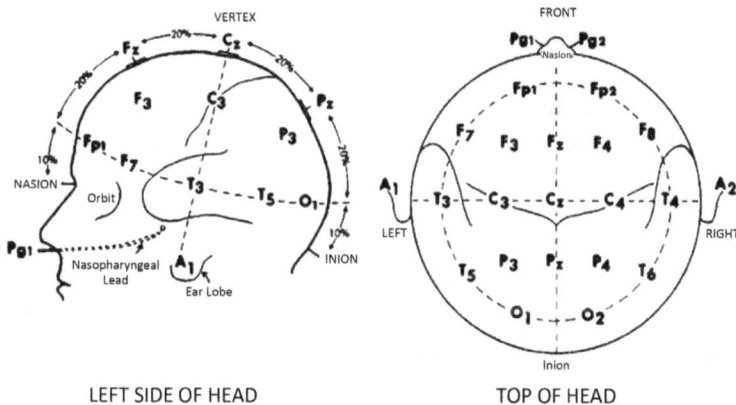

Figure 2.2: Positions on the scalp on the left side of the head corresponding with the 10/20 Placement System. Positions on the scalp on the top of the head corresponding with the 10/20 Placement System. Reprinted from: Syakiylla Sayed Daud, S., & Sudirman, R. (2016). Artifact removal and brain rhythm decomposition for EEG signal using wavelet approach. Jurnal Teknologi, 78. https:// doi.org/10.11113/jt.v78.9460

What to expect from a training session:

The treatment or training is non-invasive as mentioned earlier and is generally free from the side effects that can often follow from medication. Generally speaking, the immediate after effects are pleasant. With normal power training one generally feels a difference for between 2-24 hours. The carry over effect becomes progressively longer until it becomes permanent. One of the first things that are normally reported to shift is the quality of sleep. After a training session one generally feels alert and calm, and of course this varies according to the particular protocol, one falls asleep more easily and one wakes up feeling rested and alert. Sleep is a very important marker of brain regulation and when sleep improves there are usually many other aspects of the dysregulated brain that fall into place.

Common side effects that would occur if the frequency that is being enhanced is too high for the particular brain would be the presence of agitation, problems with sleep onset, heightened activity, loud unmodulated voice, tension in the neck and shoulders, burning eyes, itchiness, irritability, hot flashes, abdominal burning, headache, fidgeting, tense jaw, fast heart rate, skin crawling feeling, acting out behavior, increased worrying, increased appetite, impulsiveness, aggressiveness, agitation, emotional detachment, physical tension, obsessive or compulsive behaviors, anger, vivid dreams or nightmares, tics or nervous habits and stuttering. These symptoms would generally last for up to 24 hours.

Common symptoms that would occur if the frequency band being enhanced during treatment would be too low for the particular brain to achieve a state of improved regulation would be tension in the neck and shoulders, pressure behind the eyes, grogginess, sadness, spaciness or fogginess, headache, fidgeting, belching, inappropriate anger, difficulty waking, incontinence, whining, difficulty maintaining sleep, fatigue, depression, emotional over sensitivity, night terrors, sleep walking, low blood sugar symptoms and snoring.

Some of the symptoms of training at a too high frequency or training at a too low frequency are the same. The therapist needs to consider all the information pertaining to the client's discomfort in order to ascertain if the reward frequency is either too high or too low. These symptoms could last up to 24 hours.

It is important to provide accurate feedback to the therapist so that he or she can make appropriate changes in placement areas, training time or frequency bands. Therapists usually request feedback after every session in terms of specific markers that are indicators of brain regulation. Often feedback from teachers and other role players is also requested.

When other forms of neurofeedback training are involved – other than amplitude training – the after effects are different and often not as immediate. The therapist will indicate when the feedback report is required. Personally, I request a feedback report 24 hours. after power training sessions and on the third day after live Z-Score training sessions.

Although there is separate section in this book dedicated to case studies from my own practice as well as from other experienced therapists in South Africa, I just wish to provide a few snippets from reports of people of what to expect from the treatment or training program.

I am currently on a book sabbatical in a remote region in the North Eastern furthermost part of Namibia in what used to be called the Caprivi. I am in a tent on the banks of the Kavango River – a beautiful river that never runs dry. Birdlife is prolific and there is an abundance of game, including elephants, hippos, buffalo all the cat species and most antelope species, a truly magical space. What is the relevance of this you may wonder! Bear with me. I met one of my clients here yesterday. I am 2 800 km away from my practice to give you an idea of the likelihood of that happening. I believe that things unfold as they should so I don't question these things too much. This client, a gifted sixty-year-old opera singer, happens to be one of the clients of whom I requested a short testimony of sorts if they would want to share their experience of the results of the neurofeedback intervention. Angelique did not finish her report in time before I left on my sabbatical. We made an arrangement that she would send a message as soon as she had completed the report and I would then make an arrangement to access the internet which is not freely available here in the wilderness.

So there she was in the dining room of the lodge that I frequent now and then for dinner. After the shock of the coincidence was processed, I was introduced to her husband who promptly asked me if I had received Angelique's report yet. I smiled at her and waited. She said that she had planned to set aside time on a few occasions to compile a report on where she was at and what her life was like now. Every time, she said, she felt that she never wanted to revisit that time of darkness again. She wants to enjoy her new joy filled life to capacity. She also mentioned that she wouldn't have believed, prior to neurofeedback, that it would be possible for her to be able to sit in peace next to this magnificent river and experience such quiet contentment. She continued to describe the magnificence of the buffalo, the beauty of the surroundings with such heartfelt gratitude that three friends who were with me, commented on their experience of the joy she emanated.

Angelique was severely depressed when I met her. She was overwhelmed by the day to day responsibilities and locked herself away in her room often when it was expected of her to interact with others. There truly was no joy in her life. She received no other intervention that could have caused or contributed to the transformation of her experience of life and none of the circumstances in her life have changed. She ascribes the change in her mood and experience entirely to the neurofeedback treatment.

Neurofeedback has the potential of improving the regulation in the brain to the extent that it can bring relief to a myriad of negative symptoms that originate in the dysregulated brain.

2.3 Definitions of EEG and QEEG

The brain is an electro-chemical organ. The electrical and chemical aspects of the brain are related and inseparable. The main focus of medical science has mainly been on the chemical aspects of the brain and ways to alter the functioning of the brain through chemical interventions such as the use of medication. Technology has made it possible for clinicians to access the electrical activity of the brain and modulate the functioning of the brain by using this neuromodulatory technology. The electrical activity is measured by the use of the EEG.

In this section, the EEG and QEEG are discussed and defined. These two tools are to be distinguished from neurofeedback. Neurofeedback is the process or therapy by which the electroencephalogram and the quantified electroencephalogram are influenced and changed.

The electrical activity in the brain is reflected by the electroencephalogram. Sensors are placed on the scalp and task specific sensitive amplifiers record the activity. Hans Berger – as mentioned earlier – was the first person to publish such a recording. All the common brain rhythms namely – delta, theta, alpha, beta and gamma had been identified and named within 10 years after the publication of the first EEG in 1929 (Berger, 1929).

Micro voltages are produced by neurons in the upper layers of the cerebral cortex. The cerebral cortex contains the outer information processing layers of the brain and is divided into the frontal, parietal, temporal and occipital lobes. The predominant signals are produced by giant pyramidal cells organized in layers.

The EEG is a core tool used by neurologists and even psychiatrists. Wave forms are inspected, and abnormalities are identified from the raw EEG. Epilepsy is one of the most common diagnoses following the inspection of the EEG by a medical specialist. Transient events such as a spike and wave activity may be observed that is indicative of seizure activity. The EEG is a useful indicator of some aspects of brain functioning but is, according to Thomas Collura (2014) not a direct measure of information processing. The EEG is also not the activity of the brain. The presence of a particular rhythm indicates that the brain is in an idling or relaxing state. A certain rhythm may also be an indication of a certain area that is "offline" so to speak. An excess of slow brain wave activity in the frontal lobes for instance, indicate inactivity of the frontal lobes. An EEG is often also requested by a neurologist after a head injury and stroke. In these cases, other scans are usually also requested. The neurofeedback practitioner's interest lies in normal EEG waves and variations on normal EEG waves.

The display of the EEG is in the form of a wave like line. Specific frequency bands can be filtered out of the raw data to view separately. The different frequency bands have different names and characteristics. They are separated and named in terms of their frequency (cycles per second) and their morphology or appearance.

A measurable EEG signal is the result of numerous cortical cells firing in unison. The cells are activated, excited, or depolarized in unison which provides, what Thomas Collura (2014) refers to as a "consensus potential". The potential viewed from the scalp is very small when the cells behave independently when they are in an excited or active state. The measured potentials are a result of the normal activity of the brain. These consequences in the form of measured potentials, help us understand and diagnose what is happening in the brain. The example that Collura uses to describe this phenomenon is clear and succinct: The measured potentials of the brain cells is like the vibration on the hood of a car with a running engine and gives us information about what is happening inside the car.

In the course of the brain's normal activity, it puts certain areas in a state of activation and others in a state of deactivation. The modulation of these states, produce the waxing and waning visible in the EEG which as a reminder, is a result of cortical cells firing in unison.

There are many billions of neurons in the cortex or the outside layer of the brain. These neurons are organized into functional groups that are also interconnected. Cortical regions are thus interconnected and connected with sub-cortical brain structures as well. When measuring brain wave activity it is important to consider the fact that approximately 50% (Collura, (2014) only of the recorded activity arises from the brain cells beneath the particular sensor that has been placed on the scalp. It is also important to

57

remember that the activity measured by sensors at certain placement areas has been affected or spread by the skull and the brain by what is called volume conduction. Any brain activity is reflected at more than one site simultaneously.

Neurofeedback practitioners observe the EEG waveforms and electrical frequency patterns that are distinguished with the purpose of designing a treatment plan and making protocol decisions that meet the objectives of the client and to improve regulation which finally results in improved self-regulation.

On the following page is an example of an EEG Recording.

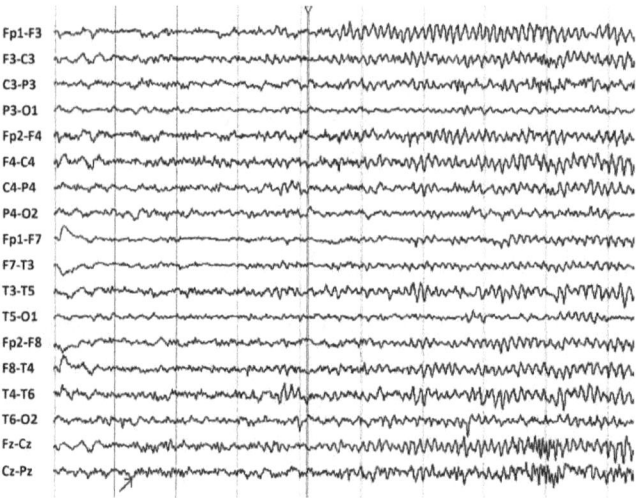

Figure 2.3: EEG recording. Reprinted from: Glass, H. C., Prieur, B., Molnar, C., Hamiwka, L., & Wirrell, E. (2006). Micturition and emotion-induced reflex epilepsy: Case report and review of the literature. Epilepsia, 47(12), 2180-2182. https://doi.org/10.1111/j.1528-1167.2006.00859.x

2.3.1 Frequencies and Waveforms

Below is a description of bandwidths that have been identified in terms of particular characteristics. The morphology of a brainwave as well as its cycles per second or 'hertz', abbreviated as Hz, define it. Location and amplitude are also further distinguishing factors. The different bandwidths correspond with certain states of consciousness and age groups.

According to Collura (2014) EEG rhythms result from rhythmic potential variations driven from action potentials from the lower brain via the reticular activating system (RAS). The RAS influences the neuronal mass that starts cortical activity. According to Collura, the cortex only has an intrinsic rhythm of 40 Hz. He suggests that the cortex ought to be thought of as having many groups of neuronal masses that are ready for activation but do not generate rhythms unless stimulated from what is referred to as "pacemaker sites" such as the amygdala, hippocampus, hypothalamus and the reticular activating system (RAS). Until recently, it was believed that certain rhythms originate in the cortex.

Delta

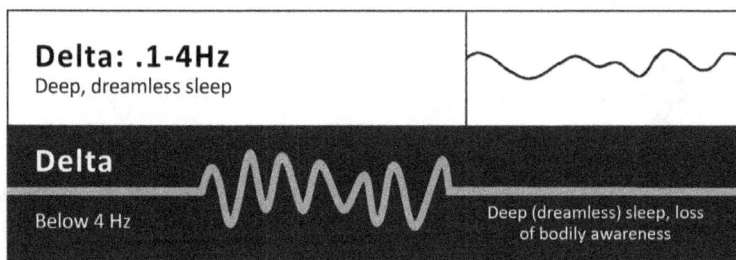

Figure 2.4: Delta brainwaves

Brain waves that make 0.5–3.0 cycles per second (Hz) and have the morphology of delta waves, is known as delta brain wave activity.

Characteristics

This brain wave activity appears to coincide with periods of reduced activation of the cortex (less pyramidal cell neuronal activity). Delta brain wave activity is normal during sleep with all age groups. During deep sleep, more than half the brain wave activity is delta activity. Delta is the dominant frequency in the brains of children ranging from birth to approximately six months.

Higher amplitudes than normal are often observed with cognitively handicapped children and children with learning disabilities and with people of all ages that have suffered damage to the cortex due to open or closed head injuries.

New research also indicates that high amplitudes of delta are often present in the EEG's of individuals that have suffered early childhood trauma.

High amplitudes of delta during wakefulness, is also associated with low arousal. Delta plays an important role in the immune system.

Research shows that excess delta activity is associated with memory problems, schizophrenia, and epilepsy.

Eye blink artefact also shows up in the delta frequency band. When delta frequency is being inhibited or down trained, it is important that the therapist is certain whether the delta is true delta activity or whether it is possibly due to eye movement. Low amplitudes of delta are associated with a diminished capacity for sleep.

Theta

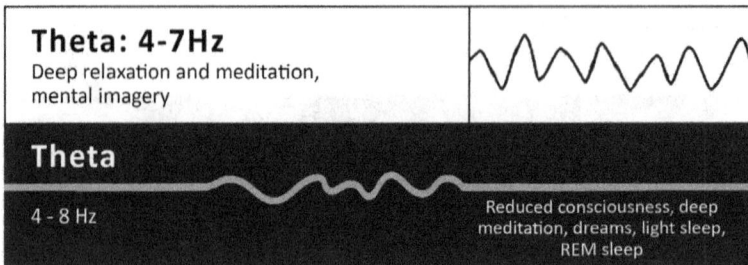

Theta: 4-7Hz
Deep relaxation and meditation, mental imagery

Theta

4 - 8 Hz

Reduced consciousness, deep meditation, dreams, light sleep, REM sleep

Figure 2.5: Theta brainwaves

Brain waves that produce 3–7 or 4–7, or 4–8 oscillations per second (Hz) and have the morphology of theta, is theta brain wave activity.

Origin

Some researchers are of the view that theta brain wave activity appears to originate mainly from the thalamus and the septal area in the limbic system. Others are of the opinion that theta brain wave activity in humans originates in the cortex. According to Collura (2014), lower frequency theta waves are produced by reverberation between the cortex and sub-thalamic nuclei. Neuroscience researchers distinguish between hippocampal theta rhythm observed in the hippocampus of numerous species of mammals and cortical theta rhythm originating from the cortex.

Characteristics

Theta is associated with the retrieval of memories. It has an effect on impulse control. Theta is the dominant frequency from the age of six months to approximately six or seven years. The theta brain waves become more dominant in the EEG of older children and adults when they become drowsy and are not actively engaged in the stimuli from the environment. Thinking creative thoughts is possible in a dominant theta state. Theta is also referred to as the transition frequency and occurs at the point where the theta and the alpha amplitudes intersect. During alpha/theta training this process is referred to as a crossover which potentially leads to recall of suppressed memories and significant associations and insights.

Excessive theta in the front-central area of the brain is a reliable biomarker for attentional problems. A significant percentage of the Attention Deficit Hyperactivity Disorder population, more so with the subgroup with the mainly inattentive presentation, have a high theta/beta ratio in the frontal lobes.

The amplitude of theta brain wave activity changes according to a 24-hour cycle. In other words, it has a diurnal rhythm unrelated to most external and internal factors other than fatigue. There are slight variations amongst individuals, but mostly the highest amplitudes are detected at 11:00, 13:00 and 15:00.

Research shows that an excess of theta can be associated with ADHD, Schizophrenia, memory problems and Tinnitus.

Low amplitudes of theta are associated with a diminished capacity to experience emotions and a lack of sense of self. The main focus of all the trauma related work in neurofeedback is currently based on the lack of the sense of self (Fisher, private conversation, 30 December 2018). The lack of the sense of self due to trauma can result in a person being hypervigilant and consequently feeling anxious and exhausted.

Alpha

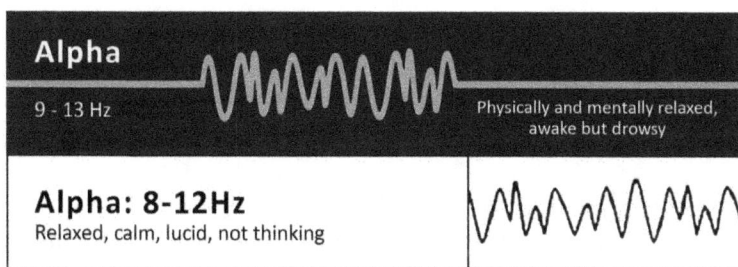

Figure 2.6: Alpha brainwaves

Typical morphology of alpha brainwave
Brain waves that produce 8–12 cycles or oscillations per second (Hz) and have the morphology of alpha, are alpha waves. Alpha has a distinct regular sinusoidal form.

Origin

The reticular activation system is, according to Collura (2014) the main generator of the alpha rhythm which was previously believed to originate in the thalamus. According to Steven Warner (2013), alpha is reported to be derived from the white matter of the brain.

Characteristics

Alpha is the dominant frequency in roughly 90% of people when their eyes are closed. Alpha is considered to be indicative of a resting state. The alpha frequency has been the focal point of a lot of research during the past decade. Alpha is generally the dominant frequency in the EEG recorded over the central region of the brain when the person is daydreaming and/or when the mind feels to be at rest. The alpha amplitude ought to differ significantly between when the eyes are closed and when the eyes are open (the alpha arrest reaction is discussed below). The alpha amplitude is increased during meditation and is associated with a calm, relaxed open focus. There are a variety of exercises suggested and available to increase the alpha amplitude in order to reduce stress and anxiety and induce a tranquil mental state. Alpha is also the dominant frequency when one watches television or when one has calm and free flowing thoughts. Asymmetry of alpha in the frontal lobes is associated with depression. The amplitude of alpha in the right frontal lobe ought to be higher than the alpha amplitude of the left frontal lobe by a specific margin. When there is more alpha activity in left frontal lobe, it may be a cause of depression. Other research findings are mentioned below.

Increased alpha is detected during and for approximately a few days after smoking marijuana.

Although too low amplitudes of alpha are typically associated with anxiety and nervousness, as paradoxical as it seems, too high amplitudes of alpha measured over certain regions of the scalp, can also lead to anxiety and other symptoms of discomfort. Research findings are mentioned below.

High alpha (11–12 and even 11–13 Hz) is distinguished from the broader alpha bandwidth. During the high alpha dominant state, the mind and the body is calm, but also ready. From this dominant state one has the ability to respond accurately and quickly to a wide variety of stimuli. This state is often described as "the zone" and is an important factor in peak performance training, whether it is mental or sport related peak performance. Enhancing 11–13 Hz is a very common protocol used in peak performance training. Collura (2014) refers to the alpha state as "an active but idle" state.

Since the work of Dr Neils Birbaumer on the importance of training larger pools of neurons, secondary synaptic training has also been included in peak performance protocols recently. This will be discussed further in the section on peak performance.

Low alpha, (8–10 Hz) is distinguished from the broader bandwidth of general alpha. To be more precise, it actually refers to that bandwidth that is below the individual's own peak frequency. The peak frequency can become lower with age and also with cognitive deterioration. The individual's specific peak frequency in the alpha bandwidth with the eyes closed has been linked with cognitive potential. The higher the peak frequency the higher the potential as a rule of thumb. When the peak frequency is higher than 12 Hz it can however be as problematic as a peak frequency that is too low (S. Fisher, personal communication, December 30, 2018). These brains, according to Fisher, are driven brains. Such high peak frequencies are also common to sociopaths.

Alpha brain waves, like theta waves also show diurnal variations in amplitude. The alpha amplitude tends to be higher in the vicinity of 11:00, 13:00 and 15:00. Fatigue may have an influence on the amplitudes, but not other factors such as digestive processes.

When a process called alpha blocking or the alpha arrest reaction does not occur when a person opens his eyes, it may be indicative of either hypo- or hyper- arousal. When a person closes his/her eyes, the absence of visual stimuli ought to cause the brain to be in a relaxed or idling state resulting in higher amplitudes of alpha. When the eyes are opened and the visual cortex gets stimulated, the alpha amplitude ought to reduce which indicates higher activation of the cortex. A hypo- aroused person would typically have unusually high alpha amplitude when the eyes are open which would result in less alpha blocking. A hyper-aroused person on the other hand would typically have higher alpha amplitude when the eyes are closed which would result in a smaller difference in the EO and EC conditions as well.

A low alpha amplitude during the eyes closed condition, can by the same argument be indicative of hyper-vigilance, difficulty in allowing the brain to rest and anxiety.

Research shows that an excess of alpha can be associated with ADHD, OCD, and autism. A deficit of alpha can be associated with anxiety, schizophrenia, memory problems and tinnitus. A low alpha peak frequency can be associated with ADHD. Decreased alpha has also been associated with impulsivity with explosiveness.

Beta and Gamma

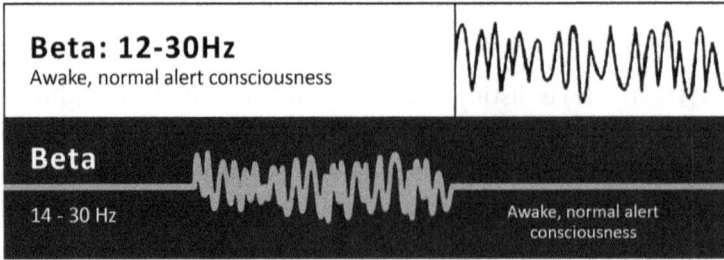

Figure 2.7: Beta brainwaves

Typical morphology of beta brainwave

Beta activity is a broad bandwidth of which different sub-divisions used for different purposes exist. Generally, all brain wave activity higher than 12 Hz (for some purposes 12 Hz brain wave activity is included in the reference to the beta bandwidth) is referred to as beta activity. For the purpose of this book, beta indicates brain wave activity from 12–35 Hz and gamma indicates EEG activity of 36– 42 Hz. Beta and gamma activity is considered to be fast brain wave activity and are discussed together for that reason and also for the fact that there is very limited information available on gamma brain wave activity.

In *The Neurofeedback Book*, Michael and Lynda Thompson (2015), divide the beta bandwidth into the sensorimotor rhythm (13–15 Hz), (others identify 12–15 Hz as belonging to this sub-group of beta activity), low beta (16– 20 Hz), high beta (which includes all beta spindling) that usually occurs at above 20 Hz and sheer rhythm (38– 42 Hz). Others use the following sub-divisions in the beta bandwidth in QEEG reports:

Beta 12–20 Hz, described as small fast waves associated with concentration and mental activity.

High beta 20– 30 Hz, described as fast waves associated with worry, anxiety, and over-thinking.

Low amplitudes of beta 1 are associated with a diminished capacity for a moderate external focus required for driving for instance. Low amplitudes of beta 2 on the other hand are associated with a diminished capacity for intense external focus which is required for academic success. Low amplitudes of beta3 activity are associated with a diminished capacity for hypervigilance.

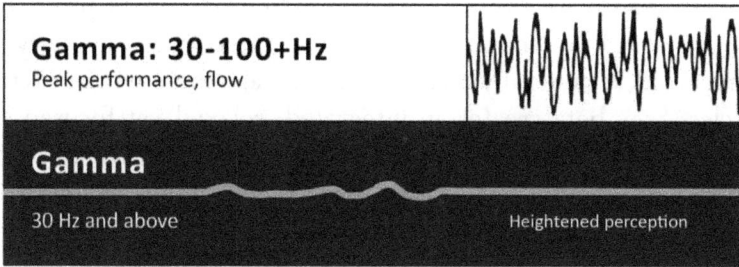

Figure 2.8: Gamma brainwaves

Typical morphology of gamma brainwave

Gamma 30–100 Hz, are fast waves originating from the thalamus which move from the back to the front of the brain and back again 40 times per second. Although the exact function of gamma is not yet known, neuroscientists are of the opinion that these very fast brain waves are able to connect information from all areas of the brain. This frequency appears to have a dominant role in peak performance. For the purpose of this book, we'll be referring to low beta (13–15 Hz) which is also referred to as high alpha; midrange beta (15–18 Hz); high beta (18–30 Hz) and gamma (36–44 Hz).

Characteristics

Beta activity is generally indicative of an alert, problem-solving state during which the individual is thinking logically.

Beta reflects desynchronized active brain tissue, according to Warner (2013). Beta usually has symmetrical distribution in the left and right hemispheres. Beta amplitudes ought to be higher on the left side of the brain than on the right. Asymmetry of beta in the right hemisphere is associated with anxiety. Hyper- coherence of beta can also be indicative of anxiety and the presence of panic attacks and anticipatory anxiety.

A dominant frequency in the beta band may indicate an excess of norepinephrine.

Increased beta at Fp2 and F3 may offer a clue to suppression of feelings and emotional flatness.

The presence of 12–15 or 13–15 Hz activity, used to be known as the sensorimotor rhythm, is very important across the sensor-motor strip of the brain. Barry Sterman named this sub-set of the beta band in 1967 and determined the importance of this bandwidth. The waveform has a distinct spindle-like appearance. This rhythm is known as the resting rhythm of the motor system and is very often enhanced in neurofeedback protocols. The amplitude of this frequency band is at its highest when the body is still. When enhanced, it generally results in mental alertness without tension in the muscles. Low beta creates an integrated, relaxed yet focused state of being. According to Steven Warner (2013), low beta is inhibited by motion and restraining the body can result in higher amplitudes of low beta. The waveform of this frequency in other areas of the cortex is different in appearance.

Midrange beta (15–18 Hz) is associated with heightened awareness of self and the surroundings, alertness without agitation.

Beta 16–20 Hz is, according to the Thompsons (2015), is referred to as "problem- solving beta". When a person focusses on solving a particular problem, an immediate increase in 17 Hz activity can generally be noted.

Muscle artefact often shows up in the high beta range.

High beta is associated with feelings of alertness, efficient problem solving, anxiety, rumination and activation of the mind and the body. Hyper-coherence is associated with feeling overwhelmed whereas hypo-coherence in this bandwidth is associated with feeling immobilized.

Beta spindling refers to bursts of beta which mostly occur at frequencies higher than 20 Hz.

Some of the activity in the gamma range (36– 44 Hz) is associated with intensely focused attention. It is possibly the 40 Hz activity that enables the brain to consolidate when having to process information from its different regions. When gamma brain wave activity is enhanced through training, it appears to result in improved memory and learning.

The sheer rhythm (38– 42 Hz) was named after David Sheer who did important work with enhancing 40 Hz activity in the 1970's (see Bird et al., 1978ab). It is important not to include this particular bandwidth in any inhibit when doing neurofeedback.

2.4 Abnormal EEG Patterns and Unusual Waveforms

Abnormalities in EEG patterns are mostly beyond the scope of practice of most neurofeedback practitioners unless the neurofeedback practitioner is also a neurologist. The neurofeedback practitioner is however familiarized with the main abnormalities in EEG patterns in their original didactic training and more advanced neurophysiology training before certification so as to be able to identify these patterns and make necessary referrals when appropriate.

2.4.1 Abnormal EEG Patterns Associated with Epilepsy

The most common abnormal EEG patterns that the neurofeedback practitioner will probably come across, is the spike and wave pattern in the EEG associated with epilepsy. The epileptiform activity may however also be present in other disorders.

The abnormal EEG pattern may present during a seizure (*ictal*) or between seizures (*inter-ictal*). The observed abnormality may furthermore be *localized* or *generalized*. There are different theories on the origin of and dynamics involved in the spike and wave appearance of the epileptiform activity. The *center-encephalic* theory explains that thalamic projections are involved, but this theory has since been elaborated on and modified and it appears that the reticular formation and the cortex are involved in seizure activity.

The cause of epilepsy is often unknown. Brain injury, stroke, brain tumors, infections of the brain and birth defects are among some of the factors that can cause epilepsy. A small proportion of cases are linked to genetic mutations.

In focal epileptiform activity, the neurofeedback practitioner will see localized spikes and sharp waves from a few neighboring electrodes. According to the Thompsons (2015), this irregular activity may be surrounded by irregular slower waves or followed by an after-going wave. There are many disorders that may show epileptiform activity.

There are very many different kinds of seizures. Seizures can be divided into the *generalized* and *partial* seizure groups. The generalized seizures involve both hemispheres and the partial or focal seizures involve a single area in one hemisphere.

Another abnormal EEG pattern that the neurofeedback practitioner may come across is the EEG pattern associated with *absence* seizure. It has a characteristic 3 Hz high amplitude spike and slow wave activity. The mainly inattentive presentation of the ADHD population probably shows a higher incidence of this occurrence simply because those with absence seizures are often misdiagnosed as ADHD sufferers.

Following is a figure of a typical 3 per second spike and wave pattern associated with absence-seizures.

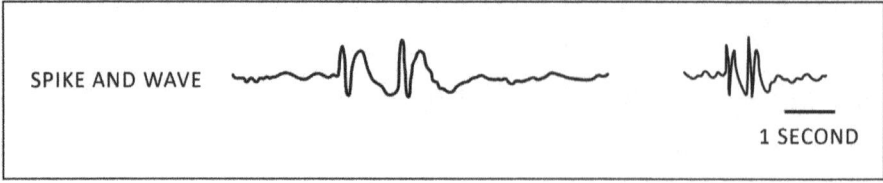

Figure 2.9: Spike and wave pattern associated with epilepsy.

The figure on the following page illustrates the EEG pattern of a person during a tonic seizure followed by an illustration of the EEG pattern during a tonic-clonic seizure. Pay attention to the spikes with following slow waves.

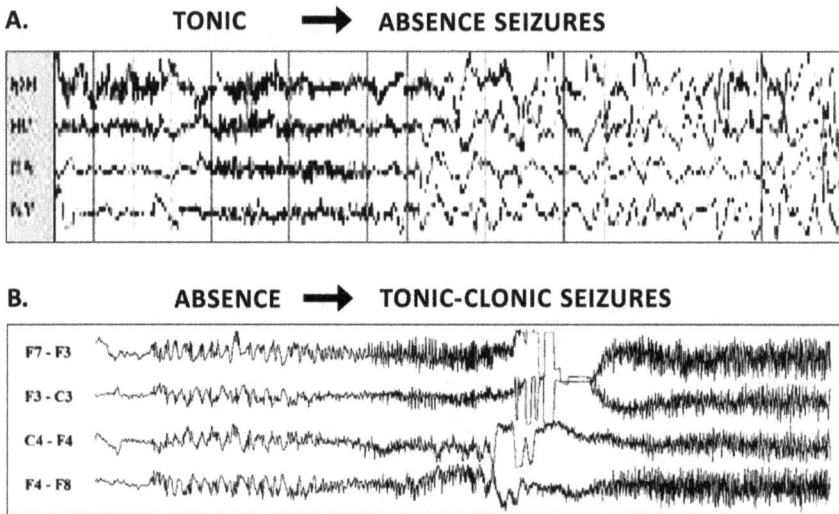

Figures 2.10A and 2.10B: Tonic and tonic-clonic seizures. Reprinted from: Fan, D., Duan, L., Wang, Q., & Luan, G. (2017). Combined effects of feedforward inhibition and excitation in thalamocortical circuit on the transitions of epileptic seizures. Frontiers in Computational Neuroscience, 11, 59. https://doi.org/10.3389/fncom.2017.0005

Non spike and wave abnormalities may also present in some seizure disorders. Bursts of rhythmic slow waves may be present in temporal or frontotemporal areas.

To complicate matters a bit further, just a reminder that spike and wave patterns are sometimes present with no relation a seizure disorder.

The QEEG report will usually indicate when there is epileptiform activity present and whether a referral to a neurologist for further investigation is advisable.

Those of us, who started out with neurofeedback in South Africa about two decades ago, were petrified of going anywhere close to a brain in the presence of epileptiform activity or where there was a diagnosis of epilepsy. When we came across anything that resembled the possibility of seizure activity, we would make long distance calls to our mentors in the USA and contacted anyone who could possibly offer reassurance and advice. I am of the opinion that the newly trained neurofeedback practitioners are still very hesitant to approach a client with a seizure disorder despite all the research and teachings that we currently have free access to. Today there are many neurofeedback practitioners that specialize in the treatment of epilepsy. I wish to remind all neurofeedback practitioners that still feel hesitant and fearful in the face of epilepsy, that probably the most significant work in the field that caused the original interest in neurofeedback to spread like wildfire, was Barry Sterman's work in the late sixties based on decreasing the paroxysms of unusual EEG activity by enhancing the SMR activity which resulted in the wide spread use of neurofeedback as an intervention for epilepsy (see Egner & Sterman, 2006). According to the available research, the current statistical rating of neurofeedback as an intervention for seizure disorders is level 4, which means that it is efficacious and statistically significantly equal or superior to another treatment with established efficacy.

I have anecdotal evidence from my own practice of the success of neurofeedback in this regard.

2.4.2 Lambda Waves
These waves are saw-tooth shaped and found in the occipital region. These are only considered abnormal when they are markedly asymmetrical. The abnormality will then be on the side with the lower amplitude.

2.4.3 Mu Rhythm
These waves are usually found in the 7–11 Hz bandwidth and have the appearance of alpha waves. The presence of this rhythm is mostly detected at C3 and C4. Mu is blocked when making a fist on the opposite side of the recording. Mu waves ought to be distinguished from central alpha in the treatment of ADHD. Other than the "fist test" one can also request the client to close their eyes and to then open them during which time the therapist would be able to observe the alpha blocking or ART (alpha arrest response). Mu waves have a pointed top and rounded bottom or the other way around, whereas alpha has a distinct sinusoidal appearance.

2.4.4 Spikes

The amplitude of a spike is higher than the amplitude of the background waves. They have a sharp appearance (like a spike) and have a very short duration of between 20 and 70 milliseconds.

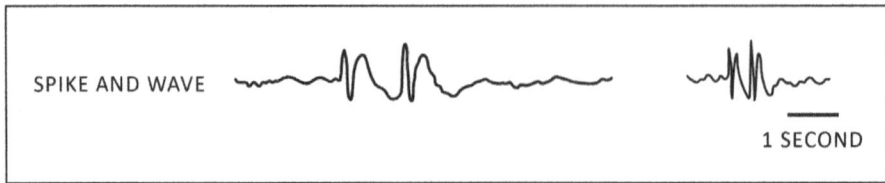

Figure 2.11: Spike and wave pattern.

It is very important to be able to distinguish between an ordinary spike and seizure activity. In seizure activity the spike is followed by a slow wave.

2.4.5 Sharp Waves

Sharp waves are less pointy than spike waves and have been compared in appearance to the tip of a pencil in *The Neurofeedback Book* (Thompson & Thompson, 2015).

2.4.6 Sharp Transients

Infrequent bursts of sharp waves are called sharp transients. This kind of activity may occur between seizures but are mostly referred to as being non-specific. When these complexes last for a few seconds without symptoms associated with a seizure they are referred to as a sub-clinical electrographic seizure.

2.4.7 Paroxysmal Discharge

One or more waves that stand out from the rest of the EEG are referred to as a paroxysmal discharge. They usually begin and end abruptly. They are often observed when a person is drowsy.

2.4.8 Sleep Spindles, V-Waves and K-Waves

Neurofeedback practitioners do not generally work with sleep patterns in the EEG. On occasion however, during alpha/theta training sessions a client may fall asleep.

Sleep spindles look like low beta (12–15 Hz) spindles and are observed more frequently over the central regions.

V-waves are negative and have extremely high amplitudes of up to 250 microvolt. They last for only up to 200 milliseconds. K complexes are detected during phase 2 sleep and are also negative, sharp, and last longer than V-waves.

2.4.9 Square Waves

Square waves have the appearance of theta or delta waves with faster, lower amplitude beta waves riding on top.

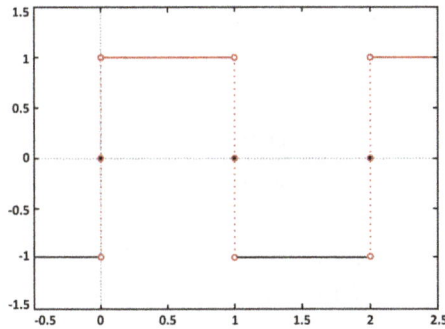

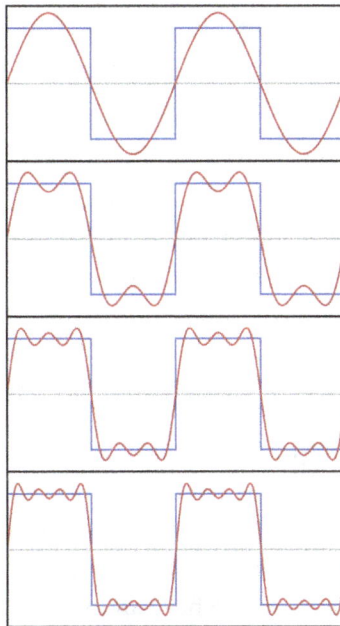

Figure 2.12: Square waves. Reprinted from: File: Fourier Series.svg. (n. d.). In Wikipedia. https:// commons. wikimedia.org/wiki/File: Fourier_Series.svg

2.4.10 Localized Slow Waves

Brain wave activity lower than 8 Hz may be indicative of a localized lesion for example a stroke, migraine transient ischemic attack, mild head injury or a large infolding of the dura mater separating the cerebellum from the cerebrum. Delta would then often be surrounded by theta and would not respond to opening the eyes or hyperventilation.

2.4.11 Bi-Laterally Synchronous Slow Waves

When bilaterally synchronous slow waves are observed in an alert adult, they could be indicative of midline structural damage. In children who are drowsy, these brain waves are normal. FIRDA or frontal intermittent delta activity (3 Hz) is seen in some who have absence seizures.

2.4.12 Generalized Asynchronous Slow Waves

Generalized asynchronous slow waves are regarded to be the most common EEG abnormality. This brain wave activity is normal in individuals that are sleepy and in children that have fever. These waves occur over both hemispheres and are slower than 8 Hz. A neurologist ought to confirm that there is no associated abnormality.

2.4.13 Continuous Irregular Delta

Irregular delta is seen with lesions affecting the white matter of the brain.

2.4.14 Abnormal Beta

When beta activity is asymmetrical it is abnormal on the side with lower beta power if the difference is more than 35%. Decreased beta is sometimes seen during a migraine attack. Isolated reduction in beta is viewed by neurologists as being indicative of local brain damage.

2.5 Ratios of Frequency Bandwidths and Asymmetry

Ratios compare the distribution of frequency bandwidths at a given site. The amplitudes of the different frequency bands of the brain wave activity are less significant than the ratios of the amplitudes of the bandwidths in relation to one another. Some individuals have higher amplitudes of all the frequency bands than other individuals. Some have an overall "flat EEG". Such an EEG displays low amplitudes of all bandwidths.

The best researched ratio is probably the theta-beta ratio, pioneered by Lubar et al. (1995b). A number of conclusions have been drawn from theta-to- beta ratios. The most significant is probably that a theta-to-beta ratio greater than 3:1, constitutes a slow wave disorder (Demos, 2005).

Theta-to-beta ratios decrease with age. The largest theta-to-beta ratios are found at Cz or Fz whereas the smallest ratios occur on the temporal lobes. The ADHD population generally have a larger theta-to-beta ratio than the general population. There are however also other ADHD sub-groups that have higher beta and alpha amplitudes were the theta-to-beta ratio is not higher than 3:1. According to the research done by Dr Robert Chabot from New York University, ADHD sufferers can be divided into subgroups based on their EEG (Chabot et al., 2005; Chabot & Serfontein, 1996). According to his research, 47% of the ADHD population have excessive theta activity in the resting brain, 31% have an excess of alpha power, 7% have an excess of beta activity and 15% of the ADHD population have normal EEGs. The group with the excess beta activity may be the group that respond poorly to stimulant medication.

High theta-to-beta ratios at the frontal lobes indicate problems with attention and executive functions.

The following ratios are expected in a normal EEG:

- The beta amplitudes measured at the frontal sites, F7 and F8 should show higher amplitudes on the left than on the right. A difference of more than 35% can be problematic and beta ought to be enhanced on the side with the lower amplitude.

- Alpha amplitudes measured in the frontal lobes on F3 and F4, show a lower amplitude on the left (F3) than on the right (F4). The difference ought not to be greater than 50%. Alpha that measures higher on the left is often associated with depression.

- Amplitudes of theta ought to be or less equal measured at T3 and T4.

- In the normal EEG, measured along the central strip on Fz, Cz and Pz, anterior beta is expected to be higher than posterior beta. Posterior alpha is expected to be higher than anterior alpha and anterior theta is expected to be higher than posterior theta.

- Symptoms ought to always be considered in conjunction with EEG information.

- Lower SMR and beta amplitudes in relation to theta amplitudes are not an unusual phenomenon in ADHD. Unusually low SMR amplitude is not an unusual phenomenon with Parkinson's disease sufferers according to the Thompsons (2015).

* Beta 23–36 Hz power is generally lower than beta 15–19 Hz power.

2.6 QEEG (Quantitative Electroencephalogram)

A QEEG is a 19 channel EEG recording which is then quantified in terms of certain markers. The individual's EEG is compared to one or more normative databases. Deviances from the normative database are presented as quantified information. Regions that are dysregulated can be identified by the QEEG. In neurofeedback there is a general movement away from an implicit systems theory approach during which protocols based on one channel training where the strategic placement of a single electrode can affect an entire system, to a more QEEG based or location-based approach. As mentioned elsewhere in this book in the chapter on the evolution of neurofeedback, the reader is reminded that the systems approach is still very much in use with successful outcomes and is being revisited by many researchers. Many experienced clinicians have an approach in which they collect as much information about the functioning of the individual's brain in terms of symptoms as well as very technologically sophisticated quantified information and then masterfully blend the information to determine a training path which often includes both approaches.

Some clinicians do only QEEG guided neurofeedback. Clinicians new to the field of neurofeedback may also probably feel safer with a QEEG report in hand that dictates a training path. Personally, I request a QEEG when there are particular complicating factors such as traumatic brain injury or when a client responds differently to the anticipated outcome of a specific protocol. I need to add here that due to our circumstances in South Africa, the neurofeedback practitioners had to make do without QEEGs for an extended period of time. During that period, we possibly developed an acute sense of awareness of our client's symptoms and other related skills associated with intuition and sensitivity that hopefully turned us into better therapists for it.

I possibly would not have had the courage to voice this opinion had I not been in the company of the best regarding this opinion. I regard Sebern Fisher as one of my most appreciated mentors, although I have only had the privilege of attending one of her workshops in person. Sebern Fisher (2014) writes, "There is no easy way to understand why a Q-recommendation fails. The brain is too complex, and the desire to quantify it is, understandably, great. The Q feels to me like looking at the sky through Galileo's telescope when we need something even more advanced than the Hubble. We are, I think, at the kinematics stage in QEEG-that is, describing what we see happening but not yet knowing what forces are actually at play. Our understanding is Newtonian when it needs to be quantum." Having said that, all the practitioners will know that the connectivity measures provided by the QEEG provides such important information that we would not have had access to. All practitioners will also agree that the protocol recommendations provided in the Q-reports are spot on sometimes. A further significant advantage is that therapists can embark on the newer, technologically advanced paradigms such as multi-channel training and training involving live data bases which is probably not to be recommended without the detailed information provided by the QEEG reports.

The QEEG report will also be more helpful and even essential to one client base more so than to another. Some practitioners work almost exclusively with pathology. According to Joseph Guan (2017) research suggests that QEEGs have a high level of reliability. He voices his opinion on the value of the QEEG as follows: "of all the imaging modalities, the greatest body of replicated evidence regarding pathophysiological concomitants of psychiatric and developmental disorders has been provided by EEG and QEEG studies". A brief discussion on the information provided in a typical QEEG report, follows:

A 19-channel resting state EEG gets recorded for the Eyes Open and the Eyes Closed condition. The recording gets artifacted with advanced software and epileptiform activity is identified by an Epileptiform Episode Detection algorithm. The data is compared to an age and gender appropriate database and deviances are indicated.

The profile report provides a comprehensive report on the relation between the client's brain activity profile and her/his symptoms indicated on standardized online questionnaires. The one section of the report indicates the correlation between the individual's EEG results and the client's symptoms as well as the EEG biomarkers for psychopathology and arousal. The biomarker match section indicates the correlation of the individual's EEG with the biomarkers (based on scientific evidence) for ADHD, Depression, Anxiety, Autism Spectrum Disorder, Schizophrenia, Memory Disorder, Insomnia, Dyslexia, Tinnitus and OCD. Epilepsy, Substance Use Disorder and TBI are not depicted because these disorders have not been reliably associated with biomarkers. Certain deviations in neural oscillations have been related to different psychopathologies indicated on the EEG Biomarker scale section. Excess theta and alpha power as well as deviant

75

beta power have been associated with ADHD. Frontal alpha asymmetry is a marker for depression. Excess delta power is associated with TBI and memory disorders. The EEG biomarker scales are graphical representations of the correlation between measures of neural activity pathology and neural activity arousal.

In the next section of the profile report, the activity and connectivity of certain Resting-State networks are assessed. The relevant networks are The Default Mode Network, The Dorsal Attention Network, The Emotion-Regulation Network, The Sensory-Motor Cortex, The Memory Network and The Visual Cortex. Where there is deviant activity within any of these networks, the brain areas involved as well as the Brodmann areas are indicated.

The reports also include Z-scored absolute power maps and coherence and phase connectivity measures. Areas in which the brain are deviant from the normative database in this section of the report are also indicated with the associated brain areas, Brodmann areas and symptoms associated with the defect. Classical amplitude training protocols based on the findings as well as recommended Z-score training protocols are suggested. The level of scientific support available to support the findings as well as the specificity of the degree of the deviance and the data quality is indicated for all the identified biomarkers.

There are other data bases and types of QEEG reports available than the type discussed here that include Event Related Potentials and different normative databases. At this point in time, however, I am not aware of any validity debates or concerns about the accuracy of the information. The only aspect of the QEEG reports that is ever in question to the best of my knowledge is the fact that the protocol recommendations, albeit apparently justifiable and valid, don't have the expected outcome. The individual response to training or treatment remains unpredictable – more so with complicated issues than with straight forward cases and the neurofeedback practitioner should remain ever vigilant of all symptoms.

Chapter 3

Brain Basics and Neuro-Anatomical Structures

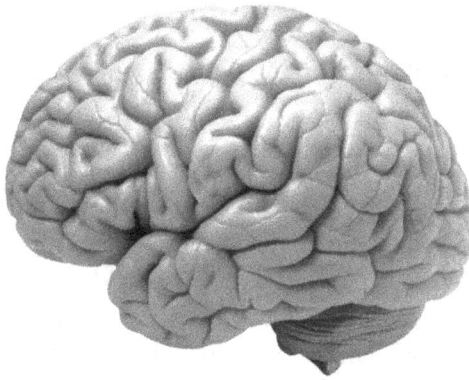

Figure 3.1: The natural brain

The purpose of this chapter is to provide the reader with basic information of the brain and an overview of the neuroanatomical structures. More detailed knowledge of neuroanatomy and neurophysiology of the brain is required for Board Certification of neurotherapists. This overview is presented in terms of how the neuroanatomical structures pertain to the EEG and certain behaviors.

The brain is a wonderfully interesting, vulnerable, and complex organ that literally governs every movement and every thought and every feeling we experience or express. The brain floats inside fluid in the skull. Daniel Amen, in one of his webinars compares the consistency of the brain with that of butter and Harry Kerasides (2017), who wrote extensively on concussionology, compares the consistency of the brain with that of something between peanut butter and memory foam. Despite its protection in the very hard skull, it can be easily affected by trauma to the head. The most vulnerable areas of the brain are probably the frontal and the parietal lobes (illustrated below) due to their proximity to the skull.

The brain of a healthy human adult comprises approximately 2% of the average body weight and uses 20% of the oxygen we breathe and uses 20% of our energy. It needs sufficient blood flow and sufficient oxygen to function. Both Daniel Amen and Harry Kerasidis emphasize the importance of the conscious control we can have on the health of our brain by consciously eating the right food, getting enough sleep, exercising enough, drinking enough water and avoiding toxic and harmful substances. Neurofeedback practitioners have at least a basic knowledge of healthy lifestyle principles and either offer basic guidelines in this regard or make appropriate referrals.

3.1 Three Main Parts of the Brain

The brain is organized into three main sections: the forebrain, the midbrain, and hindbrain.

The cerebral cortex is grooved and contains sulci and fissures. The fissures are large folds in the cortex and the sulci are shallower grooves. The fissures divide the brain into lobes and hemispheres. The tissue between the sulci is called gyri. The gyri are the convolutions or ridges of the surface of the cerebral hemispheres and are separated by fissures or sulci. The brain also consists of billions of specialized cells which are referred to as neurons and glia. The neurons transmit the signals between the cells and the glia regulates homeostasis and provides support and protection to the function of the neurons. The brain probably contains 100 billion neurons and ten times more glial cells.

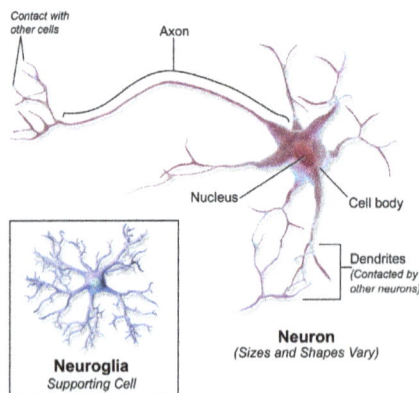

Figure 3.2: Neural tissue. Reprinted from: Blausen.com staff. (2014). Medical gallery of Blausen Medical 2014. Wiki Journal of Medicine, 1(2). https://doi.org/10.15347/wjm/2014.010

Some of the main anatomical structures are illustrated in the following figure:

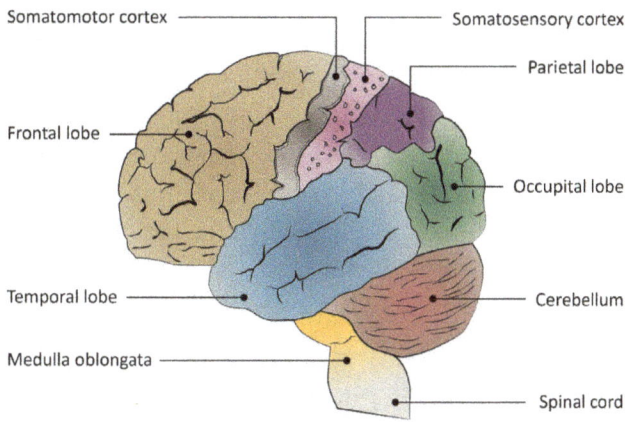

Figure 3.3: Anatomical structures. Reprinted from: File: Cerebrum lobes.png. (n. d.). In Wikipedia. https:// commons.wikimedia.org/wiki/File:Cerebrum_lobes.png

The cerebellum of the brain is involved with voluntary, physical movements, posture, balance, coordination and with the facilitation of the role of the prefrontal cortex (PFC) in assisting with judgement and impulse control. Damage to the cerebellum leads to motor coordination difficulties and difficulties with learning (to be distinguished from learning difficulties due to dyslexia or dyscalculia).

The brainstem is at the base of the brain and is continuous with the spinal cord. Signals from the brain to the body are relayed through this section of the brain. Heart rate, respiration and blood pressure are regulated by the brainstem.

3.2 The Left and Right Hemispheres

Another and better-known division of the brain is the division of the cerebrum or the forebrain, which is the largest area of the brain, into two symmetrical cerebral hemispheres, the left hemisphere and the right hemisphere. The hemispheres are covered by the cerebral cortex and contain the basal ganglia and the limbic system. The two hemispheres are associated with specific characteristics, which lead to the popular tendency of brain profiling that most readers would have heard of. People often want to know whether they are left or right brain dominant. The characteristics of the two hemispheres are provided purely from a neurofeedback point of view. The hemisphere characteristics can be relevant to protocol decisions as well as symptom tracking and the understanding of reactions to protocols.

The left hemisphere is mostly the dominant hemisphere. It is associated with analytical thinking patterns during which a complex process is broken down into its individual components. It is focused on detail. The thinking processes associated with the left hemisphere are logical, sequential, and linguistically based. The left-brain dominant people are good at math and analytical reasoning. The left-brain processes one word and one concept after the other. It perceives, understands, or comprehends, stores information in memory, formulates opinions and expresses the insights and knowledge in language, and stores verbal memories. Beta activity is usually higher in the left hemisphere and theta activity is mostly more or less equal between the two hemispheres.

Thinking processes associated with the right hemisphere are holistic and spatial. Puzzle building skills, hearing the musical chord, insight and intuition abide here. The right hemisphere can read facial expressions, find, and remember places, understand vocal intonations. Creativity is also associated with the right hemisphere as well as empathy and a concept of self that develops early. The right hemisphere synthesizes or combines components into an integrated whole and then experiences the process in its entirety rather than in detail. The experience and expression of anger, rage, anxiety, and mood regulation reside here. Alpha activity is mostly higher in the right hemisphere.

3.3 Basic Terminology Used in the Description of Areas and Regions in the Brain

Certain terminology has been standardized to rule out any error in specifying areas and regions of the brain. Over and above the terminology used to name the lobes, deeper structures and Brodmann areas, directionality and sections also need to be specified to be able to understand and interpret scans with cross sections for instance and also to enable succinct communication amongst clinicians.

The first terms to be discussed are, anterior or rostral, medial, posterior, superior or dorsal, inferior or ventral. These terms pertain to specific areas or regions of the brain.

Anterior or rostral

Anterior means front. The anterior or rostral part of the brain is the area behind the forehead.

Medial

The medial part of one's brain is located in the middle of the head in the area of the crown of the head and includes the entire middle section of the brain.

Posterior

The posterior part of the brain is located at the back of the head.

Superior or dorsal

Both these terms indicate the top. The Thompsons (2015) suggest that one uses the analogy of a fish and reminds oneself of the dorsal fin of a fish). This term can also mean back. If you were to think of a fish once again, the top of the fish is also the back of the fish.

Inferior or ventral

The inferior or ventral surface indicates the under surface. Ventral can also indicate the front. The opposite of dorsal is ventral. If dorsal indicates the back, then ventral indicates the front.

Lateral

A lateral perspective is a perspective from the side – either the right or the left side.

Sections of the brain

For the comprehension of brain related imaging studies, it is essential to be able to distinguish between *coronal* (also referred to as transverse sections), *horizontal* and *sagittal* sections. In neuroimaging techniques, the structure and other components of the central nervous system are imaged.

Coronal or **transverse** sections are sections across the brain from the front (prefrontal cortex) to the back (cerebellum) in a **vertical plane.** The sections will then be "slices" from the dorsal surface (top) down to the ventral surface (down) made across the brain from front to back.

Horizontal sections are "slices" from the top of the brain to the bottom of the brain made from a **horizontal** plane. The first "slice" would then lift off the top of the brain.

Sections or "slices" made from a **vertical** plane moving from the left temporal lobe to the right temporal lobe or vice versa, are referred to as *sagittal* sections.

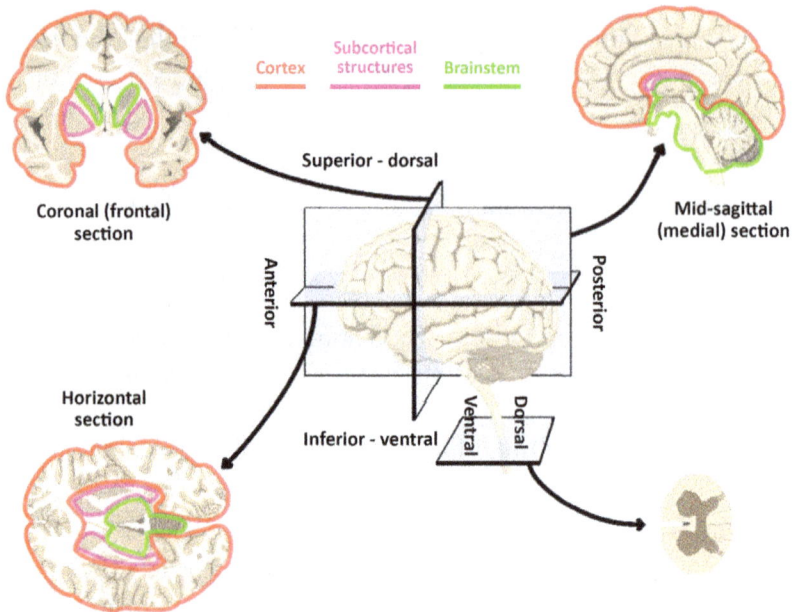

Figure 3.4: Illustration of different areas and sections of the brain. Reprinted from: One Class. Boston University. (n. d.). Chapter 3 – Structure of the nervous system. https://oneclass.com/textbook-notes/us/ boston-u/cas-ps/cas-ps-231/436013-phys-ch-3docx.en.html

More terminology

Gyrus
A gyrus is a broad ridge of cortex.

Sulcus
A sulcus is a dip or valley in the cortex.

Fissure
A fissure is a very deep dip or valley, like for instance, the longitudinal cerebral fissure that separates the two hemispheres.

Dura mater
The outside layer of the connective tissue that covers the brain and separates the cerebellum and cerebrum is referred to as dura mater.

Tentorium

It is a large infolding of dura mater separating below from the cerebrum above.

Grey matter

The grey matter in the brain consists of the cell bodies of neurons, the unmyelinated axons and dendrites of the neurons, glial cells, and other types of support cells.

White matter

The white matter in the brain consists mainly of those areas that have myelinated axons. The myelin sheath of nerve fibers causes the white appearance of the white matter. White matter is less dense due its fat content. Myelinization allows for faster transmission of nerve impulses and is only completed during the second decade of a person's life. The right hemisphere contains more white matter than the left hemisphere.

3.4 The Lobes of the Cerebrum, Deeper Structures and Cortical Surface Areas

3.4.1 Lobes of the Brain

The cerebrum can furthermore be divided into lobes, comprising of the frontal lobes, temporal lobes, parietal lobes, and occipital lobes, differentiated by their location and functions.

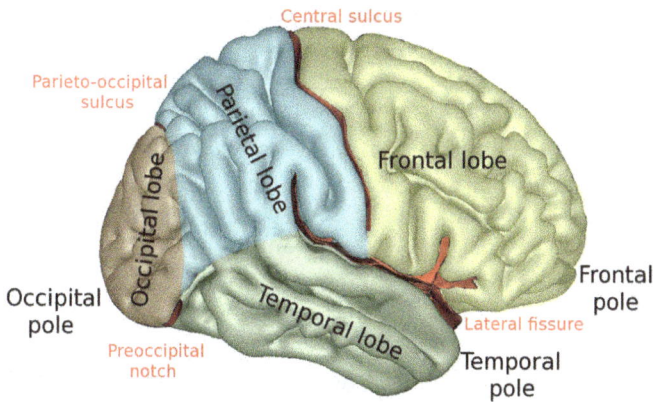

Figure 3.5: Lobes of the brain. Reprinted from: File: LobesCapts.png. (n. d.). In Wikipedia. https:// commons. wikimedia.org/wiki/File: LobesCapts.png

The lobes can be subdivided into regions of interest that can be divided even further into Brodmann areas that enable, what Gracefire (2017) refers to as "tailored selections of cortical areas for training". Brodmann areas are divisions of the cortex into voxels based on the structure and organization of cells that enable accurate selection of regions of interest involved in particular functions. Advanced software enables clinicians to target specific Brodmann areas in the treatment protocols.

A description and functions of the division of the cortex into broader regions of interest follows after which there is a description of the more refined division into Brodmann areas.

Frontal lobes

The frontal lobe is the largest of the four major lobes and is located at the front of the brain near the forehead. It takes up one third of the total brain. The paired lobes, part of the cerebral cortex are known as the left and right frontal cortex. The frontal lobes are involved in motivation, memory, motor function, language, problem solving, judgement, impulse control, spontaneity as well as in social and sexual behavior. The frontal lobes have been described as the "control panel" of our personality and our ability to communicate.

The frontal lobe can be divided into the motor cortex, (sub-divided into the *primary motor cortex, premotor cortex,* and *Broca's areas*) and the prefrontal cortex (sub-divided into the **dorsolateral area** of the frontal lobe, **anterior cingulum** of the frontal lobe, and the **orbital area** of the frontal lobe).

The main function of the *motor cortex* is to control voluntary movement, including the movements involved in speech, writing and ocular movement.

The *primary motor cortex* sends commands to the neurons in the brain stem and spinal cord, involved in specific voluntary movement. In each hemisphere the opposite side of the body is represented (motor homunculus).

The *premotor cortex* controls the planning of movement. Movement programs related to previous experiences are automated and harmonized and stored.

Broca's area is considered to be the center for the production of speech as well as language processing, comprehension and writing. The electrode placement area on the scalp to train Broca's area based on the 10–20 system is F7.

The Prefrontal Cortex (PFC) is located in the front part of the frontal lobe. It is considered to be the most advanced part of the human brain. It receives information from the limbic system and acts as a mediator between cognition and feelings through a set of executive functions necessary for controlling and regulating behavior. This area of the brain is involved in decision making, impulse control, working memory, attention and establishing goals.

Problems pertaining to this area will include impulsivity, procrastination, poor decision making and lack of goal setting. Under-activation of the left prefrontal cortex may lead to depression and over-activation of right prefrontal cortex may cause anxiety.

The electrode placement areas on the scalp to train the prefrontal cortex based on the 10–20 system include, Fp1, Fp2 and Fp.

The *dorsolateral area* of the frontal lobe is one of the most recently developed areas of the human brain. It establishes connections with other areas of the brain and transforms the information into thoughts, decisions, plans and actions. This region is involved in attention, working memory, short term memory, metacognition (self-analysis of cognitive activity), problem solving, the ability to adapt to new situations and planning.

The *anterior cingulum* of the frontal lobe is involved in motivational processes.

The *orbital area* of the frontal lobe, known as the *orbitofrontal cortex (OFC)* is a prefrontal cortex region in the frontal lobes of the brain involved in cognitive processing and decision-making. It is located right above the orbits or eye sockets with many connections with sensory areas as well as with limbic system structures. It consists of Brodmann areas 10, 11 and 47. This region is also thought to be relevant to adaptive and goal-directed behavior. The OFC has been the focus of many research studies recently.

The electrode placement areas on the scalp to train the OFC based on the 10–20 system is Fp1, FPz and Fp2.

Temporal lobes
The electrode placement areas on the scalp to train the temporal lobes based on the 10–20 system are: T3, T5, T4 and T6.

The temporal lobes are involved in auditory processing, language, memory, mood stability and temper control. Due to their position in the brain the temporal lobes are prone to accidents in contact sport and other activities. Injury to the temporal lobes can result in aggressiveness and temper problems as well as problems with memory. Without clear left temporal lobe dominance, stuttering and dyslexia may occur.

Women have up to 30% more inter-hemispheric connections and therefore they understand emotions better and manage dyslexia better.

Parietal lobes

The electrode placement areas on the scalp to train the parietal lobes based on the 10–20 system are P3, Pz and P4.

The parietal lobes are involved in sensory perception and processing, sense of direction, and spatial relations. Cognitive processing and attention are also relevant to this area of the brain. According to Steven Warner (2013), the parietal lobes solve the problems that the frontal lobes conceptualize. The parietal lobes generally get affected quite soon with Alzheimer's disease, which results in people getting lost and not being able to find their way.

According to Harry Kerasidis (2017), problems in these regions can also lead to inaccurate interpretation of body perception.

Precuneus

The precuneus is part of the superior parietal lobe in front of the occipital lobe. It is also described as the medial area of the superior parietal cortex. The precuneus is on the medial surface of both hemispheres. It is involved with episodic memory, aspects of consciousness, self-reflection, and visuospatial processing. The precuneus is one of the least accurately mapped areas of the cortical surface (Cavanna & Trimble, 2006).

Inferior Parietal Lobule

The inferior parietal lobule is one of the three divisions of the parietal lobe. The inferior parietal lobule of the left hemisphere lies at a key location in the brain at the junction of the interpretation of sensory information, language, mathematical operations and body image – all functions associated with this region of the brain (Geschwind, 2011).

Superior Parietal Lobe

The superior parietal lobule contains Brodmann areas 5 and 7. This brain region is involved with spatial orientation and receives a lot of sensory input from a person's hand as well a visual input. The superior parietal lobule is also involved with other general functions of the parietal lobe (Koenigs et al., 2009).

Occipital lobes

The placement of the electrodes on the scalp to train the occipital lobes according to the 10–20 system is O1, Oz and O2.

Vision and visual processing are controlled in the occipital lobes. Procedural memory, dreaming and visual perception are also associated with the occipital lobes. In addition, the occipital lobes are also involved in the process of color perception, finding objects in the environment, reading, writing and spelling.

According to Warner (2013), over activation of the occipital lobes may be indicative of brain stem problems.

Cuneus

The cuneus is a smaller lobe in the occipital lobe. The cuneus receives visual information from the same-sided superior quadrantic retina. The cuneus is important in basic visual processing. The cuneus is known as Brodmann area 17 (Haldane et al., 2008).

3.4.2 Deeper Brain Structures

Basal ganglia

The basal ganglia are a group of subcortical nuclei which are situated at the base of the forebrain. Basal ganglia are strongly interconnected with the cerebral cortex, the thalamus and the brainstem and other brain areas. The basal ganglia are associated with voluntary motor movements, procedural learning, habit learning, eye movements, cognition, and emotion.

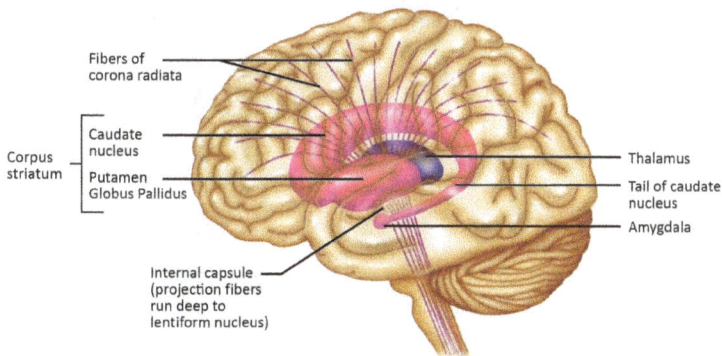

Figure 3.6: Basal Ganglia. Reprinted from: FLIPHTML5. (2009). CNS – composed of the brain and spinal cord cephalization. https://fliphtml5.com/trvn/opyy/basic/51-88

The main components of the basal ganglia are the **striatum** (both the dorsal striatum and the ventral striatum) **globus pallidius, ventral pallidum, substantia nigra** and the **sub-thalamic nucleus.** The dorsal striatum comprises the caudate nucleus and putamen whereas the ventral striatum includes the nucleus accumbens and the olfactory tubercle. The largest component of the basal ganglia is the striatum (dorsal and ventral) which receives input from many brain regions beyond the basal ganglia, but it only sends output to the other components of the basal ganglia. The pallidum receives input from the striatum and sends inhibitory output to a number of motor related areas. The substantia nigra is the source of the striatal input of dopamine which has an important role in the basal ganglia. The sub-thalamic nucleus receives input from the striatum and cerebral cortex and projects to the globus pallidus. The basal ganglia play an important role in the decision-making process regarding which of a number of possible behaviors are to be executed. It controls the activities of the motor and pre-motor cortical areas which results in the smooth execution of voluntary movements. The basal ganglia have an inhibitory influence on a number of motor systems.

Basal ganglia dysfunction is associated with many disorders and neurological conditions such as Tourette syndrome, obsessive-compulsive disorder, addiction, dystonia, movement disorders such as Parkinson's disease and Huntington's disease. There is also evidence that over-activity of the ventral tegmental area is associated with schizophrenia (Chakravarthy et al., 2010).

Thalamus

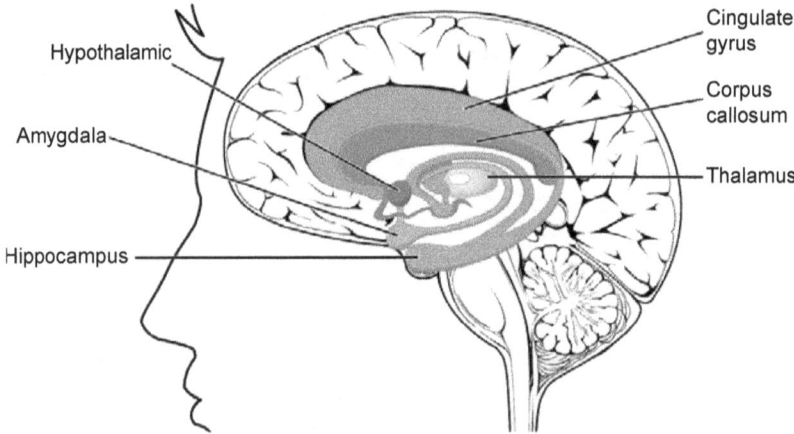

Figure 3.7: Inner structures of the brain. Reprinted from: Limbic system. (n. d.). In Wikipedia. https:// en.wikipedia.org/wiki/Limbic_system#/media/File:1511_The_Limbic _ Lobe.jpg

The thalamus is a small structure just above the brain stem between the cerebral cortex and the midbrain with extensive nerve connections to both. Its main function is to relay motor and sensory signals to the cerebral cortex. It receives sensory impulses from the body as sensations and relays these signals to the cortex. The thalamus is involved in the regulation of sleep, consciousness, and alertness. The thalamus sets the overall level of arousal or excitation for the entire cerebral cortex. It connects the sensory organs to areas of primary processing.

Hypothalamus

The hypothalamus (under the thalamus) is a small region located at the base of the brain near the pituitary gland. It regulates hunger, thirst, the pain response, pleasure perception, sex drive, sleep, the hormonal system, and the autonomic nervous system. The hypothalamus links the nervous system to the endocrine system via the pituitary gland. The functions of the hypothalamus are core to the overall state of being of the individual. This region of the brain is constantly very active.

Amygdala

The amygdala is an almond shaped set of neurons located deep in the brain's medial temporal lobe and is considered to be part of the limbic system. The amygdala is considered to be the integrative center of emotions, emotional behavior and motivation. The amygdala stores unconscious memories.

Septal Nucleus

The septal nucleus, together with the hypothalamus and the hippocampus is involved in internal inhibition and calming of the arousal level.

3.4.3 Cortical Surface Areas

Limbic System

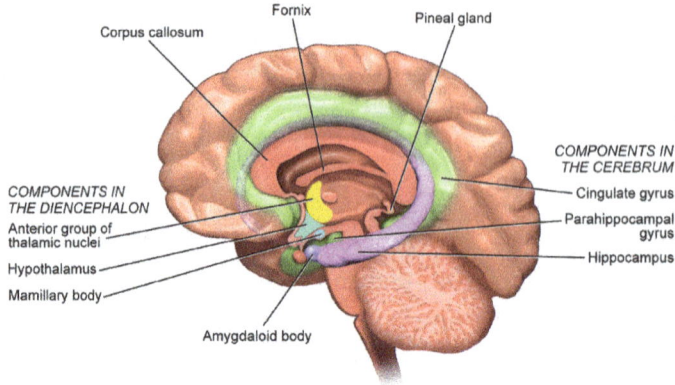

Figure 3.8: Illustration of the limbic system. Reprinted from: Blausen.com staff. (2014). Medical gallery of Blausen Medical 2014. WikiJournal of Medicine, 1(2). https://doi.org/10.15347/wjm/2014.010

The limbic lobe is the C-shape border of the hemisphere. The limbic system comprises a set of brain structures located on both sides of the thalamus, immediately beneath the cerebrum. The limbic system arches deep inside the brain, from the frontal lobes, through the parietal lobes to the temporal lobes and sets the emotional tone to be either positive and hopeful or negative and pessimistic. Emotional memories are held in the limbic system.

Gyri (Ridges of the Cortex)

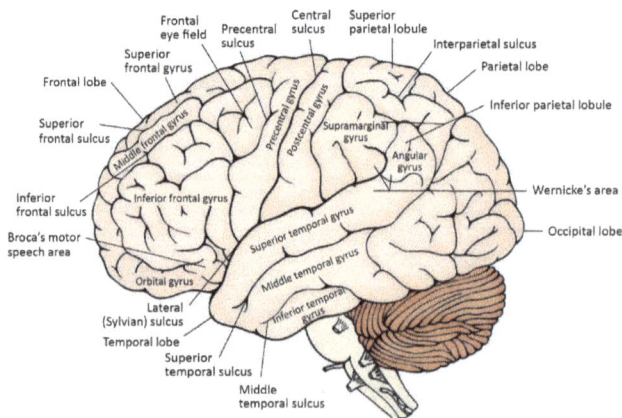

Figure 3.9: Surface areas with gyri and sulci. Reprinted from: Operative neurosurgery. (n. d.). Lateral cortical surface. http://www.operativeneurosurgery.com/doku.php?id=lateral_cortical surface

Anterior Cingulate Gyrus (ACG)

The electrode placement areas on the scalp to train the ACG based on the 10–20 system are on FPz and Fz. The cingulate cortex is considered part of the limbic lobe. It receives input from the thalamus and the neocortex.

This area runs lengthwise under the PFC and regulates our ability to shift attention, to adapt to change and be flexible in thought and reasoning. Problems in this region could cause a person being stuck in negative thought patterns or actions, argumentativeness, and causes a person to be overtly worrisome, to hold grudges and to be argumentative and oppositional. This region is considered a very important role player in emotional regulation and limbic system control. It assists the mind in letting go of concerns and helps the body to stop ritualistic tics and movements.

When the cingulate is over activated it causes OCD-like symptoms, Tourette-type symptoms and symptoms associated with ADHD.

Posterior Cingulate Gyrus (PCG)

The electrode placement areas on the scalp to train the posterior cingulate gyrus are Cz and Pz.

The PCG is closely aligned with the para-hippocampal cortices and is therefore also involved in memory and spatial orientation. The division between ACG and PCG is considered to be Cz.

Inferior Frontal Gyrus

The inferior frontal gyrus is part of the frontal gyrus of the frontal lobe. There is growing interest in the role of the right inferior frontal gyrus in terms of response inhibition. The ability to refrain from performing an action when given a signal is said to be controlled by the inferior frontal gyrus. Broca's area, important to speech production is found in the left inferior gyrus (Nolte, 2008).

Precentral Gyrus

The precentral gyrus is also known as the primary motor area or the motor strip. This region of the brain is immediately anterior to the central sulcus. It is a prominent structure on the surface of the posterior frontal lobe. It is known as Brodmann area 4. The internal pyramidal layer (layer V) contains giant pyramidal neurons or Betz cells. There is a precise somatotopic representation of the different body parts in the primary motor cortex. Voluntary movements of skeletal muscles are controlled by this area. Cell bodies of the pyramidal tract are found here. Lesions of the precentral gyrus result in paralysis of the contralateral side of the body (information available under CC BY-SA 3,0).

Postcentral Gyrus

The postcentral gyrus is a prominent gyrus in the lateral parietal lobe of the brain.

This area of the brain is also the somatosensory cortex which is the main sensory receptive area for the sense of touch. As in the case of the other sensory areas, there is a map of sensory space in this area called the sensory homunculus. This brain region encompasses Brodmann areas 1, 2 and 3. Brodmann area 3 receives the most of the thalamacortical projections from the sensory input areas (Kaas, 1993).

Superior Frontal Gyrus (SFG)

The superior frontal gyrus makes up approximately one third of the frontal lobe. The superior frontal gyrus similarly to the inferior frontal gyrus and the middle frontal gyrus, is more of a region in the frontal gyrus than a true gyrus. The SFG is located at the superior part of the prefrontal cortex. This region of the brain is thought to contribute to higher cognitive functioning including working memory. There are possibly functional sub-regions in this area. According to Li et al. (2013), the functions involved in this brain area are still being debated.

Medial Frontal Gyrus

The medial frontal gyrus is the most superior part of the medial surface of the frontal lobe and is continued on to the medial surface of the hemisphere, the medial frontal gyrus. The medial frontal gyrus is part of the prefrontal cortex. This region plays a role in executive mechanisms (Talati & Hirsch, 2005).

Middle Frontal Gyrus

The middle frontal gyrus is more a region in the frontal gyrus then a true gyrus. It makes up approximately one third of the frontal lobe. The sulci of the middle frontal gyrus have generated a lot of confusion in the literature on the anatomy of the brain. This region of the brain is part of the default network and is also involved in cognitive control, working memory, semantic processing, and reorienting of attention (Vossel et al., 2006).

Inferior Temporal Gyrus

The inferior temporal gyrus is the convolution on the temporal lobe of both hemispheres that lie beneath the middle temporal sulcus and stretches to the inferior sulcus. This region of the brain plays a very important role in the recognition of objects (Haxby et al., 2000).

Middle Temporal Gyrus

The middle temporal gyrus is in the temporal lobe of the brain and is located between the superior and inferior temporal gyri. The exact function of the middle temporal gyrus is unknown, and it has been associated with facial recognition, accessing the meaning of words while reading and also with estimating distance (Acheson & Hagoort, 2014).

Transverse Temporal Gyrus

The transverse temporal gyri are also called Heschl's gyri or Heschl's convolutions and located in the area of the primary auditory cortex hidden within the lateral sulcus. This area comprises Brodmann areas 41 and 42. Transverse cortical gyri are the first cortical structures to process incoming auditory information. These gyri do not run from front to back like all the other temporal lobe gyri, but mediolaterally, in other words, towards the middle of the brain. A study has shown that the processing rates of the transverse temporal gyri in the left hemisphere have faster processing speeds (33 Hz) compared to those in the right hemisphere (3 Hz) (Warrier et al., 2009).

Superior Temporal Gyrus

The superior temporal gyrus contains the primary auditory cortex and is located above the external ear. This gyrus is the topmost of the three convolutions or gyri in the temporal lobe. Wernicke's area is located in this gyrus in the left hemisphere with most people. Wernicke's area is the major region responsible for the comprehension of language. Emotions indicated by facial expressions are also interpreted in this region. The superior temporal gyrus comprises Wernicke's area and Brodmann areas 41 and 42 which are the primary adrenal cortex involved in audio sensations (Bigler et al., 2007).

Superior Occipital Gyrus

The superior occipital gyrus is also known as Brodmann area 19 and is part of the occipital lobe. Brodmann areas 18 and 19 together comprise the extrastriate cortex. The extrastriate cortex is a visual association area.

The functions of this area include feature-extracting, shape recognition, attention, and integration. The diverse fields that comprise Brodmann area 19 have reciprocal connections with Brodmann areas 17 and 18 as well as posterior parietal and inferior temporal areas. Area 19 receives inputs from the retina via the superior colliculus and pulvinar and may contribute to the phenomenon known as blindsight. This area is activated by somatosensory stimuli in patients that have been blind from a young age. Area 19 is therefore thought to be the differentiation point of the two visual streams namely the 'what' and 'where' pathways (Talati & Hirsch, 2005).

Middle Occipital Gyrus

The middle occipital gyrus is the major convolution on the lateral surface of the occipital lobe. The occipital lobe is the visual processing center of the brain. This gyrus is the largest gyrus in the occipital lobe. The anterior boundary of the middle occipital gyrus is the anterior boundary of the occipital lobe (SparkNotes, n. d.).

Inferior Occipital Gyrus

The inferior occipital gyrus is described as a stubby, knuckle-shaped gyrus on the lateral surface of the occipital lobe of each cerebral hemisphere, just below the lateral occipital sulcus. (SparkNotes, n. d.).

Para-Hippocampal Gyrus

The para-hippocampal gyrus is a grey matter cortical region that surrounds the hippocampus. This region of the brain is part of the limbic system. It plays an important role in memory encoding, memory retrieval and scene recognition. Damage to this area is associated with schizophrenia, Alzheimer disease and hippocampal sclerosis (Reuter, 2005).

Angular Gyrus

The angular gyrus is a region in the parietal lobe, near the superior edge of the temporal lobe and immediately posterior to the supra-marginal gyrus. This region of the brain is involved in language, the processing of numbers, spatial cognition, memory retrieval, attention, and theory of mind. This region is also known as Brodmann area 39 (IMAIOS, n. d.).

Fusiform Gyrus

The fusiform gyrus is also known as the occipitotemporal gyrus and is part of the temporal lobe and the occipital lobe. It is located between the lingual gyrus and the parrahippocampal Brodmann area 37 (Fusiform gyrus, n. d.).

Lingual Gyrus

The lingual gyrus is named after the shape it resembles, namely the tongue. This structure of the brain is involved in the visual processing of letters and the logical order of events as well as the encoding of visual memories (Lingual gyrus, n. d.).

Orbital Gyri

The term "orbital" refers to a set of convolutions on the ventral surface of the frontal lobe. The orbital gyri are located on the inferior surface of the frontal lobe. The inferior or orbital surface of the frontal lobe is concave and rests on the orbital plate of the frontal bone. It is divided into four orbital gyri by a clear H-shaped orbital sulcus. They are the medial, anterior, lateral, and posterior orbital gyri. The middle and superior gyri are referred to as the prefrontal area and the inferior gyri are referred to as Broca's area (IMAIOS, n. d.).

Rectal Gyrus

The rectal gyrus or straight gyrus is the very inferior and medial part of the frontal lobe. The gyrus rectus is known as a non-functional gyrus. The resection of the gyrus rectus is agreed to be a safe procedure to achieve a better surgical view during certain surgeries (Joo et al., 2016).

Subcallosal Gyrus

The subcallosal area is also known as the parolfactory area of Broca. It is a small triangular field on the medial surface of the hemisphere in front of the subcallosal gyrus. The subcallosal gyrus is not a cortical convolution like the other gyri but is the ventral continuation of the transparent septum. It is a slender vertical whitish band anterior to the lamina terminalis and anterior commissure (Subcallosal gyrus- An overview, n. d.).

Supra-Marginal Gyrus

The supra-marginal gyrus is part of the parietal lobe. It is also known as Brodmann area 40. This area of the brain is involved in language perception and processing. Lesions in this region may result in receptive aphasia (Gazzaniga, 2009).

Uncus

The uncus is an anterior extremity of the para-hippocampal gyrus. It is part of the mesial temporal lobe. The term comes from a Latin word meaning "hook". Although it appears to be part of the hippocampal gyrus, it is morphologically part of the rhinencephalon (Tamraz & Comair, 2000).

Insula

In each hemisphere the insula or insular cortex is part of the cerebral cortex folded deep within the lateral sulcus. The lateral sulcus is a large fissure that separates the frontal and parietal lobes from the temporal lobe. This brain region has been neglected in determining its functionality for long time and is currently believed to play an important role in what it feels like to be human. The insula appears to be involved in the experience of compassion, empathy, self-awareness, and interpersonal experience (Insula, n. d.).

Paracentral Lobule

The paracentral lobule is on the medial surface of the hemisphere and is a continuation of the precentral and postcentral gyri. It includes portions of the frontal and parietal lobes. The paracentral lobule controls motor and sensory innervations of the contralateral side. Defecation and urination is also controlled by the paracentral lobule (Conn, 2003).

3.5 The Brodmann Areas

The previous section contains a description of the Brodmann areas. The location, function and associated symptoms of deficits are discussed here for the purpose of planning training protocols. The layman may identify a particular Brodmann area that represents most symptoms of discomfort when reading the symptoms of deficit. Should the reader find this section too technical, he/she can skip it as it is more relevant for therapists.

Latest technology has made it possible to triangulate the source of the EEG activity deeper within the cortex by referencing 19 electrodes on the scalp by means of Standardized Low Resolution Electromagnetic Tomography (sLORETA) which is an inverse mathematical algorithm. sLORETA training is discussed in the section where the different neurofeedback paradigms are explained. This development has made it more important than ever that neurofeedback practitioners will familiarize themselves with the Brodmann areas which is a division of the cortex based on the structure and organization of cells that can be related to function and to the symptoms being treated with the purpose of being very specific in training deeper areas.

The Brodmann areas were originally defined and numbered by a German anatomist, Korbinian Brodmann in the early 1900's (see Loukas et al., 2011). The research was duplicated many times and follow up studies have confirmed the validity of the existence of the areas that are clearly distinguishable from one another.

Numbers are assigned to the voxels that contain an organization of cells that have a particular structure and function. The Brodmann areas are illustrated next:

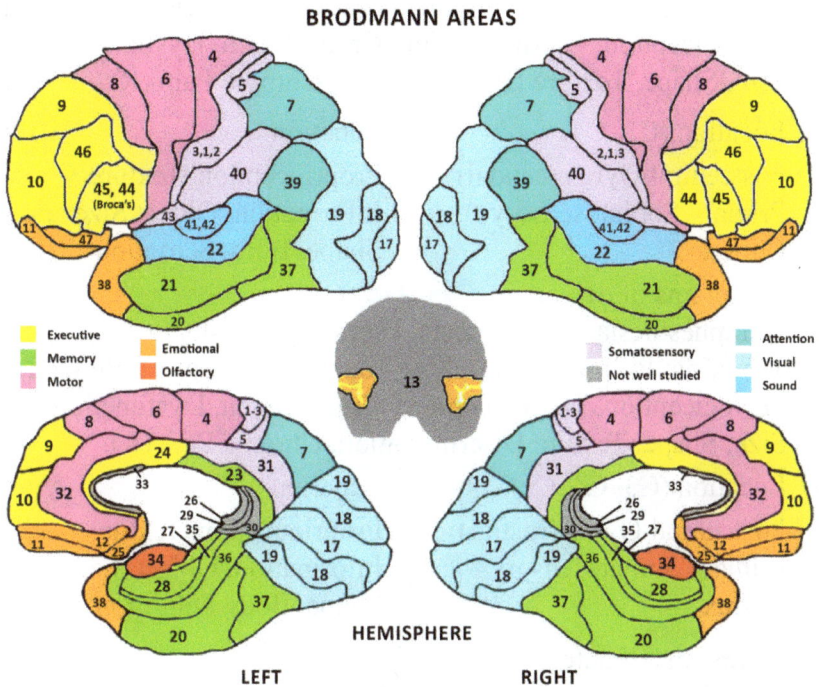

Figure 3.10: Brodmann areas. Reprinted from: Liu, Y., Liu, Ya., Wang, C., Wang, X., Zhou, P.- Y., Yu, G., & Chan, K. (2015). What strikes the strings of your heart? –Multi-label dimensionality reduction for music emotion analysis via brain imaging. IEEE Transactions on Autonomous Mental Development, 7(3), 176-188. https://doi.org/10.1109/TAMD.2015.2429580

The location, function and symptoms associated with a defect of all of the Brodmann areas are stipulated in a summary below to enable easy referencing of symptoms.

The information in brackets after "location" indicates electrode placement positions based on the 10–20 international placement system. Where

10–20- positions are not available, 10–10 placement positions have been indicated for some Brodmann areas.

No	Location (C3, C4)	Function
1	Postcentral Gyrus (middle) Primary Somatosensory Cortex	Proprioception, Texture Information, Object Size and Shape, Body sensations
	Symptoms of defect Agraphesthesia, Asterognosia, Hemihypesthesia, Loss of Vibration, Proprioception, Fine Touch, Hemineglect, Reduction in Nociception, Thermoception, Crude Touch, Dysfunction in Size, Shape, Texture Discrimination, Chronic Pain (R)	

No	Location (C3, C4)	Function
2	Postcentral Gyrus (caudal) Primary Somatosensory Cortex	Proprioception, Texture Information, Object Size and Shape, Body Sensation
	Symptoms of defect Agraphesthesia, Asterognosia, Hemihypesthesia, Loss of Vibration, Proprioception, Fine Touch, Hemineglect, Reduction in Nociception, Thermoception, Crude Touch, Dysfunction in Size, Shape, Texture Discrimination, Chronic Pain (R).	

No	Location (C3, C4, Cz)	Function
3	Postcentral Gyrus (rostral) Primary Somatosensory Cortex	Proprioception, Texture Information, Object Size and Shape, Body Sensation
	Symptoms of defect Agraphesthesia, Asterognosia, Hemihypesthesia, Loss of Vibration, Proprioception, Fine Touch, Hemineglect, Reduction in Nociception, Thermoception, Crude Touch, Dysfunction in Size, Shape, Texture Discrimination, Chronic Pain (R).	

No	Location (C3, C4, Cz)	Function
4	Posterior Frontal Lobe Primary Motor Cortex	To plan and execute movement
	Symptoms of defect Poor Motor Control, Touch Recognition Problems, Paralysis	

No	Location (Pz)	Function
5	Superior Parietal Lobule Somatosensory Association Cortex	Somatosensory and association
	Symptoms of defect Impaired Somatosensory and Spatial Perception, Pain, Fibromyalgia, Balance Problems, Touch Recognition Problems, Decreased Tactile or Skin Sensitivity, Blurred Vision	

No	Location (Fz, Cz)	Function
6	Frontal Cortex, Premotor and Supplementary Motor Cortex	Planning complex, coordinated movements
	Symptoms of defect Hyperactivity (R), Blurred Vision	

No	Location (P3, Pz, P4)	Function
7	Parietal Cortex Somatosensory Association Cortex	Convergence of vision and proprioception, visiomotor coordination
	Symptoms of defect Easily Distracted, Poor Comprehension, Difficulty with Social Cues (R), Dyslexia (L), Dyscalcula, Agnosia, Aphasia, Focus Issues, Obsession, Fibromyalgia, Impaired Spatial Perception, Decreased Tactile or Skin Sensitivity, Denial (R), Insensitive to Others' Emotional Expressions (R), Facial Recognition Problems, Space/Orientation Problems (R), Poor Social Skills (R)	

No	Location (F3, Fz, F4)	Function
8	Frontal Cortex Frontal Eye Fields	Non-tracking, Voluntary Eye Movements; Control of Visual Attention, Motor Planning, Mood Control.
	Symptoms of defect Deviation of the Eyes to the Ipsilateral Side, Hyperactivity (R), Executive Function Problems, Tactile Agnosia, Impulsive, Oppositional, Depressed (Sad and Blue), Poor Social Skills (R)	

No	Location (F3, Fz, F4)	Function
9	Frontal Cortex Dorsolateral Prefrontal Cortex	Working memory, Cognitive flexibility, Planning, Inhibition, Abstract Reasoning
	Symptoms of defect Executive Function Problems, Concentration Problems, Impulsive, Oppositional, Anger Control Problems, Depressed (Sad and Blue), Failure to Initiate Actions, Obsessive Thoughts about Self, Multitasking Problems, Self-Esteem Problems (R), Poor Social Skills (R)	

No	Location (FP1, FPz, FP2)	Function
10	Prefrontal Cortex Anterior Prefrontal Cortex	Strategic Processes, Memory Recall, Some Executive Functions, Executive Emotion and Planning
	Symptoms of defect Executive Function Problems, Compulsive Thoughts or Behavior, Impulsive, Oppositional, Concentration Problems, Amnesia, Aphasia, Anger Control Problems, Low Motivation, Mood Swings, Delusional, Failure to Initiate Actions, Obsessive Thoughts about Self, Multitasking Problems, Self-Esteem Problems (R), Poor Social Skills (R), Slow Thought, Easily Confused	

No	Location (FP1, FPz, FP2)	Function
11	Frontal Cortex Orbitofrontal Area	Planning, Reasoning, Decision making
	Symptoms of defect Executive Function Problems, Disturbances of Mood or Thoughts, Impulsive, Oppositional, Apathy, Mutism, Aggression, Compulsion, Self-Image Issues, Derealization, Anger Control Problems, Low Motivation, Mood Swings, Delusional, Obsessive Thoughts about Self, Multitasking Problems, Self-Esteem Problems (R), Poor Social Skills (R), Slow Thought, Easily Confused	

No	Location	Function
13	Insular Cortex Rostral Frontal Cortex	Primary Emotional Sensation

Symptoms of defect
Progressive Non-Fluent Aphasia, Addiction, Anxiety Disorders, Emotional Dysregulation, Oppositional Panic, Persecutory Delusions, Fibromyalgia, Low Motivation, Migraines, Chronic Pain (R), Obsessive Thoughts about Self, Self- Esteem Problems (R), Poor Social Skills (R)

No	Location (O1, Oz, O2)	Function
17	Posterior Occipital Lobe Primary Visual Cortex	Visual Sensations, Pattern Recognition, Processing Information about Static and Moving Objects

Symptoms of defect
Cortical Blindness, Impaired Visual or Spatial Perception, Slow Reading, Letter Perception Problems (L), Blurred Vision

No	Location (O1, Oz, O2)	Function
18	Lateral Occipital Lobe Secondary Visual Cortex	Visual Integration

Symptoms of defect
Impaired Visual or Spatial Perception, Slow Reading, Agnosia (R), Denial (R), Letter Perception Problems (L), Blurred Vision

No	Location (T5, T6, P3, Pz, P4, O1, Oz, O2)	Function
19	Dorsolateral Occipital Lobe Associate Visual Cortex	Visual Perception

Symptoms of defect
Easily Distracted, Impaired Visual or Spatial Perception, Slow Reading, Dyscalcula, Dyslexia (L), Agnosia (R), Denial (R), Letter Perception Problems (L), Insensitive to Others' Emotional Expressions (R)

No	Location (FT9, FT10)	Function
20	Inferior Temporal Lobe Inferior Temporal Gyrus	Memory, Auditory Processing

Symptoms of defect
Story Memory and Sequential Memory Problems

No	Location (T3, T4)	Function
21	Middle Temporal Lobe Middle Temporal Gyrus	Memory, Auditory Processing and Language
	Symptoms of defect Auditory Sequencing Problems, Receptive Language Problems (L)	

No	Location (T3, T4)	Function
22	Superior Temporal Lobe Superior Temporal Gyrus	Auditory Processing, Contains Wernicke's Area
	Symptoms of defect Auditory Sequencing Problems	

No	Location (Pz)	Function
23	Posterior Cingulate Ventral Posterior Cingulate Cortex	Spatial Memory, Configural Learning, Maintenance of Discriminative Avoidance, Learning, Memory Retrieval, Emotional Salience
	Symptoms of defect Alzheimer's, Autism Spectrum Disorders, ADHD, Depression, Schizophrenia, Easily Distracted, Impaired Spatial Perception, Short-Term Memory Problems, Slow Thought, Easily Confused	

No	Location (F1, F2)	Function
24	Ventral Anterior Cingulate Ventral Anterior Cingulate Cortex	Regulating Blood Pressure and Heart Rate, Reward Anticipation, Decision- Making, Empathy, Impulse Control, Emotion, Error Detection and Conflict Monitoring, Registering Physical Pain

No	Location (Pz)	Function
31	Posterior Cingulate Dorsal Posterior Cingulate Cortex	Somatosensory
	Symptoms of defect Impaired Somatosensory Perception, Loss of Visual Imagery, Attention Problems	

No	Location (FPz)	Function
32	Dorsal Anterior Cingulate Dorsal Anterior Cingulate Cortex	Motor Planning
	Symptoms of defect Impaired Motor Control, Depressed (Sad + Blue)	

No	Location	Function
33	Mesial Anterior Cingulate Part of the Anterior Cingulate Cortex	Unclear
	Symptoms of defect Hyperactivity (R), Easily Distracted, Short-Term Memory Problems, Hyperfocused, Obsessive, Low Motivation, Impulsive Disturbances of Image / Awareness, Depressed (Sad and Blue), Failure to Initiate Actions, Multitasking Problems.	

No	Location	Function
34	Superior Mesial Temporal Lobe Dorsal Entorhinal Cortex	Olfactory
	Symptoms of defect Ipsilateral Anosmia, Impaired Olfactory Perception	

No	Location	Function
35	Mesial Temporal Lobe Perirhinal Cortex	Memory
	Symptoms of defect Impaired Memory	

No	Location	Function
36	Mesial Temporal Lobe Ectorhinal Area	Memory
	Symptoms of defect Impaired Memory	

No	Location (T5, T6)	Function
37	Posterior Temporal Lobe Fusiform Gyrus	Memory
	Symptoms of defect Impaired Memory, Slow Reading, Letter Perception Problems (L), Receptive Language Problems (L)	

No	Location (FT9, FT10)	Function
38	Anterior Temporal Lobe Tempo- ral Area	Emotional Regulation, Auditory Pro- cessing
	Symptoms of defect Alzheimer's Disease, Temporal Lobe Seizures, Impaired Emotional Regulation, Anger Control Problems, Delussional, Auditory Sequencing Problems, Insensitive to Others' Emotional Expressions (R), Receptive Language Problems (L)	

No	Location (T5, T6)	Function
39	Lateral Parietal Lobe Angular Gyrus	Language, Number Processing, Spatial Cognition, Memory Retrieval, Attention
	Symptoms of defect Semantic Aphasia, Gerstmann Syndrome, Fibromyalgia, Migraines, Slow Reading, Difficulty with Social Cues (R), Dyscalcula, Dyslexia (L), Agnosia (R), Denial (R), Letter Perception Problems (L), Insensitive to Others' Emotional Expressions (R), Receptive Language Problems (L), Facial Recognition Problems, Spatial Orientation Problems (R), Poor Social Skills (R)	

No	Location (P3, P4)	Function
40	Temporo-Parietal Lobe Supramarginal Gyrus	Somatosensory
	Symptoms of defect Fibromyalgia, Migraines, Slow Reading, Difficulty with Social Cues (R), Dyscalcula, Dyslexia (L), Agnosia (R), Denial (R), Letter Perception Problems (L), Insensitive to Others' Emotional Expressions (R), Receptive Language Problems (L), Facial Recognition Problems, Spatial Orientation Problems (R), Poor Social Skills (R)	

No	Location (C5, T8)	Function
41	Superior Temporal Lobe Auditory Cortex	Auditory Sensation, Language Processing
	Symptoms of defect Impaired Auditory Perception, Difficulty with Social Cues (R), Migraines, Slow Reading, Letter Perception Problems (L), Receptive Language Problems (L), Spatial Orientation Problems (R)	

No	Location (T3, T4)	Function
42	Superior Middle Temporal Lobe Auditory Cortex, Wernicke's area	Auditory Sensation, Language Processing
	Symptoms of defect Impaired Auditory Perception, Slow Reading, Letter Perception Problems (L)	

No	Location	Function
43	Superior Middle Temporal Lobe Primary Gustatory Cortex, Wernicke's Area	Somatic Sensation, Language
	Symptoms of defect Migraines, Chronic Pain (R), Receptive Language Problems (L)	

No	Location (F5, FC6)	Function
44	Lateral Posterior Frontal Lobe Pars Opercularis, Broca's Area	Executive Functions
	Symptoms of defect Impaired Executive Functions, Chronic Pain (R)	

No	Location (F7, F8)	Function
45	Lateral Posterior Frontal Lobe Pars Triangularis, Broca's Area	Executive Functions, Moods, Language
	Symptoms of defect Executive Functions Problems, Compulsive Thoughts or Behaviors, Delusional, Lack of Empathy	

No	Location (F3, F4, F7, FP1, FP2, F8)	Function
46	Dorsolateral Frontal Lobe Dorso- lateral Prefrontal Cortex	Executive, Mood, Language, Attention, Working Memory, Self-control
	Symptoms of defect Lesions Result in Impaired Short-Term Memory, Difficulty Inhibiting Responses, Organization and Relevance Problems, Executive Function Problems, Oppositional, Compulsive Thoughts or Behaviors, Concentration Problems, Anger Control Problems, Mood Swings, Delusional, Obsessive Thoughts about Self	

No	Location (F7, F8)	Function
47	Ventromedial Frontal Lobe Pars Orbitalis, Inferior Frontal Gyrus, Broca's Area	Executive, Emotion
	Symptoms of defect Executive Function Problems, Compulsive Thoughts or Behavior, Delusional, Executive Function Problems, Lack of Empathy	

Neurophysiological Basis of the EEG; the Role of Neurotransmitters; Instrumentation; Electronics

I always find it interesting that some clients have a clear desire to understand as much as possible about the training process with a clear preference to detail whereas others don't wish to attempt to understand the underlying dynamics of the processes involved, at all. Initially I assumed that males with an engineering background would generally be skeptical of the process until they understood the scientific basis of neurofeedback. It turns out that I was wrong. A person's career profile does not determine the level of his quest for knowledge.

During the first five years or more of having integrated neurofeedback into my practice I felt the need to have to validate neurofeedback by memorizing and quoting many research studies and by offering elaborate technical information. Of course, I understand that those attempts at validating an already validated, solidly scientifically based process were fear based. We don't enjoy the unconditional acceptance and positive preconceived opinions of clients that the mainstream medical practitioners encounter, but we need no longer and should not feel the need to justify our field of expertise. Those attempts detract from the client's needs. This serves as a reminder that the therapist needs to remain tuned into and focused on the client's experience and needs as far as it is possible. The client will indicate how much or little technical, clinical and research information they want. When I am not certain, I ask if the person would want a detailed or nutshell version of an explanation of various components of the underlying dynamics.

Should you be one of those people who require a mere overview of a process rather than an in-depth analysis, you may want to just scan the rest of this chapter. Those readers who would want more information than what is within the scope of this book in terms of the main topics addressed in this chapter, I trust that you will be well enough equipped with links, authors and key words after having read this chapter to be able to do more in depth research.

Part One

4.1.1 Neurophysiological Basis of the EEG

The function of neurons is to communicate with other neurons. There is both chemical and electrical transmission of information. Some types of neurons are excitatory and some are inhibitory. For the purpose of neurofeedback, we are mainly interested in the electrical relay of information.

The brain consists of a network of neurons that are interconnected, which, have control properties involved in the production and maintenance of certain mind states or states of consciousness and the transition between these states. It was Weiner in 1948 that discovered that the control systems either maintain states in the face of changes or cause change based on goals (see Collura, 2014, p.47). Neurofeedback is a process by which goals are established by which the brain learns new ways in which to self-regulate, thus causing change.

According to the Thompsons (2015), "The EEG is generated by the synchronous activity of postsynaptic inhibitory and excitatory potentials involving large groups of cortical pyramidal cells".

The neuronal circuit of the cortex consists of six layers of cells. The layers are named and illustrated on the following page.

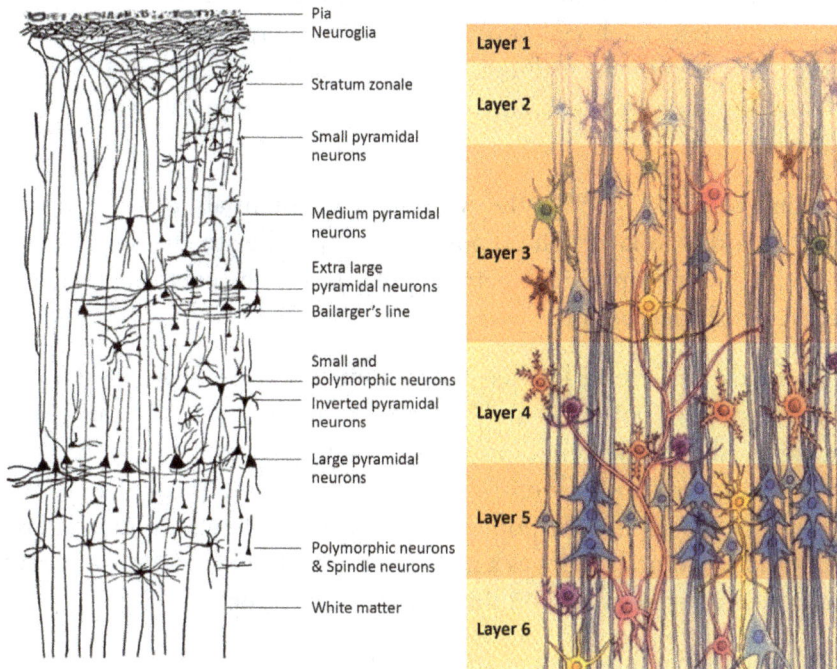

Figure 4.1: Layers of cells in the cortex.

The pyramidal cells are excitatory white cells, the granular cells are grey and can be either excitatory or inhibitory, the stellate cells are excitatory and the basket cells are inhibitory.

Layer two receives input from other cortical association areas and from non-specific thalamic nuclei and the reticular formation. Layer four is the main input area and receives afferents from the primary sensory and other input systems. Inputs from other cortical association areas, non-specific thalamic nuclei as well as from the reticular formation, enter mainly layer two. Layers three and five are the primary output layers (Szentágothai & Hamori, 1969).

The neurotransmitter of the pyramidal cells is glutamate. The stellate cells are excitatory and the basket cells are inhibitory.

Pyramidal cells are specialized neurons whose dendrites can produce action potentials. Dendrites normally produce excitatory and inhibitory slow potentials which summate at the axon hillock to produce action potential. The pyramidal cells are thus mainly the cells that produce the electrical activity recorded from the scalp.

109

The pyramidal cells are in the upper layers, the layer referred to as layer 1V, of the cortex. Each cell produces an extremely small current flow in its immediate region, according to Collura (2014) but there is also current produced throughout the brain due to a phenomenon known as volume conduction.

According to Fisch (1999), the postsynaptic potentials of the pyramidal cells form a dipole layer. The dipole layer is parallel to the surface of the cortex and projects opposite electrical polarities to the cortical surface. This process is explained below.

Dipole fields are created when many neurons depolarize in unison to produce external potential and to create dipole layers. Those reacting asynchronously are cancelled out. The postsynaptic potentials (PSP) have what is considered to be long time duration of 15–200 ms. The external potentials of the significant population of pyramidal cells in unison create the EEG. The potential changes summate and the EEG records the potential (either positive or negative) on the surface of the scalp.

Some of the dipoles are not oriented parallel to the surface and the activity from those dipoles can be hidden in a fissure or sulcus and a sensor placed directly above it will not read the activity whereas a sensor placed a distance away from the activity will read a percentage of it. A considerable amount of the cortical surface is in the folds or sulci of the cortex. For this reason, Baehr et al. (2001) and others are of the view that some dipoles are best recorded with a bipolar montage. Consequently, some practitioners would do asymmetry training for depression with a bipolar two channel hook-up at F3-Cz and F4-Cz.

According to Collura (2014), the role of local synchrony in the generation of EEG rhythms is so profound that less than 5% of the pyramidal cells in the brain can be responsible for 90% of the EEG recorded signals. This fact makes it very probable for the brain to be able to alter its EEG when certain patterns and rhythms are being rewarded.

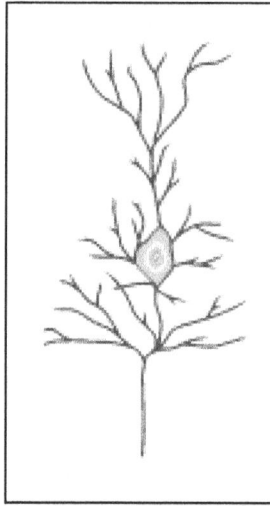

Figure 4.2: Pyramidal cell.

There are four prerequisites to the production of sufficient electrical activity: These conditions involve **directionality, synchronicity, proximity**, and **valence**. The pyramidal cells need to be lined up perpendicularly. In other words, they must be parallel to the scalp. Because of the irregular gyration or undulation of the cortex, they are not always perfectly lined up, but at least relatively so. If they were not lined up they would have no contribution to the EEG. Secondly, there has to be simultaneous firing and discharge at the synapses of the axons which are connected to the dendrites of the pyramidal cells. The thalamus is the main structure involved in controlling the rhythm of the firing of the pyramidal cells. Thirdly, the firing cells have to be in the same area (within a cluster or macrocolumn which is a group of cells several millimeters in diameter, six layers deep containing pyramidal cells, stellate cells and basket cells). The same thing must be happening at precisely the same area (proximal or distal). Fourthly, the valence has to be the same for virtually all of the pyramidal cells within a special cluster. They must have either an excitatory or inhibitory PSP. These four conditions are the prerequisites for being able to detect an electrical charge and record it as an EEG from the scalp.

Inhibitory cells in the cortex, such as basket cells, cannot meet the above conditions and do not contribute to the EEG directly, but they have an influence on the pyramidal cells.

The action potentials, as opposed to the PSPs, have a short duration of one millisecond and do not contribute to the EEG significantly. The EEG

111

is portrayed as voltage versus time. The voltage is the potential difference between at least two locations or electrodes.

A brief overview of the electrical and chemical processes involved in action potentials will follow:

There is a critical change that occurs at the axon hillock which is about moving from a resting level of approximately 70 microvolt to what is called the threshold of excitation at 55 microvolt. This occurs when the depolarizing changes summate to the point where the potential at the axon hillock is changed sufficiently to above 10 microvolt. The membrane then suddenly loses its charge and an action potential is produced and sent along the axon to the next synapse. A temporary reversal in charge occurs along the cell membrane to approximately 110 microvolt and lasts for 1millisecond. This sudden change causes a similar change in the adjacent membrane which causes current to be propagated down the axon. The membrane of the adjacent cell suddenly becomes a thousand times more permeable to sodium than in the resting state. Because there are two gateways to sodium, the propagation down the dendrite is unidirectional. The first gate way opens immediately when activated by an appropriate chemical or electrical charge and the second gate is regarded to be a slow gate which closes shortly after sodium enters the cell and remains closed until its resting state is achieved again. The resting state is achieved by the active sodium pump removing sodium from the interior of the cell until the cell achieves the negative resting potential. A second depolarizing stimulus cannot open this gate before the negative resting potential is reached. The time during which a stimulus cannot open the gate is called the refractory period. The result of this process is that the current can only be sent or spread in one direction down the axon.

The cycle involved in the cell membrane affecting the permeability of potassium (K) and sodium (Na) is known as the *Hodgkin Cycle*. The sodium-potassium pump uses energy (Adenosine Triphosphate (ATP), is used for intracellular energy transfer) to maintain a resting potential.

Potassium flowing out of the cell assists in the repolarization phase. Action potentials are very brief local events and are not reflected in the EEG.

However, EEG is the result of the activity of many brain cells and the existence of a particular frequency does not mean that there is an oscillator in the brain at that frequency. Linear analysis assumes that there is one oscillator and one measurable output, but the EEG is more complex than that. The output is not necessarily proportional to the input from the main source, which makes it non-linear.

The EEG has non-linear components but is not random. The output is thus not in a uniform relationship to the input, as the EEG frequency wave has a specific origin or starting point and does not change its origin in an unpredictable manner. It may originate in the thalamus and then gets influenced and changed by a number of variables such as chemistry, electrical activity, blood flow in the immediate environment of the wave and so on.

The EEG is a sum of different rhythms produced at different frequencies by different generators located in different cortical areas. The driving rhythm is from deeper structures such as the thalamus. Although the cells in the sub-cortical regions do not contribute directly to the electrical potential that we measure in the EEG, they do influence the pyramidal cells. The thalamus for instance, sets specifically theta, alpha, and SMR or low beta, rhythms. The function of the thalamus in this regard has been likened by the Thompsons (2015) in *The Neurofeedback Book*, to a radio station that sends signals to relay stations over the entire cortex. The EEG contains information on brain function and it can provide information on deeper cortical structures through a mathematical process, LORETA in which the source of the measured activity can be estimated.

Much of the activity between the neurons is inhibitory which results in a controlling influence on the excitatory activity arbitrated by the pyramidal cells.

The interaction between the thalamus and the cortex is very important in the creation of the measurable EEG signals from the scalp. The thalamo-cortical projections are projected to virtually all areas of cortex.

When through neurofeedback, we encourage a specific rhythm to increase, the inhibitory influences at the thalamic level are reduced to allow the cortical rhythm to be expressed. Neurofeedback therefore actually influences areas deeper than those reflected in the EEG. The process of neurofeedback is a process by which the brain determines how to achieve predetermined goals and those means are not limited to the brain locations that are being monitored.

Localized brain activity can appear dispersed on the scalp due to *volume, conduction* and *spreading*. This is not because of diffuse activity of the brain. When the EEG is interpreted it is important to look for the spreading which is referred to as a ' field'. According to Collura (2014), any brain event is reflected at more than one site on the scalp. When the sensor is placed near the generator it will be read as a maximal signal, but that signal will appear at other locations although in decreasing magnitude depending on the distance from the generator. As mentioned before, Collura (2014) is of the view that approximately 50% of a measured signal can be considered to originate from tissue immediately beneath the recording sensor. The remaining signal is measured from adjacent sites.

The following concepts of neuronal dynamics are relevant to understanding the underlying dynamics of the EEG and the regulatory abilities of the brain: **cyclic patterns, inhibition**, and **inter- connectivity**.

Groups of neurons produce measurable potentials in the form of the EEG. The brain is a complex and hyper-connected system that relies on extensive communication between the different sections and regions. Subgroups of neurons have the ability to isolate themselves, that was referred to as lateral inhibition (Lateral inhibition, n. d.).

The billions of neurons organized into functional groups and networks undergo rhythmic activity at frequencies between one and 100 per second. These rhythms refer to the external measurable potentials within the EEG range. The underlying neuronal activity occurs at thousands of cycles per second. These networks are warned then activated and then released in coordinated activity of different regions that is visible in rhythmic patterns characteristic of particular regions. This cyclic activity produces the waxing and waning of the activity measured from the scalp. When we examine the EEG, we can establish the dominant rhythm and determinate the degree of activation of the region.

Over the entire cortex there is, what Collura (2014) refers to as a repetitive, cyclic pattern of activation that involves the thalamus and the particular region of the cortex. In a phenomenon known as thalamo-cortical reverberation, the alpha rhythm as well as the low beta rhythm is created. The Theta rhythm also originates here but according to Collura (2014) this happens according to a slightly different process.

Faster frequencies are the result of cortical-cortical reverberations produced by shorter-range connections between cortical sites. The cyclic, rhythmic activity visible in the EEG gives an indication of the activation and deactivation of the area.

Connections through the thalamus to the cortex will according to the Thompsons (2015), lead to feedback from the cortex through the basal ganglia, which will select one response and inhibit other response systems. The thalamus then sends specific instructions to relevant related areas in the cortex. According to Thompson and Thompson (2015), neurofeedback to a particular site on the scalp will influence the entire cortical-basal ganglia-thalamo-cortical network.

The concept of inhibition is fundamental to understanding the EEG (Collura, 2014). It is through the control of inhibition that the brain can manage to regulate and process information. Lateral inhibition between areas in close proximity is essential for processing of sensory input.

Inhibition is very important in thalamo-cortical regulation. The lateral nuclei of the thalamus project from the outer regions of the thalamus to the nuclei. The nuclei then project to the cortex. The laminar nuclei of the thalamus use GABA to provide the key regulatory function. When a particular rhythm is measured from the cortex, it is accompanied by a relaxation of the inhibitory influence of the laminar thalamic nuclei. The expression of a rhythm is thus also the expression of a relaxed inhibition from the region (Collura, 2014).

When a particular rhythm is rewarded and enhanced in neurofeedback, the main mechanism at work is the reduction in the inhibition at a thalamic level and thus allowing the cortical rhythm to be expressed.

Cyclic activation and inhibition, is, according to Collura (2014), a key aspect of a healthy neuronal network.

4.1.2 Overview of the Role of Neurotransmitters in the Transmission of Signals

A very brief overview of the role of neurotransmitters is provided.

The main focus of neurofeedback is on the electrical activity in the brain, whereas other modalities focus mainly on the chemical component of brain activity. The two components are, as mentioned earlier, interconnected, and intertwined.

The information on how many neurotransmitters have been discovered varies. According to the Thompsons (2015) in *The Neurofeedback Book,* more than 250 neurotransmitters have been identified.

It is mostly the receptor site that determines whether a transmission will be excitatory or inhibitory. Receptor sites respond to neurotransmitters that are specialized chemical substances that transmit signals from one neuron to another. *Acelylcholine* is the most common neurotransmitter, in the central nervous system, it can be either excitatory or inhibitory. Acetylcholine is the main neurotransmitter of the *parasympathetic* division of the autonomic nervous system. In Alzheimer disease, this neurotransmitter is deficient. This neurotransmitter is involved in the recording of memories in the basal forebrain and the hippocampus. It also plays a part in attentional processes controlled from the reticular activating system Acetylcholine is also involved in the control of sleep cycles.

Three other groups of neurotransmitters have been identified namely norepinephrine, dopamine and serotonin.

They are three neurotransmitters in the *biogenic amines* (catecholamines, which are hormones produced by the adrenal glands) subgroup. Norepinephrine and dopamine are derived from the amino acid *tyrosine*. Serotonin is derived from *tryptophan* which is also an amino acid. Dopamine is generally *excitatory* whereas serotonin is mostly *inhibitory*.

Norepinephrine is both excitatory and inhibitory and is the central neurotransmitter of the *sympathetic division* of the autonomic nervous system. Norepinephrine is released during the experience of stress and is probably part of the fight and flight response. Norepinephrine is also associated with fear, anxiety, and probably manic experiences. Norepinephrine deficiency is associated with depression and an excess of norepinephrine has been linked with mania. Norepinephrine gets depleted in persons that suffer chronic stress.

Serotonin (5-hydroxy-trypamine, 5-HT) is produced in the brain stem. Serotonin is involved in the regulation of mood, the sex drive, appetite, and plays a role in sleep onset. Serotonin is a precursor for melatonin which is important in certain biological rhythms. Low levels of serotonin is associated with depression, obsessive compulsive disorder and with aggression. The SSRI (serotonin reuptake inhibitors) group of medications have a good effect when serotonin levels are deficient.

The hallucinogenic affects produced by LSD and mescaline (a naturally occurring psychedelic) is probably, according to the Thompsons (2015), due to binding to dopamine receptors. Schizophrenia is also associated with an excess of dopamine. Parkinson's disease on the other hand is associated with dopamine deficiency.

The second group of neurotransmitters is the *amino acids*. The two inhibitory neurotransmitters in this group are GABA (gamma amino butyric acid) and glycine. The excitatory neurotransmitters in the amino acid sub- group are glutamate and aspartate.

GABA is the most important *inhibitory neurotransmitter* in the *central nervous system*. When a neuron is stimulated a feedback loop is activated to prevent or inhibit that neuron from firing continuously. GABA is mostly deployed to inhibit the repeated firing of the neurons and is therefore known as the braking system of the CNS.

The group of medications known as anxiolytics as well as alcohol and barbiturates activate the responses of the GABA receptors which then creates the effect of the substance.

Glycine is detected in the spinal cord and the lower part of the brain stem. A glycine blocker is released in tetanus which then results in the continuous contraction of muscles.

Glutamate, an excitatory neurotransmitter in the amino acid group, is involved in the process called Long Term Potentiation (LTP) when there is excessive activity across synapses and the post synaptic cell changes. These changes are essential to the storage of memories. This process of changes that occur in post synaptic cells is one of the possible explanations of why a few sessions of neurofeedback training can have lasting effect on the CNS.

Aspartate is also an excitatory neurotransmitter in the amino acid group of neurotransmitters. Aspartate is often combined with minerals as a dietary supplement. It is available as copper aspartate, iron aspartate, magnesium aspartate, manganese aspartate, potassium aspartate, and zinc aspartate. In low concentrations, glutamate and aspartate excite virtually every neuron in the CNS (Dingledine et al., 1999; Rojas & Dingledine, 2013).

The third group of neurotransmitters is *neuropeptides*. These neurotransmitters are short chains of amino acids. The interaction between sensory and emotional responses is influenced by the neuropeptides.

Substance P is involved in the perception of pain. Measurements of substance P taken from the cerebral spinal fluid is used for research in the dynamics involved in fibromyalgia.

The *endorphins* are also neuropeptide neurotransmitters. They are regarded as natural analgesics and also as euphorics. These neuropeptides function at the same receptors as heroine and morphine and are found in the limbic system.

Neuropeptide Y (NPY) is another neuropeptide found in the hypothalamus and is thought to be relevant to food intake and in eating disorders.

Part Two

4.2 Instrumentation and Electronics

4.2.1 Introduction

The core of neurofeedback involves measuring the EEG signal from the scalp. It is therefore essential to understand the origins of the EEG signal and how the measurement from the scalp reflects brain activity. In the previous chapter we looked briefly at how the brain produces measurable electrical potentials that can be measured from the scalp. The signals that are measurable from the scalp are a thousand times weaker than the signals produced by the brain. On the scalp, we measure the signal in microvolts. In order to be able to measure and interpret these very small potentials, it is essential that the measurements will be very accurate. The type of amplifier that is suitable for this type of measurement is a differential amplifier. A differential amplifier measures the difference between two sites and amplifies that signal and produces the amplified difference signal as the output.

In neurofeedback we use the potential difference between a positive and negative electrode as a measure of the amplitude of the EEG signal.

4.2.2 Direct Current (DC) and Alternating Current (AC)

Current is the rate of electron flow through the conductor and is measured in amperes. It therefore measures the rate of transfer of electric charge from one point to another. Electrical charge refers to the negative charge carried by electrons.

Direct current is the current there is in a battery-operated flashlight for instance. Relevant measures involved in the calculation of current are potential difference measured in volts, current measured in amperes and resistance measured in ohms. The relation between the three concepts was expressed in the following equation by George Ohm in 1826: Potential Difference (V) = Current (I) x Resistance (R).

Alternating current is the current from a wall plug and the current that is measured by the EEG. The calculation involved here includes impedance instead of resistance. Impedance can be defined as "resistance to alternating electrical flow", (Thompson & Thompson, 2015). Impedance, like resistance, is measured in ohms. The relevant equation in the calculation of **Alternating Current (AC) is: Voltage (V) = Current (I) X Impedance (z).**

Capacitance is an important factor in calculating impedance. As frequency increases, impedance decreases. A standard measurement is important for generalization in communication and standardization. When measuring impedances from the electrode sites, the current is at 10 Hz to approximate a common EEG frequency. The current flows from the selected electrode/s through the scalp to all other electrodes connected to the meter.

The impedance at each electrode site should be as low as possible. Impedance readings should be lower than 5 kiloohms (kohms) with a difference of less than 1 kohm between electrodes. Most modern amplifiers have a built-in impedance check and all devices should meet electronic standards in terms of safety that determine that the amount of current involved in the impedance check is completely within safe limits. It is possible that a person will feel at the most a slight tingling sensation.

4.2.3 The Differential Amplifier

The amplifier receives input from the positive active electrodes and from the negative reference electrode and measures the difference between these two signals. The polarity of the second input is reversed so that the currents are subtracted.

The amplifier amplifies the difference between the active and reference electrode, measured in microvolts, by more than 100,000 times. The other signals are not amplified. Changes in the signals to each input are amplified to the same degree but in opposite directions referenced to the ground of the amplifier.

Common mode rejection is applied in that all inputs that are the same in amplitude, phase, and frequency, are eliminated. Any voltage from an external source such as an air conditioner will have the same frequency, amplitude and "in phase" on both wires and will thus be cancelled out and not amplified. The EEG signals will be different at the different sites and will be amplified. This is a unique and essential feature of the differential amplifier.

When external common mode is not eliminated, it may be due to either difference in impedance between the relevant electrodes or due to a poor ground connection. When there is a sudden increase in 60 Hz or in 50 Hz in South Africa, it is usually because of the fact that one electrode has come loose.

It is very important to equal impedances at all electrode sites so that an external interference will appear the same when the active and reference inputs are compared by the amplifier, otherwise these external interfering signals will not be rejected by the amplifier.

4.2.4 Filters

There is a high pass filter, also known as a low frequency filter and a low pass filter, also called a high frequency filter. Some systems also have a notch filter which is used to filter out a narrow band of activity. These two filters of the amplifier are important in minimizing the distortions. The filtering is done differently with different systems. In most modern equipment, filtering is done in the same box that does the encoding.

High pass or low frequency filter: the function of the high pass filter is to reduce the amplitude of the waves that come in at a frequency below its cut off. It allows, in other words, waves that are above its cut off, to pass through. The frequency of the low frequency filter is normally set at somewhere between 0. 5 and 2 Hz.

Low pass or high frequency filter: the function of the low pass filter is to allow waves to come through below its cut off point. A low pass filter used to be set at 32 Hz but since the interest in gamma frequencies have increased, these filters   are usually set at higher frequencies in modern equipment. Electrical activity or interference from lights, computers and extension cords is usually very regular and shows up at 60 Hz in some countries and at 50 Hz in other countries.

4.2.5 Sampling

The original EEG is a continuous wave form in analogue format. The encoder is an analogue to digital converter which changes the alternating analogue current to digital form that the computer can process. This happens through a process called sampling. The continuous wave gets broken up into tiny parcels. This is done by an A/D converter which stands for Analogue to Digital converter.

Fast sampling is essential for receiving accurate information. The maximum frequency that can be concerted is based on the Nyquist principle. This principle indicates that the maximum frequency that can be reconstructed in a filter equals half the sampling frequency. For a 20 Hz frequency, the sampling rate must then be at twenty times per second.

The higher the sampling rate of the system you are working with the higher the frequencies of the activity you can view. Some older systems used to have lower sampling rates such as 128 samples per second, but modern equipment has much faster sampling rates.

When a sampling rate is too slow the analogue signal will appear to be running at a slower frequency than what it actually is. This concept is referred to as aliasing. A slow sampling rate can, as an example, make Sheer rhythm appear as low beta rhythm.

4.2.6 Digital Filtering

Digital filtering, according to Collura (2014) is a technique that uses computational techniques to process a signal and to produce an output that consists of only selected frequencies. The output is then a narrowband or filtered signal. A digital filter passes certain EEG frequencies and reduces others. Typically, filters have a bandwidth of at least 3 Hz.

4.2.7 Finite Impulse Response (FIR)

The FIR filter, according to the Thompsons (2015), "computes a moving average of digital samples". The number of points which are averaged is referred to as the order of the filter.

4.2.8 Infinite Impulse Response (IIR)

The Infiniti system uses this filter. This type of filtering results in a sharper 'cut off" at the beginning and the end of a bandwidth. It is a faster filter and is said to have less shoulder at the single hertz in at the beginning and at the end of specified frequency band.

4.2.9 Fast Fourier Transform (FFT)

The FFT is the most common method of QEEG analysis. It is a fast version of the Fourier Transform which was developed by Joseph Fourier in the 1950's. A signal is multiplied by a sinewave at a particular frequency and a cosine wave at the same frequency. The two results are averaged over time and combined to produce an estimate of the power and phase of the signal (Collura, 2014). The FFT provides a much faster cut off than the FIR filter according to the Thompsons (2015) but it relies on mathematical calculations that require more time. The EEG is mathematically expressed as an average voltage for a specific frequency over a specified time, called a spectrum.

In order to ensure that the frequencies are properly represented in an FFT analysis, the sampling has to occur at least twice the highest frequency rate in question. However, according to Collura (2014) this does not render adequate visual representation of the signal and therefore much higher sampling rates (1 024 samples per second or higher) are applied in QEEG's and neurofeedback.

4.2.10 Joint Time Frequency Analysis (JTFA)

The JFTA filtering method is similar to the FFT method in that it makes use of sines and cosines. It is different in that it does not use a fixed epoch size. Collura (2014) explains that the intermediate results are passed through a low pass filter that produces a slow-down estimate of the frequency content while it does not require the signal to slide into a fixed epoch. Changes in the EEG are reflected as estimates very rapidly because data can be compounded at every data point.

While FFT emphasizes the data in the middle of the epoch, JFTA emphasizes the most recent data. JFTA is computed up to 256 times per second, while FFT computes eight times per second.

4.2.11 EEG Sensors and Montages

4.2.11.1 Sensors

Sensors serve the purpose of sensing the voltage on the surface of the skin. There must be a good connection to the skin after proper preparation of the area with mostly an abrasive gel and a conductive gel or paste. The gel or paste is the electrolyte that conveys the signals or EEG currents. There is an array of caps, bands, and other equipment available to attach the EEG sensors and hold them in place.

Different practitioners prefer different types of sensors for different reasons. When clinicians use more sensors they may prefer to hold them in place with a head band whereas this may not be necessary for one or two channel training scenarios.

All sensors other than silver chloride sensors have a metallic connection which is not suitable to DC as well as low frequency training in, for instance, ISF. Silver chloride and carbon sensors do not block direct current or very low frequencies. Sensors made of tin (Sn) are economical and used often. They are suitable for general QEEG work. Gold sensors (Au) are the preferred choice of many practitioners. The sensors are usually gold plated and they are durable and have good noise performance. Some prefer silver (Ag) sensors but these appear to be sensitive to high frequency noise.

Silver chloride is regarded as an ideal sensor material and can also be used with DC and low frequency work. Silver chloride sensors are also least susceptible to noise. There are two different ways of manufacturing silver chloride sensors. According to the one method, a silver- or silver-plated disc is covered with silver chloride. The silver chloride may, however, wear off over time. Another method is to produce the sensors from silver chloride directly. Silver chloride is a chemical compound with the formula AgCl which converts to silver when heated. AgCl is a powder in its native form. A powder consisting of silver and silver chloride is pressed into a disc, using a process called "sintering". These sensors are referred to as silver/silver chloride sensors, Ag/AgCl. These sensors are readily available at a relatively low cost to those practitioners in countries that do not need to import them. They are suitable for most applications.

4.2.11.2 Montages

There are different ways of looking at the data provided by the EEG in terms of using different reference points. Generally, the ear lobe or the scalp over the mastoid bone behind the ear is used as a reference point for the active electrode/s because of the relative neutrality of these points in terms of electrical signals.

A referential montage is one in which the ear lobe or the scalp over the mastoid bone is used as a reference point. One can then assume that the recorded activity is from the site/s where the active electrode/s has/have been placed.

A common electrode reference montage is a montage in which a linked ear reference is used. During full cap assessments this is usually the preferred montage. Some systems have a built-in linked ear reference that determines the way in which the recorded signals are interpreted or processed.

Laplacian montage (also referred to as the common average reference montage) is one in which the active electrode is referenced to the average of the electrodes immediately surrounding it.

In a sequential (bipolar) montage, the electrodes are referenced to each other. The same recorded data can be recalculated and processed in terms of different montages as a means of confirming the accuracy and appropriateness of the inferences drawn.

The choice of montage usually depends on the goals of the recording. Neurologists mostly use sequential and also Laplacian montages. These montages are particularly good for analyzing localized activity pertaining to a lesion for instance.

The common reference montage is better suited for detection of widely dispersed activity and for analyzing asymmetry. A sequential montage may for instance reflect a lower theta amplitude than what would be reflected with a referential montage due to the fact that theta is widely spread activity. By the same argument, the beta amplitude with a sequential recording may be higher than the value registered with the referential montage.

4.2.12 Artefact (The Effects of Electrical Current, Physical Factors and Medication on the EEG)

4.2.12.1 The Effect of Electrical Current on the EEG

The problem with interfering signals during EEG recordings and neurofeedback sessions is not less of a problem with modern equipment than what it used to be with older equipment. The manufacturers of the different neurofeedback systems attempt to minimize artefact (the recorded activity that is not of cerebral origin be it from either physiologic or extraphysiologic origin).

It remains a factor to consider. Precautions ought to be taken to minimize artefact and the neurofeedback practitioners need to be able to distinguish between EEG signals and artefact.

There will be 50 Hz or 60 Hz activity coming from different electrical sources in your practices. There can be transmissions from radio stations that are conducted by the electrode wires. Static electricity is another source of interference. Lights can transmit current as can the proximity of your body with the client, create current.

To minimize the interference of electrical current on EEG signal. it is important that the electrode wires and sensors will all be of the same material. Electrodes should also be cleaned after each session according to the prescribed method for the particular material. Loose wires can be braided to ensure that the effect on the signal will be equal and thus cancelled out. Avoid using extension cords. Ensure that there is no electrode movement. Jars with conductive paste should not be left open for extended periods.

4.2.12.2 The Effects of Physical Factors on the EEG

Other than electrical interferences with the EEG signal, there are also other influences on the EEG recording that need to be identified.

Eye blink artefact affects the delta amplitude because eye blinks and eye movements mimic delta. Muscle artefact ought to be distinguished from high beta activity. Take note however that it is not advisable to include 39 – 41 Hz activity in an inhibit band in an attempt to exclude muscle artefact. The importance of the Sheer Rhythm in attentional processes, identified by David Sheer, has been established. A muscle inhibit of 45 – 58 Hz can be helpful. An inhibit band of 22 – 32 Hz discourages anxiety and rumination, but also discourages EMG (electromyography).

According to the Thompsons (2015), a regular artefact observed at 1 Hz, is probably not due to eye artefact but to electrical activity related to the regular contractions of the heart. It presents as a regular wave with a frequency of one cycle per second. Teaching the client, the diaphragmatic breathing technique (six breathing cycles per minute) may reduce heart artefact.

Tongue movement and swallowing also mimic delta activity.

Drowsiness may produce spike like activity but mostly drowsiness appears to be an excess of theta or alpha.

4.2.12.3 The Effects of Medication and Other Substances on the EEG

Many medications and addictive substances have an effect on the EEG.

The main underlying principle of the effects of medication on the electrical activity on the brain involves a reciprocal effect between alpha and beta. A stimulant would generally result in an increase of alpha when taken by a person with low arousal who would mainly have low beta amplitude. The effect of a stimulant on a person with a relatively normal level of arousal associated with good regulation ability will be a decrease in the alpha amplitude. It has become increasingly clear over the past decade that individuals respond differently to medication. "Personalized medicine" has for this reason, become a popular approach. The information below therefore pertains to averages and is based on three main sources of information namely *The Neurofeedback Book: An Introduction to Basic Concepts in Applied Psychophysiology* (Thompson & Thompson, 2003, 2015), *Electroencephalography: Basic Principles, Clinical Applications and Related Fields* (Niedermeyer & Da Silva, 1999, 2005), and the online questionnaires of Neuro 100.

Benzodiazepines, barbiturates and *tranquilizers* have an effect on beta higher than 20 Hz. The amplitude of the specified frequencies increases when the client uses medication from these groups of medication. The trade names of different medications differ in different countries. It is the responsibility of the neurofeedback practitioner to become acquainted with the common brand names of medications belonging to the different groups of medication that are prescribed often. Medications from these groups may also result in the slight decrease of the alpha amplitude.

Neuroleptics are said to increase alpha power and reduce beta power according to Hughes and John (1999).

Marijuana causes a prominent increase in the alpha frequency band on the day after the intake.

The use of *alcohol* increases beta higher than 20 Hz and decreases alpha.

Cocaine and *methylphenidate* (the active ingredient in Ritalin and Concerta) increase beta and alpha and reduces theta and delta power slightly. The effects of the stimulants on the neurotransmitters is according to Amen (1998) more drastic than the effect on the electrical activity in the brain.

The effects of *morphine, opiates,* and *heroin* result in immediate increase in alpha amplitudes and a subsequent reduction in alpha during the euphoric stage. The use of these substances is also associated with an increase of REM sleep which results in vivid dreams and hallucinations.

Caffeine and *nicotine* reduce the alpha and theta amplitudes according to the Thompsons (2015). Usage of these stimulants is generally associated with mental clarity.

The different groups of *anti-depressant medications* have different general effects on the EEG. The one common factor is that they probably all decrease alpha power. The evidence is, however, not conclusive.

The *tricyclic anti-depressants* tend to increase sleep spindles and cause asynchronous slow waves with spike and wave discharges. They decrease the alpha amplitude and possibly decrease beta power as well.

The *SSRI's* (*Serotonin Reuptake Inhibitors*) increase beta power and possibly decrease alpha.

Phenothiazines, Haloperidol and *Rauwolfia* derivatives possibly decrease alpha power and produce asynchronous slow waves.

Lithium causes generalized asynchronous slowing, an increase in theta and beta power and a decrease in alpha power.

Antipsychotics cause an increase of power across all the frequency bands except gamma which decreases.

Olanzapine often prescribed for bipolar disorder causes an overall slowing of the EEG and seizure activity have been mentioned as a possible side effect.

Antibiotics generally cause an increase of slow wave activity. Antihistamines also cause an increase of low frequency activity.

Anticonvulsants cause increases in delta and theta amplitudes. The long-term effect of anticonvulsants is a decrease in alpha peak frequency and increased delta and theta power.

Toxic substances will also have an effect on the EEG. A specialist has to be consulted in such cases.

Withdrawal from medications may result in generalized epileptiform activity. A referral to a neurologist is recommended when generalized epileptiform activity is observed.

Chapter 5

Evolutionary Developments in Neurofeedback

5.1 Background Information

In this chapter we'll be taking a look at the process of change and development that neurofeedback has undergone since it became solidly established as a viable alternative intervention for mainly only a few disorders. We will be following the neurofeedback journey from one channel power training to two and four channel power training, alpha/theta training to sLORETA, Region of Interest (ROI) training, to Surface live Z-score feedback (PZOKUL), Infra Slow Frequency training (ISF) to sLORETA ROI live Z-score feedback (ZBRAUL), to additional Z-plus feedback with PZMO and PZME..

As mentioned in the introduction to this book and in chapter 1 that dealt mainly with the history of neurofeedback, the work of Dr Barry Sterman and Dr Joe Kamiya independent of one another in different parts of the United States, captured the attention of many in the healthcare professions. The fact that the brain can be taught to change its behavior had, as it has now, potential implications that cannot be fathomed yet.

Over and above the positive effects of the increase of the amplitude of what became known as the sensory motor rhythm over the sensorimotor strip has on the dysregulated brain with a higher tendency to seizure activity, many other benefits of increasing SMR were noticed and researched. By 1972, Dr Sterman had produced 150 research papers on the results of EEG biofeedback.

A following significant beacon and milestone in the evolution of neurofeedback, was the work of Dr Joel Lubar, Professor Emeritus of the University of Tennessee pertaining to his investigation of the effects of enhancing fast brain wave activity and discouraging or inhibiting slow brain wave activity on a population of ADHD sufferers. His work on EEG

Biofeedback for the treatment of ADHD started in the 1970's (Lubar & Shouse, 1976; Lubar & Lubar, 1984; Lubar et al., 1995ab). Neurofeedback as an intervention for ADHD formed the backbone of the potential clinical applications of this form of brain training that changes the electrical activity of the brain. This was probably the first turning of the head by the mainstream medical fraternity away from chemically based interventions to interventions based on the electrical activity in the brain. The EEG was well established as a diagnostic tool, but it stopped there. The knowledge that the chemical and electrical activity of the brain was completely intertwined was also well established. Approaching intervention and attempts to change the functioning of the brain by starting to untie the knot from the other end, was simply not considered.

So, there it was: the functioning of the brain can be changed by changing the electrical activity. Not only that, but that: individual brains can be taught, through a totally non-invasive intervention, to facilitate those changes through a basic process of conditioning.

And as with all change, there were some that embraced it – and those who feared it. The few that embraced the changes grew into many more, based initially on mainly anecdotal evidence following the initial research papers on the efficacy of EEG Biofeedback in the treatment of seizure activity and for ADHD. As the supporters and the body of forward-thinking individuals grew, the research started growing and efficacy levels of neurofeedback as a viable intervention for many disorders started shifting from level 1 through to level 4 for many disorders. Meta-analysis by groups of international researchers provided unequivocal evidence of the success of neurofeedback as an intervention for many causes of discomfort.

The initial neurofeedback protocols were all based on one channel power or amplitude training and most of the current research is still based on one to four channel amplitude training.

In amplitude training, a unidirectional increase or decrease in selected bandwidths is the treatment goal. Those goals can now be guided by a QEEG or based on a combination of the analysis of symptoms, collateral information, various assessment outcomes with the QEEG, or they can be based on protocols that have been standardized or suggested by anecdotal evidence.

The didactic course that was initially compiled for the training of healthcare practitioners who wished to include neurofeedback as an intervention to their practices, did not include training in QEEG analysis. The course was compiled by individuals who wanted to establish some kind of blueprint and standardization of basic processes for the way forward in this rapidly expanding field of EEG Biofeedback or neurofeedback. The establishing of forums for discussion and of mentoring programs relied mostly on caring and sharing individuals who came from different fields of expertise and shared the common goal of wanting to validate and promote neurofeedback and the broader modality of biofeedback.

Sue and Siegfried Othmer were among the first clinicians that started training clinicians in the 1980s in the application of neurofeedback following the success they had had with training their son with seizure disorder (Othmer & Othmer, 2017). This led to wider clinical applications in private practices. After the Biofeedback Certification International Alliance was founded in 1981, the didactic training of neurofeedback practitioners became standardized according to the Blueprint of Knowledge. EEG Spectrum became one of the main training organizations in the field of neurofeedback and psychologists, physicians, therapists and other healthcare practitioners who were interested in including neurofeedback in their practices were trained around the world. Some healthcare professionals were trained as trainers and trained other practitioners in their own countries according to the provided Blueprint of Knowledge. There were other companies and associations promoting different systems that were involved in the training of practitioners as the field and the available equipment, expanded.

The didactic training included teachings on the history, terminology and concepts relevant to EEG, the underlying learning paradigms, instrumentation, neuroanatomy, neurophysiology, disorders with illustrations of EEG findings and treatment, the criteria for the levels of efficacy and research design. A lot of time was spent on the practical process with the instrumentation available at the time and all the clinicians brought their own experience and specific skill sets to the table. Specific amplitude training protocols researched by the forerunners in the field, were discussed and used in the private practitioners' practices under supervision. Mentoring sessions, forum discussions and the interaction of clinicians at clinical interchange conferences lead to more and more protocols being used.

The initial protocols that were used were the protocol of Barry Sterman on C3 and C4 for seizure disorder, Joel Lubar's protocol for ADHD on Cz, Joe Kamiya's alpha protocol, Peniston and Kulkosky's alpha-theta protocol for addiction, the protocol of Margaret Ayers for brain injury, Howard Benson's protocol for relaxation, Brownback-Mason's protocol of raising theta in multiple personality disorder and Hanselmeyer's protocol of rewarding alpha for peak performance. Documents of protocol recommendations were compiled and discussed and articles were published by experienced clinicians on the success of new protocols that were continuously being added to the documents with suggested protocols. Although QEEGs were available earlier, it was only during the last twenty years that technology progressed sufficiently to support brain mapping adequately and make the compilation of normative databases possible which is the cornerstone of the QEEG. In the compilation of a QEEG, the EEG is compared to a control group or normative data base.

So if during the initial years of neurofeedback, the protocols were not guided by a QEEG, what were the protocol decisions based on? The initial EEG research, the clinical skills of experienced practitioners, vigilant tracking of symptoms after treatment sessions, the understanding of the arousal model in relation to the functioning of the autonomic nervous system, the gracious sharing of success stories, a thorough understanding of the science behind the process and thorough assessments, were all skillfully and artfully combined by the neurofeedback practitioner to make protocol decisions and adaptions in protocols when necessary.

We will now take a look at the foundation of neurofeedback which is basic one channel power training.

5.2 Power or Amplitude Training

In one channel power training, an active sensor is placed on a certain position on the scalp based on the 10–20 or 20–20 system. One electrode is placed as a reference on the ear (if it is a clip-on electrode) or on the mastoid and one electrode serves as the ground and is placed on the other ear or mastoid. The electrodes are connected to an amplifier in the appropriate way. The reference electrode is usually placed on the same side as the active electrode and the ground sensor is placed on the ear or behind the ear on the opposite side of the active sensor.

The placement of the active electrode is based on the protocol decision of the clinician.

The clinician specifies which frequency bands are to be rewarded and which frequency bands are to be inhibited on the particular software that is being used. Although it is possible to specify more than one frequency band to be rewarded and two or more to be inhibited with some systems, the most common application of single channel power training is to specify one reward bandwidth and two inhibit bandwidths. The visual and auditory feedback is produced by the system when the EEG meets the predetermined goals.

The two factors that are being measured to determine change are amplitude and frequency. Amplitude indicates the amount of power contained in a signal whereas the frequency indicates the speed of the signal, in other words, the amount of time the signal moves up and down in a second. The frequency gives an indication of the tasking state being observed and the amplitude indicates how the tasking states are being prioritized, according to Gracefire (2017). When there is an excess or a deficit of an amplitude within a frequency range and that amplitude does not shift, it is indicative of a central nervous system that is finding it difficult to shift and regulate arousal responses.

To date most experienced clinicians have developed location-based training protocols based on the experience of decades. These protocols demonstrated that individuals respond differently to different frequencies and different locations. The dynamics of the local systems and the influence and contribution to the entire complex system being the brain, is recognized and implemented in conservative amplitude training, according to Soutar (2017). Amplitude training is considered a very reliable and conservative approach by many researchers and clinicians. According to Soutar (2017) amplitude training alters the other dimensions of measurement but at the brain's own discretion and pace.

Many clinicians continue to use single channel amplitude training which is currently still the main focus of most research studies in terms of efficacy investigations (Soutar, 2017). The more complex methods demand higher levels of training in the technological aspects of the software programs as well as a background in mathematics and science that many clinicians find intimidating. Consequently, many clinicians are staying with one channel power training. The research in neurofeedback has firmly established the efficacy of this paradigm. Specific protocols have been defined that can be used safely and successfully. Some of those protocols are specified below. Recent developments in neurofeedback involving more sophisticated software and different paradigms and approaches have the potential of reducing training or treatment time. There is no conclusive research evidence to this effect yet, but the anecdotal evidence from individual practitioners across the world who have endeavored to stay up to speed with   all new developments, appears consistently positive according to Soutar (2017). The different approaches and paradigms as they have developed over time are discussed below. We will discuss these, commencing with single channel amplitude training after we have taken a look at the arousal model.

The arousal approach in neurofeedback is differentiated from an approach which is focused on specific regions of interest. Viewed very broadly, arousal levels are generally increased by doing training of the left hemisphere and arousal is lowered by right hemisphere training.

Many clinicians consider the principles of the arousal model when they make protocol decisions involving surface amplitude training. It is therefore relevant to include an overview of the arousal model. It is also important to be reminded that the arousal model is not an outdated model that has been outranked by later theories. The research referred to in this regard is deliberately recent and current.

All who have studied psychiatry and psychology will be familiar with the basics of the arousal model. The principles of this model have been well established for decades. It was Barry Sterman who, in 1996, first incorporated the principles of the arousal model into the modality of neurofeedback. Sterman observed during his research that repeated induced changes in the sensory motor rhythm (SMR) correlate with changes in the striatum (Sterman & Egner, 2006). Sterman indicated that three systems of brain activity influence thalamic generation of the EEG at the scalp. He specified the vigilance system, the sensorimotor system, and the cognitive integration system.

In 1999, Evans and Abarbanel noted that Sterman's theory did not indicate the significance of the limbic oscillatory activity in the production of the EEG. Kirk and MacKay (2003) specify mechanisms by which low frequency theta activity related to emotional processing is shifted through arousal mechanisms to higher frequency theta involved in memory. Research showing the relationship between attention and emotion very concisely further documents the EEG changes that correlate with arousal. Emotion and cognition are interconnected at the neurophysiological level and this fact has direct implications for psychology and for neurofeedback, according to Soutar (2017).

Specific networks become available at each different and specific level of arousal. According to the Yerkes-Dodson law, which was established in 1908 (Yerkes & Dodson, 1908) and formulated by Diamond et al. (2007), performance is arousal dependent as Sterman's original theory stated. Various tasks call forth different levels of arousal and recruit different neuronal networks. Simple or familiar learned tasks require lower arousal and complex or new tasks require more arousal. Buckner et al. (2008) verified this fact in their work involving the Default Mode Network. Research study by Diamond et al. (2007) has specified that learning consolidation is arousal dependent. Soutar (2017) mentions that given the efficacy, reliability and safety of amplitude training, it is justifiable to continue with the development of a one channel amplitude training perspective into a multichannel amplitude training perspective, beginning with a thorough understanding of two channel training.

Soutar (2017) mentions that, based on the work of Davidsons's research (1995), the modification of arousal appears to be mediated by the ongoing dynamic relationship between the left and the right hemispheres. The left/right dimension of training is referred to as the Horizontal Axis. Many asymmetry protocols involving the training of homologous sites like F3-F4, using two channels of EEG, developed from the work of Baehr et al. (1997) close to the turn of the millennium and the works of Rosenfeld (Rosenfeld, 1997, 2000; Rosenfeld et al., 1996) and Davidson (1994, 1995). It appears however that the dynamic of the Horizontal Axis was more complex than what was understood at the time.

Below follows a simplified version of the arousal model as it was taught to earlier generations of neurofeedback practitioners based on the prescribed Blueprint of Knowledge.

The Yerkes-Dodson law is an empirical relationship between arousal and performance. This law of arousal was developed by Yerkes and Dodson (1908). According to this law, performance increases with physiological or mental arousal. However, when arousal levels become too high, performance decreases.

There is a substantial body of research that indicates that different tasks require different levels of arousal for optimal concentration. Difficult or intellectually challenging tasks require a lower level of arousal for optimal concentration. Difficult or intellectually challenging tasks require a lower level of arousal for optimal performance than tasks that require stamina and endurance for which higher levels of motivation will be required for optimal functioning.

For familiar, well-learned tasks, performance increases as arousal increases. For complex tasks or unfamiliar tasks, the relationships between performance and arousal reverses at some point so that arousal levels that are too high, impact negatively on performance. When the arousal level is too high, the negative effect of arousal which is stress, has a negative effect on cognitive processes including attention.

A simple task, such as hitting a nail with a hammer for instance, requires an average arousal level. If the arousal level is too low, the person may start missing the nail and more hits to pound the nail may be required. A moderate level of arousal is appropriate when listening to a lecture which results in a moderate attention level. Should the arousal level be too low when listening to a lecture, the listener will become drowsy and his concentration level will be low. Should on the other hand, the listener's arousal level be too high, he will become fidgety, impatient, miss important information and tend to become distracted. Complex tasks, like playing chess, require sustained attention. Sustained attention lowers the arousal level. A high arousal level during a game of chess would result in careless or unforced errors known as commission errors. The player would probably also become restless, bored, and hyper. Optimal performance requires an arousal level appropriate to the task at hand. The arousal level ought to be flexible. Flexible arousal levels are essential for optimal performance and adaptability. When a person is chronically under-aroused, he/she will have difficulty getting started in the morning and his/her performance will be sub-normal. People with a profile of being chronically under- aroused, generally suffer cognitive worry with constant fear of making mistakes. People who suffer chronic over-arousal, often battle falling asleep because it takes a long time to quiet down enough to be able to start moving into a dominant alpha state and on to a dominant theta and then delta state. People who suffer chronic over-arousal typically find it difficult to calm down when something upsets them.

There are also people who have mixed arousal symptoms. These people will sometimes be too over-aroused for the task or situation at hand and at other times inappropriately under-aroused. Performance is not optimal when the arousal level is unstable and vacillates from over- to under-arousal. People with unstable arousal levels have difficulty with maintaining a certain state of consciousness. The arousal level ought to be flexible for optimal performance as stated earlier, but it ought to fluctuate in a controllable and appropriate manner based on the situation or task at hand.

There are different measures of arousal levels – many of which are used by practitioners who combine biofeedback with EEG-biofeedback. Measures of arousal of the autonomic nervous system include heart rate, respiratory rate, blood pressure, muscle tension (EMG), galvanic skin response (GSR) which measures sweat-gland activity and emotional response and EEG (generalized over the cortex). One part of the brain can, however, be either less or more aroused than the rest of the brain. These measures are discussed in the section on the stress response and parasympathetic drive and sympathetic drive responses. The self-report of symptoms is considered by some to provide a good or even the best indication of arousal level.

It is not possible to pay attention efficiently when the arousal level is not appropriate. Neurofeedback links, so to speak, the arousal and attention system in the brain. The reticular activating system (RAS) activates the cortex by alerting it to incoming stimuli. Conflicting sensory input gets inhibited. The interplay between this activation and inhibition results in focused attention. The arousal level affects the activation and the inhibition which involves voluntary selection. Stable arousal levels are necessary for the filtering process involved in voluntary selection. One type of such filtering and voluntary selection involves auditory foreground and background discrimination. ADHD sufferers have difficulty with distinguishing between foreground and background sounds or selecting what to focus on because they cannot filter well due to arousal levels that are not optimum for the task. There are also other types of filtering that are involved not only pertaining to these particular auditory perceptions. Autistic Spectrum Disorder sufferers can mostly also not filter and distinguish between what needs to be focused on and which stimuli need to be filtered out.

The arousal model approach in neurofeedback dictates that when the arousal level is not optimum, the person will not be able to pay attention optimally which necessarily influences processing, learning and cognitive functioning in general. It is important to remember that the maturation of the frontal lobes is also very important in the process of selective attention and that the frontal lobes are generally not fully functional prior to the age of twenty-five.

The arousal level can be influenced in neurofeedback by the reward frequency. The faster the frequency band that is being rewarded, the higher the arousal level lifts. Activating the left hemisphere exerts pressure on the neural system to increase dopamine output. Reducing activation in the right hemisphere influences the neural system to decrease nor-epinephrine output (Davidson, 1995). The arousal level lowers by rewarding low frequency bands. The most common approach is to reward 15–18 Hz on C3 to lift the arousal in clients with low arousal symptoms and to lower the arousal level by rewarding 12–15 Hz on C4 with client's that suffer high arousal symptoms.

Unstable arousal symptoms which are often present in clients suffering mood disorders, bipolar disorder, migraines, rage and traumatic brain injury, are often addressed by training on both C3 and C4 separately at different frequencies or by doing an interhemispheric training where both sites are trained simultaneously at 12–15 Hz by those practitioners who follow the arousal model approach focusing on one channel amplitude training.

Many practitioners use a standardized symptom tracking form to identify the over-, under-, and unstable-arousal symptoms to assist them in their treatment plan. Many practitioners who do mainly QEEG-guided neurofeedback also have their clients complete a symptom checklist based on the arousal level symptoms. Below is a list of symptoms associated with different arousal levels. Completing such a checklist can be very insightful to clients who have not yet thought of the symptoms of their discomfort in an analytical and systematic manner.

5.2.1 Symptoms Associated with Under-Arousal

Sleep Symptoms

- Difficulty waking in the morning
- Not rested after sleep
- Frequent waking during the night
- Sleeping very lightly
- Sleeping too much
- Snoring or sleep apnea
- Night sweats (hypeglycaemia)
- Difficulty falling asleep due to a quiet, tired mind
- Difficulty falling asleep after awakening
- Teeth grinding
- Bedwetting or soiling

Attention Symptoms

- Inattentiveness
- Daydreaming
- Poor sustained attention
- Lack of motivation
- Spaceiness
- Poor concentration
- Hyperactivity (self-stimulating)
- Fidgeting
- Constant leg or hand movement
- Inattention + Impulsivity + Hyperactivity

Emotional and Behavioral Symptoms

- Excessive worry (but not rumination)
- Performance anxiety/error anxiety
- Depression (feelings of helplessness and hopelessness)
- Irritability (not aggression or anger)
- Feelings of being hurt easily, vulnerability, excessively emotional, crying often and easily
- Easily embarrassed
- Perfectionistic
- Low self-esteem
- Remorseful after tantrums
- Feelings of guilt and shame
- Withdraws when stressed
- Anxious and depressed
- Encopresis
- Bed wetting (Enuresis)
- Seasonal Affective Disorder
- Suicidal thoughts or actions
- PTSD
- Compulsive overeating
- Exceptionally low or high sexual libido

Panic Symptoms

- Chronic pain with depression
- Chronic aching pain
- Tension headache
- Low pain threshold
- Migraine
- Fibromyalgia

Neurological and Motor Symptoms

- Left-brain stroke
- Left-brain traumatic brain injury
- Right body paralysis or paresis
- Urinary incontinence
- Seizures
- Traumatic brain injury with stem injury

Immune, Endocrine, and Autonomic Symptoms

- Sugar craving (hypoglycaemia)
- Immune deficiency
- Low thyroid function
- Post Menstrual Syndrome (depression, insomnia, pain, irritability)
- Intolerant of alcohol and other sedating drugs
- Asthma
- Chronic fatigue syndrome

5.2.2 Symptoms Associated with Over-Arousal

Sleep Symptoms
- Difficulty falling asleep due to a busy mind
- Difficulty falling back asleep after awakening
- Physically restless sleep
- Nightmares
- Vivid dreams or overtly active dreams
- Bruxism (teeth grinding)
- Restless leg syndrome
- Menopausal hot flushes

Attention Symptoms
- Impulsivity
- Distractibility
- Stimulus seeking
- Many competing thoughts
- Hyperactivity (driven type)
- Fidgeting
- Constant leg or hand movement
- Inattention + Hyperactivity + Impulsivity

Emotional and Behavioral Symptoms
- Withdraws when stressed
- Anxiety (fear and physiological arousal)
- Agitated depression
- Anger
- Agitation
- Aggressive and/or violent
- Impatience
- Anxious and depressed

- Panic attacks and phobias
- Motor or vocal ticks
- OCD, obsessive thoughts, rumination
- Suicidal thoughts or actions
- Conduct Disorder
- Oppositional and Defiant behavior
- Autistic symptoms
- Reactive Attachment Disorder
- PTSD
- Compulsive overeating
- Sexual libido high or low

Panic Symptoms

- Tension headache
- Migraine
- Emotional reactivity to pain
- Chronic burning pain
- Chronic sharp or throbbing pain
- Sciatica pain
- Peripheral neuropathy
- High pain threshold
- Fibromyalgia

Neurological and Motor Symptoms

- Right-brain stroke
- Right-brain injury
- Left body paralysis or paresis
- Spasticity
- Tremor
- Poor balance

- Poor coordination

- Nervous habits

- Motor tics

- Seizures

- Traumatic brain injury with brain stem injury

Immune, Endocrine, and Autonomic Symptoms

- Hypertension

- Irregular menstrual periods, painful periods

- Heart palpitations

- Constipation (sometimes)

- Menopausal hot flushes

- PMS-agitated symptoms, rage, racing thoughts

- Intolerant to coffee and other stimulants

- Involuntary regurgitation

- Chronic fatigue syndrome

The reader will have noticed that some symptoms that have been listed as symptoms that will respond better to left-sided training (symptoms associated with under- arousal) have also been listed as symptoms that ought to respond well to right-sided training (symptoms associated with over-arousal) and in some cases will also be listed as symptoms that will respond to interhemispheric training or training on both sides of the brain separately (symptoms associated with unstable arousal) in the following section.

The indication of the symptoms by the client are merely some of the puzzle pieces that the well trained and experienced neurofeedback practitioner pieces together with all the other sources of information and information gathered from close observation and from engaging with the client to ascertain the client's experience in the process of determining, adapting and changing protocols that will best serve the goal of improved regulation.

5.2.3 Some Popular Amplitude Training Protocols

Listed below is single channel power training protocols that are used most commonly without a QEEG and often as a QEEG guided protocol as well. These protocols are based on the documents provided by the protocol panel of EEG Spectrum International according to discussions at the annual Clinical Interchange Conference. A template was created at the Clinical Interchange Conference that was to serve as a building tool to which protocols could be added according to the consensus of many experienced clinicians. The protocols listed below are based on that template which was often referred to as a work in progress. They are, however, far from random as they are based on the expert opinions and collaboration of brilliant minds and rich clinical experience. The protocols are merely suggestions of viable options by experienced and responsible clinicians. They are more appropriate to those clinicians who do not always do exclusively QEEG guided neurofeedback and to those who feel more comfortable with one or two channel amplitude or power training. Those clinicians ordinarily have a very strong symptom-based approach to training. To my knowledge the experts that served on the protocol panel during the first decade of the century still make significant contributions to the field of neurofeedback in different capacities. The team was led by Mike Cohen and members serving on the panel were Matt Fleischmann, Ed Hamlin, Joy Lunt, Michael O' Bannon, Bob Patterson and Gary Schummer. All in the neurofeedback fraternity know of the work of these big names in the field and many have had the privilege of either meeting them or of having attended their workshops, presentations, or webinars.

C3	Reward: 15 - 18 Hz	Inhibit 1: 4 - 7 Hz	Inhibit 2: 22 - 36 Hz

Symptoms: Inattentive ADHD with low energy levels and many prominent symptoms associated with low arousal as listed under 5.2.1

C4	Reward: 12 - 15 Hz	Inhibit 1: 4 - 7 Hz	Inhibit 2: 22 - 36 Hz

Symptoms: Combined type ADHD and other disorders that present with high energy levels and many prominent symptoms associated with over- arousal.

C3 - C4	Reward: 12 - 15 Hz	Inhibit 1: 4 - 7 Hz	Inhibit 2: 22 - 36 Hz

Most practitioners do not use bipolar placements with one channel amplitude training any longer. They would rather do two channel amplitude training or live Z-score training instead. There are however individuals that respond particularly well to some of the bipolar placements and some practitioners that still consider the bipolar placement options.

Below are some of the protocols that were suggested by the panel:

Symptom/s	Placements	Frequencies
Impulsivity	C4; C4 − Pz; FP1− FP2; AF7− AF8; C4−AF8	Reward and inhibit frequencies are set according to symptoms.
Lack of motivation	F3–A1	Reward: Either 15–18 Hz or 12–15 Hz
OCD and/or rumination	Fz	Reward: Either 5–8 Hz or 12–15 Hz or 15–18 Hz
	AF7–AF8	Reward: 12–15 Hz
	FP1–FP2	Reward: Either 10–13 Hz or 12–15 Hz
	T3–T4	Reward 12–15 Hz or lower
	T4; T4–Fz; T4–FP1	Reward: Either 12–15 Hz or lower
	F4–Fz	Reward: Base decision on client symptoms.

For the inhibit bands for the above-mentioned protocols, high amplitudes of slow frequencies that stand out at the training site ought to be targeted. Some clinicians prefer to target narrow bands of slow activity and others have good results with targeting wider bands of slow activity. The following commonly used protocols in power training are based on reports of clinical outcomes by licensed professionals and are organized by regions:

Central and Central-Temporal Sites

Site	Used For
C3 15–18 Hz or C4 12–15 Hz	Increasing arousal, depression, attention, ego strength
T3 15–18 Hz or T4 12–15 Hz	Stabilization and T3 can be helpful for ADHD adults
Cz 15– 18 Hz or 12–15 Hz	Similar arousal effects as C3 and C4 but often more stabilizing.
C3–C4	Stabilizing with a fairly direct impact on arousal.
T3–T4	Stabilizing and stabilized calming. This protocol is considered to be a good starting point for migraine headaches.
C5–C6	Sometimes successful for Bipolar Disorder.

Frontal (Pre-Frontal and Frontal Lobes):

Site	Used For
C3–FPz 15–18 Hz	Improved concentration and focus
FPz: 15–18 Hz or 12–15 Hz	Improved concentration and focus
Fz: 5–8 Hz; 12–15 Hz. 15–18 Hz	Rumination, OCD, Stuck thinking, motivation
C4–Fz: 5–8 Hz; 8–11 Hz; 12–15 Hz	Rumination, OCD, stuck thinking, motiva- tion.
C3–Fz: 15–18 Hz	Rumination, OCD, stuck thinking.
Cz–Fz: 5–8 Hz; 8–11 Hz; 12–15 Hz; 15–18 Hz	Rumination, OCD, stuck thinking
T4-Fz: 12–15 Hz	Rumination, OCD, stuck thinking, alcohol, and drug cravings
T3-Fp1: 15–18 Hz	Calm focus, attention, mental chatter, alertness, mood stabilization
T4–Fp2: 12–15 Hz	Calm focus, attention, mental chatter, alertness, mood stabilization
C3–Fp1: 15–18 Hz	Calm focus, attention, mental chatter, alertness
C4–Fp2: 12–18 Hz	Calm focus, attention, mental chatter, mood stabilization

F3: 15–18 Hz	Depression, mood, overly emotional
AF7–AF8: 10–13 Hz; 12–15 Hz	Impulsivity, tics
Fp1–Fp2: 10–13 Hz; 12–15 Hz	Focus, concentration, executive function
F3–F4: 12–15 Hz, 8–11 Hz, 15–18 Hz (seldom)	Fine motor coordination, control of movements, tremor, motiva- tion, depression, mood
F7–F8: 12–15 Hz switch to 15–18 Hz switch to 10–13 Hz	Speech initiation, fluency, vocal output
F7–A1: 15–18 Hz	Speech, impulsivity, could decrease intensity of emotion
F8–A2: 12–15 Hz	Speech, impulsivity, could decrease intensity of emotion
FPO2: 6–9 Hz, 5–8 Hz and lower frequencies	PTSD, hypervigilance, fear. Train for short periods
T4–F4: 8–11 Hz (Inhibit: 2–7 Hz)	Alcohol and drug cravings, reactivity
Cz–F4: 8–11 Hz	Obsessive thoughts or behavior

Parietal or Parietal Temporal

Site	Used For
C4–PZ: 12–15 Hz; 8–11 Hz	Anxiety, body tension, spatial awareness
C4–P4: 8–11 Hz	Anxiety, body tension, spatial awareness
Pz: 8–11 Hz; 10–13 Hz	Relaxation, reduced arousal as an alternative to C4, memory, pain, sleep onset, anxiety
P4: 12–15 Hz; 6–9 Hz	Mathematics, improved processing
P3–P4: 10–13 Hz; 8–11 Hz	Body tension, melting of muscle tension
P5–P6: 10–13 Hz	Possibly helpful for dyslexia
	Sensory integration, being demanding and wanting his/her own way

There are many other single channel unipolar and bipolar placements that have rendered good results and for which there is anecdotal evidence. The

QEEG-based power training protocols involve potentially any placement and any frequency. The protocols mentioned in this section are mainly symptom based protocols that have become known and used by many clinicians over the world that do not necessarily have easy access to QEEG's or who do a combination of symptom based and QEEG guided neurofeedback. Neurofeedback practitioners who have long since moved away from one channel training or power training all together, are reminded once again that most current research is still based on power training protocols and that amplitude training remains a very reliable albeit conservative approach.

Soutar (2017) is of the opinion that given the efficacy, reliability and safety of amplitude training, it makes sense to continue with developing the one channel training amplitude training perspective into a multichannel amplitude perspective but that a thorough understanding of two channel training dynamic will have to be developed first.

5.2.4 Bipolar and Two Channel Bi-Hemispheric Amplitude Training

When neurofeedback was still in its infancy, those clients who presented predominantly with what was referred to as "mixed arousal" or instability symptoms were treated with a bipolar hook up using one channel. The training often occurred over the sensorimotor strip with the placement of the active electrode on C3 and the reference electrode on C4 with a ground clip electrode on A1. The chosen specified bandwidth to reward would mostly be 12–15 Hz. A protocol in which the reward frequency would be as high as the frequency that would often be rewarded on C3 in a monopolar hook-up namely (15–18 Hz) was not recommended. Although desirable outcomes were widespread with this and numerous other bipolar protocols, concern was regularly expressed in different forums that it was not exactly clear what the activity was that was being rewarded due to the complexity of the neurophysiology involved in using an active and a reference sensor which employ a difference signal in a one channel training protocol. Whereas the initial bipolar or sequential hook-ups were done from a single channel and you could not be certain what the electrical measurements represented, most modern equipment allows for two channel feedback where the two sites are being monitored separately. The two-channel training will either involve two input jacks into the decoder with three electrodes involved in each channel (active, reference and ground) or a common reference (usually a linked- ear reference) and a common ground. With two channel training the amplitudes of the different frequency bands can be viewed and compared.

There were also many other interhemispheric and intra-hemispheric protocols suggested for addressing an array of symptoms. Many of those protocols are still being used with great success by many experienced and successful neurofeedback practitioners. One such a protocol that has received a lot of attention over the past decade owing to Sebern Fisher's wonderful work pertaining to developmental trauma, is T4–P4, rewarding 10–13 Hz and inhibiting 0–7 Hz as well as 22–36 Hz. She also suggests T3-T4 for developmental trauma as well as C5-C6, in her book, Neurofeedback in the Treatment of Developmental Trauma-Calming the Fear-Driven Brain (2014).

Sebern Fisher raises an important point regarding protocol decisions for problems pertaining to emotional regulation in her book. She reminds the reader that most of the research has been aimed at the regulation of attention, owing to the body of research on ADHD and not on the regulation of affect. The training path for the person with predominantly emotional regulation problems is often more difficult to navigate.

Some of the instability symptoms for which interhemispheric and intra-hemispheric protocols have been suggested are indicated in the following chart.

5.2.4.1 Symptoms Associated with Instability (Unstable Arousal)

Sleep Symptoms
- Snoring or sleep apnea
- Night sweats
- Bruxism (teeth grinding)
- Bedwetting or soiling
- Night terrors
- Nocturnal myoclonus
- Sleep walking
- Narcolepsy
- Sleep paralysis when awakening (still dreaming while awake)

Attention Symptoms
- Hyperactivity after sugar intake
- Hyperactivity with fatigue or sedatives
- Inattention + Hyperactivity + Impulsivity

Emotional and Behavioral Symptoms

- Withdraws when stressed
- Aggressive and/or violent
- Anxious and depressed Manic-depressive cycles
- Mood swings
- Panic attacks and/or phobias
- Encopresis
- Anorexia
- Bulimia
- Binge Eating
- Motor or vocal tics
- OCD, obsessive thoughts, rumination
- Suicidal thoughts or actions
- Rages
- Conduct Disorder
- Oppositional and defiant behavior
- Autistic symptoms
- Reactive Attachment Disorder
- PTSD
- Compulsive overeating
- Sexual libido high or low

Pain Symptoms

- Chronic aching pain
- Migraine
- Chronic burning pain
- Chronic sharp or throbbing pain
- Sciatica pain
- Peripheral Neuropathy
- Fibromyalgia

- Reflex sympathetic dystrophy
- Trigeminal neuralgia
- Chronic nerve pain
- RSD (Reflex Sympathetic Dystrophy or Complex Regional Pain Syndrome)

Neurological and Motor Symptoms

- Left-brain stroke
- Left-brain traumatic brain injury
- Right body paralysis or paresis
- Urinary incontinence
- Right-brain stroke
- Right-brain traumatic brain injury
- Left body paralysis or paresis
- Spasticity
- Tremor
- Motor tics
- Seizures
- Traumatic brain injury with brain stem injury
- Vertigo
- Tinnitus

Immune, Endocrine, and Autonomic Symptoms

- Sugar craving (hypoglycaemia)
- Immune deficiency
- Intolerant of alcohol and other stimulants
- Asthma
- Hypertension
- Skin allergies
- Menopausal hot flashes

- PMS (agitated symptoms, rage, racing thoughts)
- Intolerant of coffee and other stimulants
- Involuntary regurgitation
- Chronic fatigue syndrome
- Severe PMS (mood swings, migraines, sugar cravings)
- Irritable Bowel Syndrome
- Autoimmune disorders- lupus, diabetes, MS, rheumatoid arthritis

There is currently renewed interest in two channel training, which, according to Soutar (2017) was never explored fully when it emerged. The two-channel method was proposed by Baehr et al. (1999). The coherence method of training was proposed by Horvat (Horvat, 2009; Soutar, 2017). The QEEG guided feedback started playing a more prominent role in neurofeedback and demanded the main focus. QEEG guided neurofeedback was also strongly endorsed by the ISNR which detracted attention from further investigation of the potential gains of two channel training. The rapid development of the field into a multichannel approach dwarfed the one and two channel approaches. More and more commercial QEEG databases became available in the1990's with pre- and post- training maps becoming the new norm, although many clinicians are still using the TOVA (test of variables of attention), Beck Inventories and other assessment measures as pre- and post-measures.

It is possible that as the approach to neurofeedback became more technical, there was less focus on individual responses and other limiting factors, by possibly mostly the younger generation of neurofeedback practitioners. When things develop fast, there is perhaps more of a "skimming the surface" at high speed like a motorboat mind set at the cost of depth of perception. This is just a personal opinion that many will disagree with – which is wonderful. If everybody had one mind set, there would not have been the astonishing progression in the field. One of the reasons why I decided to write this book, as I have mentioned in the introduction, is to plead the case for not losing the detail and the individualized approach in which the entire skill set of the practitioner gets employed in the name of progress. It is so easy and even tempting to get caught up into the advanced technology which measures thousands of markers of the individual brain and compares them to mean scores, that we start equating the individual to those scores and defining the individual's experience in terms of those scores instead of observing and listening accurately. Truth remains that not all deviant scores are symptomatic as has been mentioned before and in actual fact some "deviant scores" may just be what gives the individual the edge over what he/she needs to overcome.

In his chapter titled "Perspective and Method for a QEEG Based Two Channel Bi-hemispheric Compensatory Model of Neurofeedback Training", published in *Handbook of Clinical EEG and Neurotherapy* (Collura & Frederick, 2017), Soutar mentions that it is reasonable to assume that every brain has metabolic limitations in terms of especially glycogen, glutamate and lactate, sodium and potassium. According to Niedermeyer and Da Silva (2005), the effects of hypothyroid function on the brain is well known and levels of T3 have been associated with neuronal function including enzyme production, growth factors controlling neuronal growth, production of matrix proteins, glutamate regulation and neurogenesis. Hypothyroid function manifests as slowed alpha with increased power. Attempting to down train this metabolic limitation will be futile. Despite the fact that most neurofeedback practitioners are not qualified to identify metabolic deficiencies and other factors that limit the efficacy of neurofeedback, careful observation, mindful listening and being tuned in to each individual that they are attempting to assist, will provide practitioners with many clues for adequate referrals. It is possible that when we become too focused on the sophisticated technology at our disposal, we may suggest more and more evaluations and attempt more and more training paradigms at high cost to the individual and with little success.

According to Othmer et al. (1999), a strategic intervention from a systems approach is most likely to be effective when implementing neurofeedback. They are of the opinion that accuracy in selecting a network may be more important than specificity in training and express it as follows: "An emerging network systems approach transcends simple anatomically defined distinctions regarding function such as Brodmann areas" (Nakagawa et al., 2013). The understanding of networks is still limited according to R. Soutar (2017) and it would probably be advisable to identify optimal attractor sites in meta-networks involving "Rich Club Hubs" which have a dominant influence on network activity because of the most connections with the shortest pathways between network nodes what is now, according to Soutar (2017) recognized as a "Small World' scale free network design that defines networks in general. Many of these hubs correlate closely with the 10–20 system.

In 1999 Baehr et al. suggested an asymmetry protocol in which homologous sites are trained using two channels. The sites in question were F3-F4. The goal was to increase alpha activity in the right hemisphere and decrease alpha in the left hemisphere. This potentially increases activation of the left hemisphere. Many other bi-hemispheric training homologous sites are being used by clinicians throughout the world.

In my own practice, I have witnessed much success with C3-C4, rewarding 15–18 Hz on C3 while rewarding 12–15 Hz on C4 with the same inhibits.

Coherence measures can be monitored carefully while doing two channel bi- hemispheric training. According to Laird (2012) the major functional networks are bilateral in nature. Teipel et al. (2009), mention that interhemispheric coherence is a measure of interhemispheric integrity.

Bi-hemispheric training, indirectly trains arousal. Arousal is linked to the relationship between the left and right hemisphere.

The reader will recall that according to Davidson (1995), activation of the left hemisphere causes the neural network to increase dopamine output, whereas activation of the right hemisphere encourages epinephrine output. Hemispheric balance of activity results in a general improvement of the system and can be modified by shifting to different meta-networks to address regional dysregulation. According to Soutar (2017), the training of homologous sites with two channel training, specific symptoms associated with the particular locations can be addressed while moving the system globally in a normative direction. A main goal ought to be to encourage normal asymmetry between alpha and beta. Alpha should tend to be higher in the right hemisphere and beta ought to be higher in the left hemisphere. Typically, an excess of slow wave activity will shift down as asymmetry is normalized. According to Soutar (2017), regional network dynamics is trained in the selection of bilateral networks. He suggests that the network posterior to the worst regulated network based on EEG findings) ought to be selected for initial training for the best results.

5.3 LORETA and sLORETA Neurofeedback

LORETA (low resolution electromagnetic tomography) is a mathematical procedure devised by Pasqual-Marqui et al. (1994). The quantitative data from a 19-channel recording find linear solutions for the sources within the cortex of activity at specific frequencies. It is thus a method of localizing activity in the brain. Tomography is the process by which two dimensional slices are created of the three-dimensional brain. Horizontal, sagittal, and coronal slices are presented in images that look like MRI images. According to Thompson and Thompson (2015), LORETA has been validated against MRI. LORETA is accurate for cortical locations. The sites are voxels which are three dimensional units that have specific coordinates. LORETA does not calculate subcortical sources of EEG frequencies. Roberto Pasqual-Marqui made LORETA available free of charge to practitioners and researchers. It can be downloaded.

The time necessary to compute inverse solutions is problematic. Real-time solutions with complete graphic displays, has not, according to Collura (2014) been available until recently. At the time of the publication of Collura's *Technical Foundations of Neurofeedback* in 2014, through the use of specialized hardware, sLORETA could compute inverse solutions for all voxels at all frequency bands in real time and provide immediate feedback for training according to the principals of learning through operant conditioning. LORETA-based techniques can be combined with Z-score training (to be discussed in the next section) or be used independently of Z-score training in which case the region/s of interest are specified while all 19 channels are being recorded and amperage training is done. Penijean Gracefire explains LORETA amperage training as follows in her article, "Introduction to the Concepts and Clinical Applications of Multivariate Live Z-score Training, PZOK and sLORETA Feedback", (2017): If the clinician needs to reduce theta in the anterior cingulate (or any other ROI) the anterior cingulate (or any other ROI) gets selected as the region of interest, the theta band then gets selected as the desired band. The software will then estimate the amperage of the current source density of theta in every voxel of the entire anterior cingulate. The client receives feedback when the overall running composite average of theta decreases representing a decrease of theta in the three-dimensional space in the cortex estimated to correspond with the position of the anterior cingulate. Symptoms get matched with ROI's in terms of the available literature on ROI's. She suggests a pre- and post-training 19-channel EEG recording to analyse the data with software that offers both surface and referential database analysis. Training should be limited to five to ten minutes per session and a re-evaluation should be done after no more than 10 sessions.

Gracefire (2017) specifies some of the advantages of sLORETA training as being that precise selection of EEG activity localized at a specific cortical region can be made that can potentially result in rapid changes in the EEG. The process also allows for more sophisticated protocol development and live monitoring of EEG changes in three dimensions is enabled.

Possible complicating factors have been mentioned to be that the practitioner needs to place 22 electrodes on the scalp for each training session that is both time consuming and costly. Accuracy in determining when to change a protocol is needed.

Following page are LORETA/sLORETA Regions of Interest (ROI's).

LORETA/sLORETA Regions of Interest (ROI's)

- Frontal Lobe
- Limbic Lobe
- Occipital Lobe
- Parietal Lobe
- Sub-lobar
- Inferior temporal gyrus
- Insula
- Lingual gyrus
- Rectal gyrus
- Sub-gyral region
- Subcallosal gyrus
- Superior frontal gyrus
- Superior occipital gyrus
- Superior parietal lobule
- Temporal Lobe
- Angular Gyrus
- Anterior cingulate
- Cingulate gyrus
- Cuneus
- Medial frontal gyrus
- Middle frontal gyrus
- Supramarginal gyrus
- Transverse temporal gyrus
- Middle occipital gyrus
- Middle temporal gyrus
- Orbital gyrus
- Superior temporal gyrus
- Extra-nuclear
- Fusiform gyrus
- Inferior frontal gyrus
- Inferior occipital gyrus
- Inferior parietal lobule
- Paracentral lobule
- Parahippocampal gyrus
- Postcentral gyrus
- Posterior cingulate
- Precentral gyrus
- Precuneus
- Uncus
- Brodmann areas 1–11, 13, 17–25, 27–47

5.4 Live Z-score Feedback (PZOK and PZOKUL)

In 2004, the main role players, Bill Mrklas and Tom Collura, of BrainMaster Technologies Incorporated, designed software that made it possible to provide feedback on EEG activity relative to a standard mean. The development of this approach did not only change the potential applications of neurofeedback, but also challenged what was believed to be core principles of the dynamics of brain activity. The use of Z-scores implements the concept of a normal distribution. Any measurement can be transformed to a Z-score when compared to a normal distribution of a particular population. A Z-score is a measure of the distance from a target value which is taken from a population, Collura (2014).

Thatcher described how an EEG database could be used to derive target values and applied in real time (Thatcher, 2008; Collura, 2014, p.46). The implementation of Z-scores could only happen when computers became competent enough. The first practical training in the implementation of Z-scores in neurofeedback occurred in 2008 by Collura (Collura, 2008).

The conceptual model of providing feedback in relation to a linear model that implies an increase or decrease in amplitude was not sufficient to provide multi- dimensional feedback which is required by the Z-score based feedback. PZOK was then developed which is a different and unique approach to neurofeedback. PZOK is an acronym for the percentage of Z-scores which are okay. "Okay" refers to within the standard deviation parameters that have been specified in the protocol set up. There are, according to Gracefire's (2017) explanation of this paradigm, three points of reference instead of two as is the case with amplitude training, namely the upper standard deviation threshold, the mean itself and the lower standard deviation threshold. The fact that there are more dimensions involved, implies that the information fed back to the brain in terms of every Z-score (which represents an element of brain engagement) is much more complex than the feedback provided to the brain about its own functioning in amplitude training. The brain does no longer with this new paradigm receive information pertaining to the increase and decrease in amplitudes of specified frequency bands only. It also receives information about the absolute power of all the frequency bands, the relative power scores of all the frequency bands as well as feedback on three connectivity measures, namely, phase, coherence, and asymmetry in terms of a standardized mean. The standardized mean for each score is based on an age and gender appropriate normative database.

Initially with the PZOK program, clinicians had to only change one command key to have the parameters expand away from the central mean which makes it easier for the brain to have more scores within the set parameters or another command key to bring both the upper and lower parameters closer to the central mean. The clinician would make these decisions based on the percentage of Z-scores the individual's brain manages to get within the parameters.

Mark Smith requested that the program would be adjusted to incorporate the separate control of the upper and lower parameters, which resulted in the "PZOKUL" feature of live Z-score training.

A protocol used very often for inattention with hyperactivity, is F3-F4-C3- C4 which is probably one of the protocols that was used most often at the beginning of live Z-score training and is still very popular for clients with profiles of connectivity irregularities. The connectivity fibers between the homologous sites is targeted as well as the executive function network between the frontal and parietal areas, which according to Gracefire (2017) plays a very important role in the determination of cortical resourcing strategies.

Gracefire (2017) stresses the importance of treating the individual instead of treating the map, which many neurofeedback practitioners probably set out to do initially. It can be so overwhelming to get to grips with the sophisticated software that is constantly evolving, that it may seem daunting. The main focus, despite all the changes in available aids, needs to be on the intent to address the client's discomfort.

It is also so important that the neurofeedback practitioner will remember that not all measures that are deviant from the mean are problematic. Careful tracking of symptoms remains crucially important. I always remind myself that despite the thousands of components of brain activity that are being measured in multiple channel training and the involved calculations involved in comparing all of those markers in a statistically sound manner to the mean of a very elaborate and valid database, there are still more components to the functioning of the individual that we are not measuring and that the individual is not a statistic.

According to Gracefire (2017), PZOK does not train the brain to be normal. It provides information to its own functioning in terms of numerous parameters across a spectrum of variables so that the brain can ascertain if there are ways that it can develop more efficient and flexible cortical activation patterns. PZOK training assists the individual brain in identifying areas "within its operational strategies where poor integration and connectivity between regions are effecting the efficient modulation of cortical activity and the allocation of resources."

5.5 Four Channel Assessment and Training Positions

The purpose of this section is to provide the reader with examples of protocols that have been proven to render positive clinical outcomes and also to give an indication of different approaches followed by different experienced neurofeedback practitioners. Although most protocols are QEEG guided, neurofeedback practitioners generally appreciate information on trusted protocols. Oftentimes, a specific protocol offers insight into a particular practitioner's way of thinking that broadens the perspective of the practitioner when learning about it. It is also significant to witness how the same protocol can be effective for different disorders. In the section on case studies, the reader will be provided with more case studies by experienced South African practitioners.

In his book, *Technical Foundations of Neurofeedback* (2014), Collura mentions that the mini-Q is an approach that could bridge the gap between single and nineteen channel assessments and training. By combining sites related to particular functions, particular sets of brain functions can be targeted. Collura provides eight, what he refers to as Mini-Q Positions. The functional interpretation of these positions is based on the work of Walker et al. (2007).

Position	Electrode Placement	Function
Position 1	Fz, Cz, T3, T4	Motor planning of lower extremities, sensorimotor integration, logical and. emotional memory. Secondary functions: phonological processing, hearing, ambulation.
Position 2	F3, F4, O1, O2	Motor planning of upper extremities, motor actions, visual processing. Secondary functions include fine motor coordination, mood elevation, pattern recognition, visual sensations and perception.
Position 3	C3, C4, F7, F8	Sensorimotor integration, verbal, and emotional expression, motor actions of the upper extremities, visual sensations, verbal/ sensorimotor integration, verbal, and emotional expressions. Secondary functions include alerting and calming responses, handwriting, drawing and mood regulation.

Position 4	P3, P4, T5, T6	Perception, cognitive processing, spatial relations, logical and emotional understanding, memory, perceptions. Secondary functions include spatial relations, calculations, and multimodal interactions, recognition of words and faces and auditory processing.
Position 5	Fp1, Fp2, Pz, Oz	Logical and emotional attention, perception, visual processing. Secondary functions include planning, decision-making, task completion, sense of self, self-control and route finding.
Position 5a	T3, T4, Pz, Oz	Logical and emotional memory formation and storage, perception, visual processing. Secondary functions include phonological processing, hearing, spatial relations, and visual sensation.
Position 6	O1, O2, C3, C4	Visual sensory processing and sensorimotor integration of the upper extremities. Secondary functions include pattern recognition, perception of color, movement, black/white, edges, alerting and calming responses, handwriting and logical and emotional memory and perception.
Position 7	F7, F8, F3, F4	Verbal and emotional expression, motor planning of the upper extremities, motor actions. Secondary functions include speech fluency, mood regulation and fine motor coordination.
Position 8	T5, T6, Fz, Cz	Logical and emotional understanding, memory, motor planning of the lower extremities and sensorimotor integration. Secondary functions include word recognition, auditory processing, recognition of faces and symbols, running, walking, kicking and ambulation

According to Joseph Guan (2017), Z-score training is a scientifically validated approach that makes training of connectivity much more accurate. He suggests the reading of the white paper compiled by Tom Collura and Robert Thatcher (2006), entitled "Real-Time EEG Z-score Training-

Realities and Prospects" for an in-depth understanding of the process. The following QEEG guided 4 Channel PZOK training protocols, were used by Guan (2017) in six case studies to demonstrate the efficacy of Z-score training.

The first case study is of a 5-year-old boy with a diagnosis of **Pervasive Developmental Delay.** His mother reported that her son had made tremendous progress since the onset of treatment in 2009.

The following protocols were used:

T3, T4, C3, C4	(5 Sessions)
T3, T4, Fp2, P4	(5 Sessions)
T3, T4, Fp1, Fp2	(5 Sessions)
T3, T4, F7, F8	(5 Sessions)
F7, F8, C3, C4	(5 Sessions)
T3, F7, P3, P4	(5 Sessions)
T3, T4, F3, F4	(5 Sessions)
T3, T4, P3, P4	(5 Sessions)
T3, T4, T5, T6	(5 Sessions)
T3, T4, O1, O2	(5 Sessions)
T3, T4, Cz, Fz	(5 Sessions)

The following training protocols were used on a sixty-four-year-old woman suffering **vertigo.** These protocols are from another case study by Joseph Guan (2017).

4 channel Z-score T3, T4, C3, C4	(12 sessions)
	(number of sessions not specified)

After the twelve 4 channel sessions, the incidence of the vertigo episodes was zero.

Guan (2017) also treated a seventy-seventy-year-old woman with a diagnosis of **Dementia**, without a QEEG assessment due to her resistance to wearing a cap. The following training protocols were deployed:

T3, T4, T5, T6	(20 sessions)
T3, T4, F3, F4	(20 sessions)

Significant improvement of short term memory and dissipation of depressive symptoms were reported.

A sixty-six-year-old male patient with a diagnosis of **Parkinson,** experienced significant improvement in flexibility and speech after thirty sessions of Z-score training by Guan (2017) using the following protocols:

T3, T4, C3, C4
C3, C4, F3, F4

The following QEEG guided 4channel Z-score training protocols were used on a twenty-six-year-old female patient with a diagnosis of **Bipolar Disorder.** At the onset of the neurofeedback training with Dr. Guan she was taking four different medications and was at the time of his writing a chapter in the book entitled *Handbook of Clinical QEEG and Neurotherapy* by Collura and Frederick (2017), using one medication and had healthy goals for the future. Improvements in the post QEEG were significant mainly regarding the reduction of the excess of slow brainwave activity globally. The training protocols were the following:

T3, T4, C3, C4
T3, T4, F3, F4
T3, T4, Fp2, P4

Another case study by Dr. Guan referred to in the same chapter, involves the treatment of an **Autistic** boy with Z-score training. He had severe speech and comprehension delays. It was not possible to do a pre- treatment assessment due to the fact that he was hyper-kinetic. The following protocols were used:

T3, T4, C3, C4	(5 sessions)
T3, T4, F7, F8	(number not specified)
19 Channel Z-score	(10 sessions)

The boy, had by the time of publication, started speaking in full sentences and started having conversations with his peers and parents.

According to Gracefire (2017), that which underlies the clinical success of PZOK-training is "that each brain is its own best advocate when it comes to self- regulation and repair". When, according to Gracefire (2017), a neural system has been seriously compromised by injury or disease, it may need, what she refers to as an 'extra nudge' . For this reason Z-plus was designed to offer two more options to enhance the potential of PZOK.

PZMO is a system by which the same central mean is used as a reference as is the case with PZOK. The function of the added feature is to keep track only on the variables that fall outside of the PZOK range. Those variables are the only ones for which feedback is provided. Whereas PZOK is keeping track of and providing feedback for the Z-scores inside of the set parameters of for instance −1,8 to +1,8, PZMO focusses on the Z-scores outside of those parameters. It focuses, in other words, on the outliers. This feature encourages the outlier Z-scores to become flexible.

PZME also focuses on the Z-scores outside of the set parameters. This feature also thus encourages the outlier Z-scores to become more adaptable and to move closer to the mean score. It differs from PZMO in that it is not referenced to the same mean score that PZOK and PZMO use. A running average of the outliers is averaged in real-time and that averaged score is used as the reference. When this secondary separate mean reduces, feedback is provided. The outliers (representing the poorly integrated aspects of the brain activity) are thus strongly encouraged to shift. Both PZMO and PZME are focused on the outlier Z-scores by different calculations.

5.6 19Channel PZOK and 9Channel PZOK

In 2008, BrainMaster developed 19Channel PZOK training software and the Discovery 24 EEG amplifier was released. Most clinicians were still busy coming to terms with and gaining confidence in the application of four channel training.

The idea of placing 22 electrodes on the scalp of an individual for each training session and the attempts at comprehending the effects of the overwhelming amount of information that is fed back to the brain, had many clinicians feel unease and apprehensive and unwilling to embark on this daunting journey before enough evidence was available on an intermediate step of 9Channel training.

Rutter explored the idea of determining clinical improvements of 9 Channel training with a group of 30 adults that presented with a mixture of depression and anxiety symptoms based on the Beck Depression Inventory and the Beck Anxiety Inventory. The ten candidates with the highest scores were chosen to continue.

The same protocol was used for the participants to the study irrespective of the QEEG findings. The following nine channels were chosen: F3, Fz, F4, C3, CZ, C4, P3, Pz and P4. The ten candidates received five sessions of 9 Channel PZOK training at a frequency of one per week. During week six, a follow-up QEEG was done. The temporal and occipital areas were excluded to minimize possible complications with the occipital and temporal regulatory systems that might imply the necessity of follow-up sessions. F3, F4, P3, P4 had previously provided enough anecdotal evidence to imply global clinical improvements, possibly owing to improved quadric cortical integration and "the brain creating an interactional matrix of both inter- and intra-hemispheric coordination" (Gracefire, 2017).

Out of the ten candidates, seven completed the process. Modest to average positive changes were noted in symptoms, BAI and BDI scores, and in QEEG data. Another finding from this short study was that clients who are less open and compliant to recommendations regarding exercise, nutrition, hydration and other lifestyle changes, experience slower rates of improvement.

Any number of targeted Z-scores can be included in the protocol design in Z-score training. The entire brain can be included. Any number of channels from two channels to nineteen channels can be included.

19 Channel training and 19 Channel PZOK training has since become a popular training option. According to Gracefire (2017), positive clinical outcomes and improvement in function often results from even a very elementary application of 19 Channel PZOK without any customization using a pre-structured normative reference. In more complicated cases the Z-builder option can be explored which offers the function of doing a statistical analysis of the individual EEG recording and then generating a Z-score baseline to be used as a point of reference. This option of recording a status quo can possibly be meaningful in cases of brain injury and chemotherapy. The person may want their brain function restored to where they were at prior to injury or incident. Most clinicians however prefer to do training relative to a standard population mean.

It appears that it is sometimes better to provide global feedback to the brain for the brain to be able to determine its own strategy to improve regulation. Best the practitioner bear in mind that the information fed back to the brain can be very overwhelming and that treatment periods be increased in little increments. The number of variables that the brain processes during 19 channel training is approximately 5700.

The LORETA algorithm, as discussed earlier in this section, has provided significant contributions to the field of research and also as a diagnostic tool because of the advanced imaging capabilities. The imaging resolution of the current sLORETA is 300% better than the imaging of the original LORETA. sLORETA added an invaluable dimension to PZOK training. For more information on sLORETA training options and clinical outcomes, refer to the section LORETA and sLORETA neurofeedback in this chapter.

5.7 ISF (Infra-Slow Fluctuation) Neurofeedback or ILF (Infra-Low Frequency) Neurofeedback

The author has received basic didactic training in the ILF paradigm of neurofeedback training, and she has limited experience in this paradigm.

In a chapter by Smith, Leiderman and de Vries in *Handbook of Clinical QEEG and Neurotherapy* (Collura & Frederick, 2017), Infra-Slow Fluctuation (ISF) is described as a paradigm or a form of neurofeedback training that focuses on the slowest frequencies or oscillations in the human cortex. This paradigm is to be distinguished from SCP (Slow Cortical Potential) which is addressed in the Alternating Current (AC) domain. Direct Current (DC) is necessary for accurate recording and training of ISF. Although there are, according to Smith (n.d.), correlations between SCP and ILF (Infra-Low Frequency) training, the clinical effects are very different.

Aladjalova (1957) indicated that the infra-slow band increased in amplitude when subjects were exposed to stress provoking stimuli. The theory then was that the parasympathetic, reparative response of the hypothalamus was reflected by the increase in amplitude of the infra-slow band. The implication of this research is that the efficacy of ISF neurofeedback may be based on the impact this paradigm has on the ANS (autonomic nervous system).

Research has established that the success of ILF is probably related to its effect on the hypothalamus. The hypothalamus plays an important role in emotional regulation. It is the control center for many autonomic functions of the peripheral nervous system, (Smith, n.d.). Hypothalamic hormones control pituitary hormone release which influences and manages adrenal secretion of epinephrine and neuro- epinephrine which in turn influence the sympathetic nervous system response. The HPA (Hypothalamic/ Pituitary/ Adrenal) axis has feedback loops that promote parasympathetic nervous system response.

These low frequencies of lower than 1 Hz have been proven to be associated with the coordination of neuronal network communication. Networks that regulate social, emotional, and sensory processing are involved. According to Liu et al. (2010), homologous regions are coordinated by coherent fast and ultra-slow rhythmic activity. The infra-low activity influences the excitability of the higher frequencies, according to Smith (n.d.). According to Monto et al. (2008), human behavioral performance is correlated with the infra-low fluctuations in ongoing brain activity. Broyd et al. (2011) determined that with the ADHD population, deactivations of the ILF signal does not occur in the Default Mode areas of the cortex which implies that they get "stuck" in self-referential processing. They are unable to turn off networks in the cortex when appropriate.

Latest technology, including amplifiers that are DC-coupled, simplify ISF training signals representing oscillations lower than 1 Hz and can be trained with little or no noise in the signal.

According to Smith et al. (2017), ISF training "turns on the selection of an Optimum Frequency" for each individual. The frequency is determined by identifying an autonomic response to the training during the session. Peripheral measures of autonomic function including heart rate variability, skin conductance and finger temperature are monitored and the client is observed very closely for any signs of a state shift. These signs guide the therapist to identify a state of autonomic balance for the client. The goal of the training is to train the client towards a state of optimal relaxation and simultaneous alertness.

Some of the common reactions to ISF training are, according to Mark Smith, improved autonomic functioning, reduction in pain, improved attention, and a tranquil state of mind. In the treatment of autism, research has shown improvements in the networks associated with the sense of self, productive language, sensory processing, and social behavior (Smith et al., 2017). Reduction in anxiety and improved affect regulation are also common clinical outcomes for the ASD population after ISF training. The networks mentioned above demonstrate improved information sharing in the post treatment QEEG's of the same population.

In ILF training, a bipolar placement of the electrodes is typically used and usually includes one of the temporal lobes. The other placement can be on any of the 10–20 placement areas based on the client's symptoms pertaining to arousal and attention. Theoretically, according to Smith (n. d.), brain areas that are linked in chronic automatic stress are being differentiated electrically. The non- temporal area is differentiated from the HPA distress signal.

According to Mark Smith (n. d.), although immediate results may be evident with ISF, it is important to remember that many repetitions are necessary for the new behavior to become learned behavior based on the principles of operant conditioning.

5.8 Alpha-Theta Training

Alpha-theta training involves accessing deep states and this training paradigm does have some correlation with hypnotherapy although the deeper state that the person enters is induced by the neurofeedback equipment and the particular protocol. Before I discuss the history of this training paradigm and describe the process, it is necessary to spend some time on emphasizing the importance of the environment regarding the general ambiance of the therapy room and of the importance of the neutral, calm, quiet and confident presence the therapist ought to aspire to having in order to allow the potential of this powerful process to be actualized.

The role of the therapist is central to the success of all the training paradigms we have discussed and influences the outcome of therapy in ways that we will never be able to establish accurately. In deep-state training, I believe this factor that the therapist brings to the process to be even bigger.

The alpha-theta paradigm of neurofeedback training is not, to my knowledge, applied by many neurofeedback practitioners. I base this assumption on the number of neurofeedback practitioners that use this modality in South Africa. It is a powerful and suitable aid to those therapists interested in deep-state training. This training paradigm is usually attractive to therapists that have an interest in meditation practices and possibly spiritual matters. I regard visualization exercises to be an important component of alpha-theta work but accept that not all neurofeedback practitioners necessarily feel comfortable with it.

The setting for alpha-theta work is important. A general office environment where there are usually many activities happening in the background, including ringing phones, people moving in and out of offices and traffic noise also being part of the cacophony of sounds, is not suited for deep-state work. In the general office environment there is mostly also a demand on all our other senses as well in the form of fluorescent lights, the smell of coffee and perhaps a chair that is not completely comfortable.

A chair that can be set to recline is necessary. But some chairs that have the recline function are pretty uncomfortable and leave one hanging in limbo with dangling feet. I would suggest that the chair should be tested for comfort. When you lean back in the chair you should be able to feel safe, supported, and relaxed. The training environment ought to be relatively sound proof, with soft pleasant lighting. Create an ambience in which you would feel safe and calm. During my alpha-theta training sessions, I unplug phones and make arrangements that nobody will walk past the office during the session and that should the next client arrive early, that they would wait outside. Soft, neutral, pleasant music in the background can contribute positively to the ambience and block out any invasive sounds.

At the risk of stating the obvious, advise your client to use the bathroom prior to the session. Also advise your client to arrive early so that he/she will not be flustered or unsettled on arrival. It would probably not be a good idea to have a heavy meal prior to the session that may cause discomfort when leaning back but it would not be advisable to arrive hungry either. That all basic needs ought to have been met in moderation prior to the session is possibly a good guideline to use.

One of the common applications of the alpha-theta training paradigm is for addiction. Take additional caution in advising strongly against the use of any addictive substance or any stimulant such as coffee twelve to preferably twenty- four hours prior to the training session.

I would like to share an incident that occurred during one of my first alpha-theta training sessions to illustrate a point. It was roughly 15 years ago. The access that the few of us – that had received the basic training in alpha-theta training- had to mentoring programs and clinical support groups was very limited at the time. We were pretty much dependent on our own diligence in terms of research and a good measure of courage.

I was very excited about the potential of this training method and had an ideal first client. He had responded very well to twenty sessions of SMR training on C4 and was no longer plagued by unexpected bouts of anxiety associated with a pounding heart with accompanying profuse sweating during his waking hours. He did still, however, wake up startled with a pounding heart somewhere between two and three o'clock in the mornings. I had spoken to him about alpha-theta training at length and provided him with reading matter. We had done some work on diaphragmatic breathing, some basic meditation techniques, and other relaxation exercises. The scene was set and the time was right. I took some time to prepare myself in terms of my own state of mind before the session. I took heed of the warning of the client's extreme suggestibility and openness during these training sessions, especially during the state that is referred to as a "crossover". I calmly explained the process once more while I was preparing the scalp for the electrode placements, explained what the feedback sounds would sound like and reminded the client to just trust and allow the process without attempting to achieve anything. I explained briefly and calmly the process of going beyond the mind and surrendering while exchanging control for just being.

The background music was phased out and the feedback sounds were phased in. I was sitting quietly and neutrally watching the feedback screen and the client as he became more and more relaxed. The alpha amplitude was high enough and indicated a calm resting state and then there before my eyes the cross over between the alpha and theta amplitudes happened beautifully when the alpha amplitude dropped significantly. The 15–30 Hz activity was very low. My client was officially in a crossover state and theoretically in an optimal problem solving mode from which state the brain could process whatever it was ready for to process in terms of suppressed memories that might have caused the daily startle response or whatever other layers of unresolved issues may surface. I have still not lost that feeling of awe when witnessing transformational processes in people.

And then he started snoring! Now that you did not see coming! As his snoring grew louder, my anxiety levels went higher. I remembered something about a suggestion I had read about changing the beta inhibit to a delta inhibit after cross over to prevent a sleep state. I fumbled and doubted and reasoned and suddenly saw his beta amplitude rising quite drastically and his theta amplitude dropping significantly. I realized what was happening – he was picking up on my unsettled state. I took control of it and owing to years and years of intensive meditation practice, and diaphragmatic breathing, I went into a quieter state of mind. I could read my own inner state on the client's feedback screen – there was a direct and immediate correlation. I will never forget that experience. We know these things in theory. The importance of the openness of the person in the hypnogogic state when theta amplitude is higher than alpha in the eyes closed condition is clear to us; we know how tuned in to the intuitive mind we become when we transcend the rational mind; we know there is so much beyond the rational realm that the mind can perceive of, but we need to remind ourselves of the sensitivity and the susceptibility of the human mind when we endeavor to explore this training paradigm.

The therapist that does not have that innate sense of respect, awe and appreciation for the sensitivity and vulnerability of the human spirit that may perhaps abide somewhere in the realms that our rational mind cannot access, would possibly prefer to remain on more solid and predictable ground where reason governs. It is very healthy, necessary, and balanced I believe that we are wired differently (how appropriate!) and that we have different interests and strengths. I believe that it is of paramount importance especially for therapists, to be able to define those qualities so as to be able to apply ourselves optimally to the different aspects of the service we have chosen.

Relaxation training is often incorporated with neurofeedback training. Those clients that we consider for alpha-theta training in particular, will generally benefit much from relaxation training. Autogenic training, as proposed by

Jacobson (1938), is a progressive relaxation technique that includes imagery of warmth, heaviness and the visualization of pleasant tranquil situations. It is still being taught and applied by many neurofeedback practitioners and therapists from other disciplines. Procedures involving biofeedback modalities that involve procedures beyond progressive relaxation and the underlying physiological processes involved, will consequently be discussed in the following section.

The basic underlying principles of alpha-theta training are not new. The report on Peniston's success with the treatment of alcoholics in the early 1990s was a main event in drawing attention to and interest in the training protocol that included a neurofeedback component. Peniston, according to White (1999), used a protocol including temperature training, imagery, and neurofeedback.

The goal was to increase slow brain wave activity. What is relatively new about the process is the human-machine interface. The deep relaxation state that is brought about by the alpha-theta training protocol is the same state aimed at in the relaxation psychotherapy technique used in the 60's. Tom Budzynski describes the importance of the theta state in relation to the importance of being able to rescript suggestions whilst the client is in a state of consciousness in which he does not have the ability to resist the re-scripting suggestions. Hypnotherapy focuses on this shift in state of consciousness that occurs. The stages of the relaxation technique taught to psychiatry interns in the 1960's are basically the same stages of the protocol used by Peniston to treat alcoholics (Peniston & Kulkosky, 1989, 1990). We now have the understanding that these different stages are related to specific dominant frequencies of brain wave activity which was not the inherent understanding of the techniques when taught to the psychiatry interns.

Meditators that have pursued mind states of inner focus, or contentment, have been accessing what we know as the alpha state and the theta state for centuries. "Sidi Consciousness", a state of optimal problem solving ability where there is no perception of time delay between the problem and the solution, can be compared with the concept of "Buddhahood" which refers to states of consciousness that take us beyond the limitations of our sensory perceptions. We have now brought modern technology to measure and induce mind states that the human race has probably ensued since the beginning of human history from different angles involving different rituals and practices. We probably have an insatiable need to go beyond the restrictions of the rational mind to find peace and access insights.

A main difference between hypnotherapy and alpha-theta therapy is that during hypnotherapy, the hypnotherapist gives certain suggestions while the patient is in a hypnogogic state, whereas the neurotherapist does not talk when the client is in the crossover state. (Some neurofeedback practitioners who are also psychotherapists do, however, work with imagery and suggestions during the crossover state). It is suggested that one works with scripts and visualizations that the client provides. These scripts are compiled beforehand and can include descriptions of goals the person wishes to achieve, a description of the "ideal me" with associated sensory perceptions. Anticipated reactions of others to this ideal image of the person as well as detail about the environment of this ideal state can be included in the description. Such a description and setting of goals can be done with the help of a psychotherapist if the neurofeedback practitioner is not a psychologist. This description can be read to the client by the neurofeedback practitioner during the preparation for the session that it may be visualized and focused on in the conscious mind for as long as rational thoughts remain present prior to the crossover state. The neurofeedback practitioner can gently and quietly remind the client that the mind has the ability to address the relevant issues as it sees appropriate.

The client ought to be well prepared and briefed prior to the onset of alpha-theta training. Alpha-theta training is not indicated for all clients despite the fact that there is research available on the improved integration of newly taught skills during open eyes amplitude training of ADHD sufferers when the treatment is concluded with a few alpha-theta closed eyes training sessions.

Reading matter, including research studies showing positive clinical outcomes of alpha-theta training in the treatment of what is appropriate to the client, may be presented. Discussions on expected outcomes as well as on the different applications of alpha-theta training will be appropriate. Some clients have a clear desire to take their training to the next level with alpha- theta training and others do not. The person's intuitive sensing of the possible outcomes for themselves has been found to be fairly reliable. It is important that the client that wishes to embark on the alpha- theta training journey will feel very comfortable with the process.

The client must be quite capable of implementing progressive relaxation techniques that have been practiced during open eyes amplitude training or Z-score training sessions. It is probably advisable to have completed a minimum of ten open eyes training sessions with clear improvement in overall regulation, before alpha-training is considered.

The client ought to have clear goals for the alpha-theta training program.

Some clients wish to attain personal or spiritual growth whereas the focus for others are more on the relief of discomfort associated with addiction, depression, grief, or PTSD. Alpha-theta training is also used successfully for mental and physical peak performance as well as for deep relaxation. Although there are studies available on positive outcomes for depressive clients, I have found, in my experience, that an alternating approach in which an alpha-theta training session is followed by a fast brain wave open eyes amplitude training session, has a better outcome for clients suffering depression. An approach during which the alpha-theta training session is concluded with a three minute beta training session has also been indicated to have positive outcomes.

At the beginning of the session the neurofeedback practitioner should ensure that the client is comfortable and relaxed. The client will at the onset of the alpha- theta training already be skilled in certain relaxation techniques that will possibly include some biofeedback training in respiration, synchrony between pulse rate and respiration, peripheral skin temperature, skin conductance and muscle tension which will be discussed briefly in the next section of this chapter. If the neurofeedback practitioner is not skilled in other biofeedback modalities, other relaxation and breathing exercises need to be implemented to enable the client to lower his arousal level and be relatively calm.

With the assistance of the neurofeedback practitioner the client will now proceed to visualize a relaxing, calm, and safe place. If the neurofeedback practitioner provides a description of such a place it is important to ensure that there is nothing in that scene with which the client has a negative association. I generally ask the client if he/she would want to provide me with a description of an idyllic scene beforehand or to list what he/she would want to have present in such a scene which I will then include in a description. Some people would want to be in a forest and have their favorite dog with them; some would prefer to be on a sunset beach while others would want to be in a crystal cave with their children's photos present. It happens often that a client will choose your office as the safe and calm place that you need to describe while they are doing the visualization. I am of the opinion that it is important to spend enough time on finding an ideal scene beforehand. Your experience as the therapist, while you are describing the peaceful, safe scene will determine whether the client will be able to engage with the visualization and relax or not. It is advisable for the therapist to do a meditation or relaxation exercise of sorts prior to the session so that he/she will be able to project the state of calm he/ she wishes to induce.

When the person is completely relaxed, leaning back in the chair in a totally comfortable position, with their eyes closed, the therapist reminds the client of the nature of the sounds he/she will be hearing and encourages him/her once again to just allow and trust the process. Personally I then add that the client may want to allow any thoughts or stumbling blocks or images that arise spontaneously, to surface without questioning or resisting or consciously engaging with any thoughts or images. The mind state could possibly be described as a state of witnessing awareness without judgement. The text that the client has compiled pertaining to the ideal self may then be briefly alluded to or read through in a very calm and quiet voice. At this point the client is already in a very relaxed and more susceptible state. Great caution has to be taken to honor the goals of the client and to be mindful of the dynamics of countertransference and other relevant mechanisms of defense that may be in play.

Personally I inform the client that I will not be talking at all for the following twenty-seven minutes at which point I will then indicate that there are three minutes remaining, so that the mind has the opportunity to conclude whatever processes it may be busy with. There are however different approaches. According to the Peniston protocol, guided imagery is added whilst in the crossover state. Some psychotherapists add instructions that the person is to imagine himself/ herself performing a task or being in an environment associated with something he/she may most want to change. The client is then requested to visualize changes according to a desired outcome including detailed positive reactions of loved ones and other potentially positive reinforcers.

At the end of the training session, it is advisable to phase the feedback sound out gently and phase in background music if you wish. If one uses the same music that served as background music to create the ambiance at the beginning of the session, it assists the client with re-orientating himself/ herself when he/ she comes out of the deep state. The client is then guided towards re-orienting himself/herself to his/her current environment in terms of becoming aware of his/ her body in the chair, the surrounding sounds, and any other sensations. He/she should then open his/her eyes and when the chair is changed to a sitting position, remain sitting quietly for a while. Depending on the need or the preference of the client, the practitioner will then either discuss the graph representing the session followed by a discussion of the experience the client had or in the reversed order. The way in which the experience of the session as well as the dreams and memories that come to the fore in the days that follow the training session are processed, will differ from therapist to therapist depending on the training and experience of the therapist.

Generally in alpha-theta training, the potential of the mind to process unresolved issues and also to integrate processes previously addressed in other therapies, are activated.

The added benefit the psychotherapist has of working with guided imagery with the client whilst in the crossover state as opposed to the psychotherapist working with a client in a hypnagogic state induced without the use of technology, is that brain activity related responses can be carefully monitored.

When the neurofeedback practitioner is not a registered psychotherapist or hypnotherapist they may want to work closely with such a therapist and recommend to the client that the issues that surface in dreams and conscious content during the process of the alpha-theta training, be addressed in a talk therapy.

5.8.1 Underlying Principles and Hook-up Options

The therapeutic principle underlying alpha-theta training is that during the deep state that one enters into when the theta amplitude is higher than (crosses over) the alpha amplitude in the occipital and parietal region in an eyes closed condition, content rises to the conscious mind that can be processed in the crossover state. This state has been referred to as an "optimal problem solving mode". One would ordinarily fall into sleep when the crossover occurs (as I witnessed because of the fact that I had failed to inhibit delta to prevent sleep) but during alpha-theta training, sufficient alertness is retained to prevent falling asleep which potentially results in the processing of the material that surfaces.

Alpha brain wave activity represents a bridge between internal and external attention. Theta, according to the Thompsons (2015), is a bridge between wakefulness and sleep. Both alpha and theta states are also involved in and are important to processes involving memory and reflection.

A crossover state is a state that one enters into when the high alpha amplitude associated with an eyes closed condition and a resting state, loses power and the theta amplitude gains power to the extent that the theta amplitude becomes higher than the alpha amplitude. When a person hovers in a crossover state while his/her eyes are closed he/she is capable of recovering memories, perceiving emotions associated with memories and gaining insights. The person's ability to think creatively is also said to improve. It is theorized that some childhood memories may actually be embedded in the theta bandwidth because theta is the dominant frequency between ages two and six during which time the child is generally very connected to his internal world. During this time, the child still mainly lives in a world of imagination and does generally not show signs of critical analytical thinking. This state is also referred to as a super learning state and the child is likely to accept whatever he/she is told. A person in this state is very open to suggestion. It is thus very important that the therapist will have the utmost respect for this state.

The placement of the active electrode was originally suggested by Peniston to be on O1. He did a linked ear reference and placed the ground electrode on the forehead. The placement on O1 causes practical complications. When the client is in a reclined position, electrode movement is likely.

A bipolar placement with one channel, training on Fz and T3 also holds merit according to Julian Isaacs (n. d.) but has mostly been abandoned for a two channel placement at Fz and T3.

The above protocols became less popular after a research study involving music students at the Royal Conservatoire in London involving a one channel training protocol with the active electrode placed on Pz (Gruzelier & Egner, 2004). The results showed statistically significant improvement in the emotional interpretation of the music.

A protocol that is still, to the best of the author's knowledge, used often is based on the abovementioned study. The active electrode is placed at Pz with a reference on one ear or mastoid and a ground electrode on the other ear or mastoid. Two enhance bands are set at 5–8 Hz and 8–11 Hz. An inhibit band is set to 15–30 Hz, which is changed to 2–5 Hz when the client reaches the crossover state or two inhibit bands are set simultaneously if the equipment has the capability. With three bands the thresholds are often set at 25%, 50%, 15%.

The feedback sounds are different to the typical sounds heard with open eyes training paradigms. The pitch of the two signals that represent alpha and theta respectively blend well in most systems and are proportional to the amplitude of the two respective amplitudes. The reward sound for alpha is generally at a higher pitch than the reward sound for theta. It is important that the sounds will be perceived as pleasant. The volume ought to be controlled at levels that the therapist senses as being appropriate and not too invasive.

Chapter **6**

Physiological
Responses
to Stress
and Tension

This chapter will provide a brief overview of the Autonomic Nervous System (ANS) and physiological responses to stress and tension in as far as these components pertain to neurofeedback and biofeedback measurements.

The author has limited theoretical knowledge only (as required by the BCIA Blueprint of Knowledge) of the measurement of Heart Rate, Respiration, Electro Dermal Response (EDR), Electromyography (EMG) Peripheral Skin Temperature and Heart Rate Variability (HRV) used in a stress assessment by biofeedback practitioners. As a neurofeedback practitioner, I use progressive relaxation techniques in combination with neurofeedback without instrumentation as yet. The information provided in this section (with the exclusion of the section on breathing) is based mainly on Thompson and Thompson's *The Neurofeedback Book* (2015). The main purpose of this book is to provide information on EEG Biofeedback and not on the other Biofeedback modalities. The reason for presenting basic information on the other modalities of Biofeedback is to convey the importance of the significance of these modalities and to recognize the validity of the conjuncture of neurofeedback with other modalities of biofeedback. There are excellent books and other sources available on all of the measurements of the autonomic nervous system incorporated in biofeedback training of which a very brief overview is presented in this chapter. This overview is aimed at providing the reader with a broader perspective, and may inspire other neurofeedback practitioners, as it does me, to merge the perspectives and available aids in our joint pursuit of relieving discomfort.

6.1 The Autonomic Nervous System

The autonomic nervous system is that part of the nervous system that it is not under our conscious control. It is responsible for the control of the bodily functions such as respiratory rate, heart rate, pupillary responses, sweat response, digestive processes, the gall bladder, the urinary bladder, the pancreas, the eyes, blood vessels, smooth muscles, the glands, the reproductive system and all body functions that we do not control consciously or with any effort. With biofeedback it is possible, however, to influence the ANS consciously.

The autonomic nervous system is part of the motor system. It comprises of excitatory and inhibitory nerves that are paired. The excitatory nerves are mostly part of the sympathetic system and the inhibitory nerves are mostly part of the parasympathetic system. The sympathetic nervous system is involved in processes that activate and expend energy whereas the parasympathetic nervous system is involved in processes that inhibit and also processes that produce or conserve energy (Thompson & Thompson, 2015). The sympathetic nervous system is responsible for the catabolic state associated with the fight and flight response referred to further on in this chapter, whereas the parasympathetic nervous system is involved in the anabolic state associated with rest and relaxation, also discussed further on.

The cell bodies of the sympathetic nervous system are found in the thoracic and lumber regions of the spinal cord. The axons exit through the ventral roots of the spine. The nerves of the sympathetic nervous system are motor nerves but the fibers do have some sensory nerves from the organs. The main neurotransmitter for the SNS is noradrenaline. The expenditure of energy by the SNS results   in increase in blood pressure and an increase in heart rate as well as glucose metabolism.

The nerves of the parasympathetic nervous system, exit the central nervous system in cranial nerves 3, 7, 9 and 10 and in sacral nerves 2, 3 and 4. The cell bodies of the ganglia are close to the organs they supply as opposed to the SNS with long preganglionic fibers. These nerves too, are motor nerves but do have sensory nerves from some organs. The main neurotransmitter of the PSNS is acetylcholine. The effect of the PSNS can be measured in biofeedback regarding the effect of slowing the heart rate during exhalation.

The PSNS contracts the pupils, stimulates saliva, constricts the airway, slows the heartbeat, stimulates digestion, dilates blood vessels, and stimulates the bladder whereas the SNS does the opposite. The sympathetic system causes the pupils to dilate, salivation to be inhibited, blood vessels to constrict, the airway to be released, digestion to be inhibited, the heart rate to increase, glucose release to be stimulated, adrenalin to be secreted and the bladder to contract.

6.2 An Overview of the Neurophysiology of the Stress Response

The stress response, although probably more essential to the survival of the human race when we needed to fight other clans and wild animals than what it is now, it is still functional. Over and above the fight and flight related responses caused by the SNS mentioned above that may cause a lot of discomfort, the stress response also has a protective function. The release of adrenaline when a person is stressed also promotes blood clotting which prevents extensive bleeding and causes increased blood flow to the brain and large muscle groups which may be necessary in a dangerous situation.

The stress response is designed to be a short lived protective mechanism with the function of improving the chances of survival. During the stress response there is heightened awareness, arousal, and focus. When the stress response becomes chronic, abnormal changes in the system can occur.

The stress response is controlled by interaction along the brain stem in which the locus coeruleus, a nucleus in the pons of the brainstem, plays an important role.

The interaction is along the AHPA-axis which is an acronym for amygdala, the hypothalamus as part of the sympathetic system, pituitary and adrenal. The frontal lobes also have a significant influence through the connections to the amygdala and hypothalamus.

The AHPA system can fail when it is over-stressed. Dysregulation along this axis can result in certain disorders. When the AHPA system is hypoactive it can cause anxiety, fibromyalgia, and chronic pain. The levels of the corticotrophin releasing hormone which has analgesic properties drop due to the hypo-activity of the APHA system which results in increased pain perception. Hyperactivity of the AHPA-axis on the other hand, has been associated with depression. Under section 6.3 chronic pain and the involvement of the central, peripheral, and autonomic nervous systems are discussed.

The normal response to stress involves specific processes. The locus coeruleus in the brain stem is signaled by the thalamus and the amygdala to release norepinephrine. The norepinephrine has the effect of arousing the sympathetic nervous system which results in a heightened awareness of new incoming stimuli. Blood pressure heart rate and sweating increase.

The function of the increased norepinephrine levels is to increase the levels of the adrenocorticotropin hormone released by the hypothalamus which in turn stimulates the adrenal glands to produce glucocorticoids. The cortisol counteracts the effects of the norepinephrine and epinephrine. The glucocorticoids down-regulates the corticotropin releasing hormone which then decreases stimulation of the locus coeruleus in order to decrease the release of norepinephrine. Endogenous opiates which increase pain threshold are also released. The process is one in which homeostasis is reinstated. The central nucleus of the amygdala also stimulates the hypothalamic production of corticotrophin releasing hormone and arginine vasopressin to increase AHPA axis activity. Serotonin also increases the activity of the AHPA-axis.

NE and CRH are involved in the emotional responses to stress including fear, limited affect and stereotypical thinking (Thompson & Thompson, 2015).

When the brain senses that the full stress response is no longer necessary, the activity in the AHPA-axis is dampened by the involvement of the frontal lobes and the hippocampus. The ACTH production reduces and the entire system returns to homeostasis.

When stress becomes chronic, the system does not return to resting state. CRH and NE levels remain very high which eventually decreases serotonin (5 HT) levels which can result in depression and anxiety. The lowered serotonin levels will also decrease the modulating effect of the hippocampus on the AHPA-axis which results in more anxiety which in turn dysregulates the AHPA-axis. The production of CRH will decrease and GC levels will drop. The decreased GC levels will not be able to exercise the modulating effect on the locus coeruleus by reducing the NE production. The lower NE levels results in less adaptive ability to new stressors which manifests in chronic pain disorders and fibromyalgia (Pacak et al., 1995).

Hyperactivity of the AHPA-axis results in chronic pain and is associated with many familiar symptoms often seen with clients and patients seeking psychological or neurofeedback intervention. People with a hyperactive AHPA- axis due to chronic stress display problems with sleep, are plagued by ruminating thoughts (they don't manage to get their thinking brain to rest), they have a narrow perspective, focusing mainly on their own preoccupations and concerns, and their cognitive performance is poor.

When the stress response is not normal and the AHPA-axis is dysregulated, the sleep cycle is affected negatively. The role of GABA is very important in the regulation of the sleep cycle. The influence of GABA gets affected by the dysregulated AHPA- axis. The normal function of GABA in the sleep cycle is that when GABA is activated by the cholinergic pathways from the brain stem to the thalamus and to the forebrain, it decreases the blood flow to the thalamus. It is the shutting down of the thalamus that is responsible for loss of consciousness during sleep. Another function of GABA is to dampen the norepinephrine output of the locus coeruleus. Anxiety, as we have noted, increases NE production. If the NE cannot be reduced, sleep onset will not occur. GABA also has the function of decreasing basal ganglia functions which results in muscle paralysis. Breathing continues despite the muscle paralysis. When there are high anxiety levels, muscle paralysis may occur momentarily but the person will not fall asleep.

AHPA-axis hyperactivity is, as we have seen, associated with insomnia. When a person has chronic stress, chronic pain, or fibromyalgia, he/she will probably also be suffering insomnia.

The immune response is also affected by chronic stress. The immune response is dampened by glucocorticoids and chronic stress increases glucocorticoids. The immune response is suppressed and even the size of the thymus gland may be influenced (Thompson & Thompson, 2015). This will result in a reduction of lymphocytes.

The combination of EEG Biofeedback and other modalities of Biofeedback can assist in improved regulation of responses to stress.

We will now take a look at certain physiological responses to stress that can be measured and influenced. Improved regulation of these markers with biofeedback instrumentation and some relaxation and visualization exercises without the use of technology will be discussed briefly.

6.2.1 Respiration: The Importance of Diaphragmatic Breathing

Mothers tell their children instinctively to breathe slowly and count to ten when a volatile reaction is expected or when it becomes clear that the child is stressed. Most readers will have been witness to the symptoms of a person with an anxiety or panic disorder or will have experienced changes in their own breathing patterns when they become anxious or stressed. All neurofeedback practitioners have knowledge of the importance of breathing correctly. Teaching a client to breathe correctly is not as simple as teaching the diaphragmatic breathing technique. There has to be a basic understanding of underlying physiological processes and knowledge about the potential dangers of over-breathing.

The basics of the physiology and the psychology of breathing ought to be explained to the client (Thompson & Thompson, 2015).

The person that consciously attempts to regulate their breathing to six inhalations per minute ought to feel comfortable and calm. The posture should be relaxed with the palms relaxed on the thighs. When the elbows are rested on the arms of the chairs, the trapezius (a large triangular muscle in the vicinity of the shoulder blades) will be contracted. A short guided meditation or relaxation exercise is advisable to assist the client with letting go of rumination and invasive thoughts.

Measure the number of inhalations per minute before attempting to guide the client toward changing the breathing cycle. Explain the significance of achieving respiratory sinus arrhythmia (RSA) which generally results in a mental and physical relaxed state. When a person breathes diaphragmatically and in a relaxed manner at a rate of six breaths per minute, the heart rate will follow in a sinusoidal pattern. This pattern, according to Basmajian (1989) correlates with the respiration pattern and is referred to as respiratory sinus arrhythmia.

The client then visualizes a balloon in the stomach below the diaphragm and physically places the hand firmly below the diaphragm. The inhalation will push the hand away from the stomach and inflate the balloon. The combination of the physical experience and the visualization makes it easier to correct the habit of shallow breathing. Explain to the client the significance of breathing in to the bottom of the lungs and releasing all the CO_2 with a complete exhalation. The breathing rate is controlled by partial pressure of CO_2 (pCO_2) in the blood stream. The partial pressure of CO_2 will be decreased when all the CO_2 is blown out from the bottom of the lungs. It is thus very important to blow out all the CO_2. When we are under stress our breathing becomes shallow, irregular, and faster. Should the client not feel comfortable with inhaling to the count of four and exhaling to the count of six (which is the end goal of achieving RSA synchrony), a rhythm of three seconds to inhale and four seconds to exhale can be started off with.

It is generally a good idea to do a short initial breathing exercise in your office and request of the client to practice the diaphragmatic breathing exercise for ten minutes every evening. Demos (2005) suggests that the diaphragmatic breathing can be practiced while lying down on one's back with a heavy book below the diaphragm. When one inhales into one's stomach, inflating the balloon in one's stomach, the book moves up and when one exhales, the book moves down. It is important that the client is comfortable and relaxed when doing the breathing exercise. The most difficult part is to break the initial pattern of shallow breathing which causes the chest to move up and down.

People with anxiety generally have high breath rates and forced inspiration that cause the thoracic cavity to expand (Demos, 2005). Rapid breathing can have serious consequences. When carbon dioxide is exhaled faster than what it is produced, it can lead to respiratory alkalosis which causes the blood to become alkaline (increased blood pH). Increased alkalinity from pH 7.4 to pH 7.5 can decrease blood flow by 50%. Alkalosis results in hyper- excitability and a compromise of the blood buffering system which can result in cerebral hypoxia and cerebral glucose deficit (Thompson & Thompson, 2015).

Teaching diaphragmatic breathing can result in hyperventilation. Sixty percent of all ambulance calls, according to Peter Litchfield (n. d.), are a result of over breathing. The therapist and the client ought to be aware of the dynamics of hyperventilation and have at least a basic knowledge of the physiological and chemical processes involved.

Cerebral vasoconstriction due to chemical changes involving carbonic acid and hydrogen occurs. The Bohr-effect is when there is an increased bonding of oxygen to Hemoglobin which results in poor release of oxygen. This has an effect on the release of potassium, calcium and magnesium which causes irritability of nerves and muscles. On a metabolic level, there is an increase in the release of adrenaline and noradrenaline which in turn influences the blood glucose, fatty acids, LDL cholesterol and insulin release. The long-term effect of this dynamic is that it results in coagulation and arteriosclerosis, coronary artery spasms and high blood pressure.

The early signs of the consequences of over breathing are, according to Thompson and Thompson (2015), the following:

- Light headedness
- Tingling skin
- Tightness in the chest
- Sweaty hands
- Breathlessness
- Restless mind
- Memory loss
- Sensory sensitivity (lights seem lighter and sounds appear to be louder)
- Activated startle response
- Muscle twitching

These signs are anxiety provoking and will probably cause an amplified discomfort.

The client will feel fear of losing control.

Over-breathing, according to the Thompsons (2015), can have a negative effect on cognitive skills, decision making skills as well as on concentration and focus skills. It can also affect memory and the ability to initiate tasks negatively. Motor skills can be impaired. Over-breathing can influence the EEG as well and more specifically, result in an immediate increase in theta power. Cerebral vasoconstriction and the decrease in oxygen release by the blood which is caused by over-breathing can have an effect on emotions. The client may feel apprehensive, anxious, fearful, and panicky as a result of over- breathing. It may also result in volatility and precipitate depression.

Other effects include the potential exacerbation of irritable bowel syndrome and asthma. It may also precipitate seizure activity or a migraine attack.

It is emphasized, however, that the clinical outcome of achieving RSA synchrony is very positive. The client will be able to apply this technique effortlessly and almost automatically when the need arises and prevent the anticipated discomfort precipitated by certain situations. Being able to comfortably breathe at a rate of six cycles per minute, generally leads to a sense of physical and emotional calm and has many benefits to overall physical and emotional health.

Thoracic breathing occurs in a catabolic state and is mostly associated with hyper- arousal. The catabolic state is thought to predispose the body to pathology according to the Thompsons (2015). In the catabolic state the body often shows a decrease in the production of white blood cells. There is an increase in cardiac output and blood pressure and an increased sympathetic drive which results in decreased peripheral skin temperature as well as increased sweating and increased heart rate.

The anabolic state is associated with effortless diaphragmatic breathing which reduces the sympathetic arousal. In the anabolic state, regeneration is encouraged in the body and it leads to an improvement in coronary heart disease, pain, panic, and hypertension. When the person does effortless diaphragmatic breathing and the body enters into the anabolic state, the peripheral skin temperature increases, sweating decreases and heart rate decreases.

6.2.2 Peripheral Skin Temperature

Interpreting the peripheral skin temperature in terms of a person's state of relaxation as done by biofeedback practitioners is based on the rationale that the sympathetic nervous system causes the arterial blood vessels in the finger to constrict. The finger will consequently become colder with an increased sympathetic drive when the fight and flee response is activated.

The temperature is measured by a thermistor from the pulp of the distal portion of the little finger. In a relaxed state, the temperature will be 32.8 degrees Celsius or between 94- and 95-degrees Fahrenheit.

Learning to control peripheral skin temperature does not only offer the client an additional stress marker as a reference for improved self-regulation but is also useful in the reduction of migraine headaches.

6.2.3 Electro-Dermal Response (EDR)

Skin conduction is also related to the sympathetic nervous system and can be used as a marker of stress. The sweat glands open and conductivity increases when the sympathetic drive is activated. The more sweaty the hand the higher the tension, stress or anxiety. Skin conduction is measured by measuring the very small current of electricity between two sensors. The unit in which this current is measured is micromhos.

People with extremely high arousal levels often have higher anxiety levels and therefore higher skin conductance levels. According to the Thompsons (2015), a flat, unchanging EDR may also be associated with chronic stress.

Higher EDR has also been associated with better learning of new material and improved memory recall according to research done by Andreassi (2010).

6.2.4 Heart Rate (HR)

Heart rate and blood volume are measured with a plethysmograph with a photoelectric transducer. Blood volume measurement is expressed as a percentage of the average of the difference in magnitude between the lowest point and the peak of a pulse.

Heart rate increases more with the experience of anger, fear, and sadness than with the experience of surprise, happiness, and disgust, according to the research findings of Andreassi (2010). Other findings include that heart rate increases with frustration and with a defensive reaction to rejection. When a person is able to exert control over an event, HR responses are greater.

Another very important and significant finding is that when a person breathes diaphragmatically and effortlessly at six cycles per minute, the heart rate follows in a sinusoidal pattern. This pattern, as mentioned earlier, is called respiratory sinus arrhythmia.

The heart rate is primarily governed by the natural rhythm of 60–100 beats per minute, of the sinoatrial node. The inhibition by the vagus nerve is the primary factor controlling heart rate and heart rate variability (Thompson & Thompson, 2015).

Heart rate increases with inspiration due to the sympathetic nervous system and decreases with exhalation. The control is released by the sympathetic nervous system and the parasympathetic nervous system, regulated partly by the medullary respiratory center through the vagus, takes over. This is the only measure by which the clinician can influence the activity of the parasympathetic nervous system and therefore indirectly influence the balance between the sympathetic and parasympathetic activity (Thompson & Thompson, 2015).

6.2.5 Heart Rate Variability (HRV)

In the training of heart rate variability, biofeedback practitioners teach the client to find the perfect synchrony between their heart rate variations and their breathing. Respiratory sinus arrhythmia is the variation in heart rate that accompanies breathing (Thompson & Thompson, 2015). Heart rate variability targets autonomic reactivity. Heart rate data gets fed back to the participant beat by beat during slow breathing and the participant attempts to maximize RSA in so doing, creating a sine-wave-like curve of peaks and valleys in which the goal is to match the RSA to heart rate patterns. RSA is the heart rate pattern that occurs when the heart rate increases during inhalation and decreases during exhalation. HRV biofeedback empowers clients to improve their emotional self- regulation.

It assists them in understanding their own physiological status and the relationship between autonomic functioning and overall wellbeing (Ginsberg, 2018).

During the HRV Biofeedback process, the amplitude of the heart rate oscillations increases to a significantly higher amplitude than during rest while the pattern becomes systematically more simple and sinusoidal. Most participants achieve these changes within a very short period of time – in less than a minute. The breathing rate is trained to a frequency at which the amplitude of the HRV is maximized.

RSA triggers very powerful reflexes in the body that assist with the control of the entire autonomic nervous system. A result of HRV Biofeedback training is that the baroreflex (the reflex that controls blood pressure) is stimulated which produces a high amplitude heart rate and blood pressure oscillations. According to the Thompsons (2015), this happens because of the resonant characteristics of the cardiovascular system. The processes involved are said by some researchers to include the phase relationships between heart rate oscillations and breathing at specific frequencies; phase relationships between heart rate and blood pressure oscillations at specific frequencies and then also the activity of the baroreflex and the resonance characteristics of the cardiovascular system.

The effect of the vagal afferent pathway to the frontal cortical areas is also considered by many researchers and practitioners. Stimulation of the parasympathetic reflexes occurs during HRV biofeedback and generally results in the body producing autonomic activity associated with relaxation (refer to section 6.1). The mechanism involved is referred to as "accentuated antagonism". According to Olshansky and Carnes (2008), abrupt parasympathetic stimulation will inhibit tonic sympathetic activation and its effects at rest and during exercise which is the response known as accentuated antagonism. This aspect of the parasympathetic efferent system is strengthened with HRV biofeedback training. Sympathetic output to myofascial trigger points may be inhibited during this process.

The vagal tone is prominent during rest and predominates over the sympathetic tone. The vagal system interacts closely with the inflammatory system. A study did by Nolan et al. (2012) indicated a decrease in C-reactive proteins (which are proteins involved in inflammation) in hypertensive patients treated with HRV biofeedback.

Regular exercise improves the effect of the baroreflex while the person is not exercising. Baroreflex gain is significantly increased by HRV biofeedback.

Hypertension is associated with poor heart rate variability.

On a biofeedback screen most commonly used, the client can see how the balance between the sympathetic and parasympathetic systems improves. Without parasympathetic control, the innate rhythm of the sinoartrial node would drive the heart rate at about 100 BPM. According to Lehrer and Eddie (2013), health is tightly related to oscillatory systems. Oscillations in vagal input, control oscillations in the heart rate (Thompson & Thompson, 2015).

Heart rate variability biofeedback (HRVB) is used for a variety of disorders as well as for performance enhancement (Gervirtz, 2013). Asthma, irritable

185

bowel syndrome, pain, anxiety depression, COPD, and blood pressure among many other conditions, generally respond well to HRVB.

HRV training includes training diaphragmatic breathing. The potential dangers of diaphragmatic breathing apply as discussed in the section on respiration.

6.2.6 Electromyography (EMG)

Electromyography is commonly used by biofeedback practitioners in an initial stress assessment and also as a means to improve muscle control and to teach the client to identify and change the tension in relevant muscles.

The electromyography reflects the depolarization and repolarization of muscle fibers.

Research done by Denkowski and Denkowski (1984), has proved that EMG feedback leads to a shift from external to internal locus of control which is a good indicator of lasting success. Relaxation in one muscle group does not tend to generalize to adjacent muscles.

6.2.7 Imagery

Over and above the above measurements of markers of stress and techniques taught with and without technology, imagery is also often used during neurofeedback and biofeedback training sessions.

An example of using imagery was discussed in the section on alpha-theta training. A more generalized discussion of imagery will follow.

Imagery as a therapeutic technique can aid in relaxation and the release of stress. It generally starts with a guided relaxation exercise. Therapists have different skill sets and interests and also different approaches to training. The relaxation technique or exercise can be as simple as encouraging the client to release all the muscle tension by focusing on the different muscles as guided by the therapist. It may also be a meditation exercise based on the principles of a particular meditation style. Meditation techniques will be discussed in chapter 7.

During the release of muscle tension, the client can be encouraged to visualize particular settings or circumstances that the client finds relaxing. After having allowed enough time for the client to engage with the relaxing scene, the client can then be requested to imagine a stressful scene, something that represents a crisis by the following definition of Thompson (1979): "a personally perceived adaptive incompetency". An example would be for a person that has a fear of being amongst strangers for that person to imagine approaching a group of people and becoming aware of the sensory perceptions. The changes in the stress markers that are being monitored could then be displayed to the client and as the client then switches to imagine a pleasant scene, the client can observe the stress marker measurements changing to what represents a more relaxed state as he/she gradually gains control over the physiological responses. It is important that the imagined scenes and settings will involve all the senses if possible.

The practitioner ought to proceed with caution when working with imagined scenes that cause discomfort. Some therapists will be more comfortable with using imagery than others and the preference of clients will also differ in this regard.

Making use of relaxing imagery only without alternating between positive and negative scenes and settings may be more appropriate in many cases.

6.2.8 Autogenic Training and Progressive Relaxation

The original autogenic training involved six exercises and was commonly used in Germany since the early 1930s according to Stoya (1986). The six exercises are meant to induce a sensation of limb heaviness and of limb warmth. One then progresses to diaphragmatic breathing after which follows suggestions of solar plexus warmth and of forehead cooling. The therapist does a guided relaxation exercise involving these components while remaining mindful of the client's experience so that the tempo and the imagery can be adapted to obtain optimal responses. A modern version of autogenic training involves four exercises. These four exercises focus on inducing a sensation of heaviness in the limbs, a raise in body temperature resulting in a comfortable relaxed feeling, diaphragmatic breathing and warming of the solar plexus. This process is also guided by the therapist in a calm and relaxing tone of voice.

A name associated with a popular technique called progressive muscle relaxation is Jacobson (1938). Dr Edmund Jacobson invented the technique in the 1920's in an attempt to ease the discomfort associated with anxiety for the sake of his patients. The technique is based on the premise that muscle tension is the body's psychological response to anxiety-provoking thoughts and that muscle relaxation blocks anxiety and relaxes the mind. It basically entails focusing on one area of the body, tensing the muscles, and then relaxing them. The tightening and relaxing of certain muscle groups is suggested in a specific sequence. There are many modern adaptations of the progressive relaxation technique that are being promoted by meditation, yoga, and spiritual teachers. Some suggest that the process of tightening then relaxing the muscles ought to start with the feet and then move up systematically all the way up to the shoulders, neck, and face. Others suggest starting with the face and moving down to the feet. There are also many localized versions of this relaxation technique used by speech therapists, singing coaches, physiotherapists, and occupational therapists.

Neurofeedback and biofeedback practitioners as well as psychotherapists and hypnotherapists usually use a progressive relaxation technique in combination with a breathing exercise and mental imagery.

It is important that the client's attention will be drawn to the difference between the sensations when the muscles are tensed as opposed to the sensation when they are relaxed. The client is to be made aware of the tension for a few moments when the muscle is tensed and then released and to feel the relaxation. The more comfortable the therapist is with the guided relaxation exercise the easier it will be for the client to engage with the process. When the therapist has experienced the benefits of the process and also engages in the process of the progressive relaxation while guiding the exercise, the therapist will be able to exude a sense of calm and confidence.

Once again it remains important that the therapist will be able to gauge what the needs of the client are and determine how to best serve those needs in a way that is conducive to healing.

A client comes to mind that refers to do progressive relaxation techniques in   his own time. He appreciates the research sources and YouTube videos with guided relaxation and meditation exercises I suggest which he then investigates and diligently implements. He prefers to be presented with graphs and technical information about the measurements we work with. Others, and very often it is the case with women it seems, do not want any technical information, and often wish to engage in relaxing techniques. The choice of words in any guided relaxation technique should best be neutral and devoid of any religious insinuations.

6.3 Chronic Pain from a Biofeedback Perspective

In the chapter titled "Investigating the Neuroplasticity of Chronic Pain Utilizing Biofeedback Procedures" by Stuart Donaldson, Mary Donaldson and Doreen Moran published in *Handbook of Clinical QEEG and Neurotherapy* (Collura & Frederick, (2017), it is stated that chronic pain is seen in changes occurring in the central, peripheral and autonomic nervous systems. A change in any one of these systems affects the other systems as well. The

Biofeedback practitioner can gain insight into the changes that occur in these systems. Often in mainstream medical approaches the practitioner is trained in understanding only the one system and the interrelatedness between the systems is ignored. The focus will be on reduction of pain, which is a short-term benefit whereas long term results relapse into the pain cycle. According to Donaldson et al. (2017), Biofeedback techniques and measures offer the health care practitioner with insight into the three parts of the nervous system. Treatment programs which utilize techniques from different modalities are now showing improved long-term benefits.

In his book *The Brain that Changes Itself*, Norman Doidge (2007) describes chronic pain as a negative consequence of neuroplasticity. Changes in the peripheral and central nervous systems are ascertained by SEMG (surface electromyography), QEEG and other stress profiling techniques.

Neuroplasticity refers to both synaptic plasticity as well as non-synaptic plasticity. According to Pasquel-Leone et al. (2011), this plasticity refers to changes in the neural pathways as well as changes in synapses which are a result of either changes in behavior or environment, neural processes or bodily injury. Neuroplastic changes do not only occur on cellular level and cortical level (remapping) but also in normal learning processes, performance enhancement and maturation. This neuroplasticity model provides a theoretical model to understand neurological changes that occur with chronic pain.

Chronic pain is described as being a maladaptation of the nervous system to repeated stimulation. Consequently, over time, changes occur in the nervous system. An understanding of the three branches of the nervous system – the central nervous system, the autonomic nervous system and the peripheral nervous system, as well as an understanding of how these three branches affect the functioning of one another, is necessary to examine the changes properly (Donaldson et al., 2017).

Chronic pain often involves repeated stimulation at a peripheral site which results in inflammation and noxious stimuli. A neuroplastic response at cortical level is caused which leads to changes in what Seifert and Maihöfner (2011) refer to as changes in somatotopic organization including central sensitization. Individuals experiencing complex regional pain syndrome, in the hand for instance, show diminished cortical somatotopic representation of the leg on the contralateral side as well as decreased distance between the representation of the hand and the mouth in the somatosensory cortex.

Reduction of the volume of grey matter in the prefrontal cortex and in the thalamus in the presence of chronic pain was reported by Apkarian et al.

(2004). Similar results have been reported in the presence of chronic low back pain and phantom limb pain.

The peripheral nervous system is also reported to be involved in neuroplasticity. Peripheral nerves respond to repeated stimulation by changes in dendrite growth and the spreading of axons (Donaldson et al., 2017).

Although neuroplasticity mostly has very positive implications and enhances the quality of life, the changes can be maladaptive and cause chronic pain.

Donaldson (see Donaldson et al., 2017) has developed a five-part evaluation plan for chronic pain patients in which he includes determining the involvement of the peripheral nervous system, the central nervous system and the autonomic nervous system. He has a clinic that focuses on the rehabilitation of chronic pain. He introduces the idea of trigger points, tender points and the concepts of myofascial pain syndromes and fibromyalgia. He provides his patients with pictures of what is possibly the source of pain based on trigger points and illustrations of the referred pain patterns.

Donaldson is of the opinion that providing the patients with a body diagram that indicates the front and the back of the body can be very helpful in ascertaining the role of the nervous systems in the experience of pain. He suggests that those patients that circle the entire body when they are requested to indicate the areas affected by the pain experience probably have fibromyalgia involving allodynia and hyperalgesia. People who indicate one or two sites probably have a myofascial pain syndrome involving the peripheral nervous system. The patients that indicate multiple but specific sites probably have central, peripheral, and autonomic nervous system involvement. He mentions that it is important to consider during the intake consultation that when the history is taken down in the case of myofascial pain syndrome, the development of the trigger points develop six weeks after the trauma. Donaldson considers the level of anger or rage a person feels after the onset of pain due to trauma, as a predictor of whether the person will recover from the pain or not.

Donaldson conducts a QEEG and a mini cognitive functioning test to ascertain the involvement of the central nervous system. A SEMG and a trigger point dolorimeter examination, ascertains the involvement of the peripheral nervous system and a psychophysiological stress test ascertains the involvement of the autonomic nervous system.

Central nervous system contributions to the chronic pain is considered when the person displays deterioration in memory, word finding problems, concentration and focus problems, deterioration in the ability to multi-task, changes in emotional status such as symptoms of irritability, depression or anxiety and poor results from a variety of physical therapies.

Although, according to Donaldson et al. (2017) there are no clear patterns in the QEEG associated with chronic pain, the deviances are found more often in the absolute power indicators. Deviances are often noted in Brodmann areas 21 and 23. Increased beta activity (18–25 Hz) is also often noted in the frontal areas with the fibromyalgia population. Decreased delta is often noted globally.

Increased 25 Hz activity on Cz is often noted with the myofascial population. When this activity is decreased, it usually indicates improvement in pain perception. Changes in the right hemisphere in terms of coherence and phase lag measures, generally signify improvement in chronic pain. The sites that are involved are F8, F4, C4, P4, T4 and T6.

When pain is related to trauma, Brodmann areas 21 and 23 ought to be considered in treatment protocols supported by QEEG findings.

The neuroplasticity models indicate that the brain will change in relation to external or internal stimulation. Once the changes have occurred as seen with chronic pain patients, the changes ought to be altered in order to break the reinforcement patterns that maintain the pain. The QEEG indicates which areas or pathways have been changed.

Chapter 7

The Value of Meditation and Neuro-meditation in Stress Reduction

7.1 Introduction

The potential value of meditation to overall mental, emotional, and physical health has been discussed and researched extensively over the past two decades. Meditation as a healthy daily practice is no longer, for the most part, frowned upon in western cultures. In my opinion, the fourteenth Dalai Lama's unfortunate expatriation from communist China in 1959 and his consequential involvement in western cultures, built a gentle bridge between customs and religions of the Eastern and the Western worlds.

The overall skepticism of meditation that was rampant in the latter half of the previous century, was probably fear based, as most negative judgement is, and born of ignorance. The main western religions regarded practices based on eastern customs as conflicting with and contradictory to Christian teachings. This is an interesting phenomenon though, because the lives of Christian and Catholic martyrs and saints such as St Teresa of Àvila (St Teresa of Jesus), St Francis of Assissi and even Mother Theresa (St Teresa of Calcutta) were deeply rooted in meditation practices. There are many other such examples. Meditation practices are associated with every major religion. Practitioners will probably come across clients that feel conflicted about meditation practices quite often and many who are totally ignorant or misinformed about meditation and the value it may add to their quality of life, especially if they are plagued by rumination, depression, chronic stress and attention related problems. It would not be unrealistic to estimate that far more than fifty percent of the clientele of the average neurofeedback and biofeedback practitioners fall within those parameters.

The introduction to this chapter serves as an attempt to empower the practitioner that wishes to include a form of meditation in their training protocols or wishes to introduce a suggestion of meditation as a daily practice. It also serves the purpose of providing basic information on different meditation styles to the reader who wishes to incorporate a form of meditation into their daily routine. The main reason why this chapter is relevant to this book is the fact that meditation practice can be enhanced very efficiently by certain neurofeedback protocols. When meditation is viewed from an EEG perspective, the potential value of a meditation practice to enhance and complement neurofeedback and biofeedback training protocols becomes clear. Although neurofeedback is scientifically validated, it is more than a science and therefore reference is made to spiritual and religious practices as well.

A common problem that people with the intent of incorporating a daily meditation practice into their lives have, is that they don't manage to maintain it. Individuals, who already have some type of early morning or evening ritual in place during which they take time out for themselves in an exercise or religious based hour, seem to find it easier to add a meditation exercise to the existing habit. Establishing a new habit is more difficult than adding something to an existing habit.

Another major reason why people fail to maintain a meditation practice is that they do not manage to meditate effectively and then it ends up feeling like something that needs to be endured and is dreaded. The average person from a western culture is not accustomed to quietening the mind and going beyond the rational mind into a more restful state. Most meditation courses start off with focusing on the breath. People then attempt to focus on the breathing with the rational mind which often results in an uncomfortable narrow focus during which you are constantly attempting to fight off invading thoughts. All sensations then become amplified – from the annoying sound of the mosquito in the room to the discomfort in the body due to the odd position you're attempting to sit in.

I met a guru a long time ago that taught me a simple truth. He was from India. He taught me that the mind behaves like a child. A child at a swimming pool constantly calls for the attention of the parent to witness the next dive or trick. All the parent needs to do is pay attention and give recognition. One should then also, according to the guru, afford one's mind the attention and allow it to jump around and do whatever it needs to. So before one attempts to sit down and meditate, you could go for a twenty minute walk or sit somewhere where you are comfortable and give your mind free reign to bring to the fore anything it wishes to bring to your attention. The important component of this phase of preparation for meditation is that you will just have what is referred to in many teachings on meditation as a "witnessing awareness". You do not resist or analyse any thoughts, you just witness them. You could imagine yourself being on a river bank and watching the leaves move downstream. The thoughts that enter your mind can be likened to the leaves floating by. You don't need to chase after every leaf in an attempt to catch it or rescue it. You just observe. After you have allowed your mind the freedom and have paid attention to the thoughts your mind brought into your attention for a while, the mind will now be more willing to become quiet.

This very simple exercise is often helpful to people who wake up at odd hours with a busy mind. The mind did not get a chance to process all the unfinished business of the day and awaits instruction on where to file the information or how to act on it. If a person sets aside a couple of minutes at bedtime to allow the unprocessed thoughts to surface and then discard the irrelevant ones and diarise the important ones, the mind can be more peaceful and willing to rest.

7.2 Different Types of Meditation and Research Findings

The types of meditation that will be discussed in this chapter are Focused Attention, Open Monitoring (also known as mindfulness meditation), Automatic Self-Transcending and Loving kindness / Compassion meditation as distinguished by and suggested as relevant to the practice of neurofeedback training by Jeffrey M. Tarrant. Dr Tarrant is the CEO of the Neuro Meditation Institute in Corvallis, Oregon. He wrote a chapter in Handbook of Clinical QEEG and Neurotherapy, by Thomas Collura and Jon Frederick (2017). Meditation protocols in amplitude training and LORETA based neurofeedback will be discussed. The term "neuromeditation" will be introduced. Alpha-theta training, which is a meditation-enhancing protocol that has already been discussed in chapter 5, will be alluded to.

Owing to the increase in available research on the efficacy of meditation for a host of disorders and symptoms, certain meditation programs such as for instance the MBSR (mindfulness-based stress reduction) program has become readily available in hospitals, medical centers and universities in America (Kabat- Zinn & Chapman-Waldrop, 1988).

A recent study in which changes in the brain density were studied before and after an eight week period of mindfulness-training, indicated significant increases in brain density in certain regions including the left hippocampus, the posterior cingulate cortex, the temporo-parietal juncture and the cerebellum (Hölzel et al., 2011). There is a growing body of evidence

194

provided from other brain imaging studies that prove the plasticity of the brain and significant improvements after basic, simple mindfulness meditation exercises.

In another earlier study, a meta-analysis in fact, conducted by Schmidt et al. (2004), it was indicated that mindfulness meditation training improves general well-being and leads to significant improvements in serious mental and physical health concerns including depression, anxiety, coping style, medical symptomology, sensory pain, physical impairment and estimates of quality of life. Many people really struggle with acquiring the skills that enable them to manage the mind. Over and above the recommendations made earlier in this regard, neurofeedback can be of much assistance. Both meditation practices and neurofeedback training are involved in training mental states. These two modalities can either enhance one another or be combined in treatment as interventions for ADHD, anxiety, or depression (Brandmeyer & Delorme, 2013). The meditator can be offered real-time feedback on his brainwave activity which is a direct measurement of brain state. The meditator can then begin to identify what it feels like to enter a dominant alpha brainwave state. Dr Les Fehmi patented Open Focus™ and wrote the book *The Open Focus Brain – Harnessing the Power of Attention to Heal Mind and Body* (2008), co-authored by Jim Robbins. With this book, many published articles on the topic as well as with online guided meditations and proposed exercises, Dr Fehmi made a very important contribution to the field of neurofeedback and biofeedback in terms of understanding the alpha dominant brain state. He also teaches extensively on the benefits of synchronous alpha.

It dawned on Dr Fehmi one day after having been in the field of studying brainwave activity for forty years, that relevant concepts in increasing the amplitude of alpha activity are about how you pay attention and about surrendering. Dr Fehmi observed that his own alpha brainwave activity increased when he gave up on a task he was attempting to perform. As soon as he surrendered, his alpha amplitude increased. When alpha increases, stress reduces with many associated physiological measurable changes related to the sympathetic and the parasympathetic drives of the autonomic nervous system. Alpha activity appears to be relevant to the space experience. When we imagine the space around us or the space inside ourselves or any aspect of space, alpha activity appears to increase and we become more relaxed.

Dr Fehmi distinguishes between four attentional styles. Attentional flexibility is important rather than having one particular style of attention. The attention styles are narrow focus, diffused focus, objective focus, and immersed attention. Various combinations of these attention styles are possible and are taught during workshops and are also available on the CD's that accompany Dr Fehmi's books (2008, 2010).

Narrow focus would be appropriate for instance when one has a narrow escape from a potentially dangerous situation. Had you for instance managed to evade an accident while driving, by the skin of your teeth due to having really zoomed in and acted swiftly, the narrow focus was appropriate. It would not however be appropriate or conducive to your emotional or mental health to grip on to that scenario and continue speculating how it would affect every aspect of your life and your children's lives. It would be appropriate to relax and widen your attention as soon as it would be possible. When we narrow focus onto something we "grip" onto it, to use Dr Fehmi's words, and that causes stress. He states that the nature of our world is that it is gripped, narrow focused and stress provoking. When we teach ourselves to become aware of the situation, the circumstances or the physical space around the stressful event or experience, the stress dissipates and our brainwaves change in that more alpha activity is generated.

Imagining any aspect of space diffuses the narrow focus into a diffused attention. The problem is not what we pay attention to, but how we pay attention. If we manage to master open focus in which all four styles of attention are merged, we tend to feel lighter and burdens become lighter. In many cases chronic pain reduces or vanishes. In open focus, you then develop an awareness of being aware.

Think of a recent stressful experience and allow yourself to really go into it. Pay attention to the changes in your body. Stay there for a while. Should you be able to do this short visualization, you would sense immediate changes as the sympathetic drive kicks in. You would notice muscles contracting, breathing becoming shallower, heart rate increasing and possibly also changes in skin tone response and dryness in your mouth. Dr Fehmi suggests that those changes occur based on your style of attention rather than what you are attending to. Allow yourself time to return to the present moment and relax as best you can for a minute or so.

You are going to recall that stressful event again, but this time you are going to pay attention to it differently. You are not going to cling onto it or narrow focus onto it while everything else gets excluded from your attention. Focus on the space between your eyes and the space around you and allow the memory of the stressful event to enter into your consciousness but let it enter into a space that contains other objects and thoughts. In other words, become aware of the space around or surrounding the memory. That memory is floating around amongst other things. It is not all consuming, you are not clinging to that memory or experiencing it as if that is all there is. It does not fill up your headspace. Your focus opens up to the space around it. The memory or the experience co-exists with other sensory perceptions of equal value. If you have done this guided exercise adequately you will find that your experience of the same incident or memory is now different. The incident is the same but the way in which you have attended to it is different and therefore your experience is different.

Dr Fehmi described open focus in a phone forum discussion as a state of attention in which one pays equal and simultaneous attention to all of your senses. In my consulting room I often have the clients, while they are receiving visual and auditory feedback in front of a computer, expanding their awareness by first expanding their visual field. I would encourage them to become aware of the frame of the monitor rather than just the graphics on the screen and to then systematically draw into their field of attention that which is visible from the peripheral visual field as well. Then they are encouraged to focus on the feedback sound, to incorporate that into the focus on the visual stimuli and to include background sounds as well. We then systematically include all sensory perceptions.

I often use fragments of suggested exercises by Dr Fehmi in presentations to encourage the audience to sense the experience of alpha and how that influences one's state of mind, your experience of your own body and your surroundings. My favorite exercise is the one in which one experiences the space in the distance between your eyes. It is as if one experiences the expansion of the mind and how it relaxes the mind. My morning ritual during which I prepare for the day ahead always includes a visualization of some aspect of space which straight away seems to counter the tendency of the mind to want to cling and control and ruminate.

It is often mentioned in talks and presentations that Dr Fehmi investigated different avenues in attempts to find ways in which to increase alpha brainwaves because of the benefits of alpha that have been researched widely. None of the visualizations involving looking at or visualizing calm and beautiful images or listening to different types of music rendered results comparable with the effect of visualizing space. The moment the brain engages in paying attention to space, the alpha amplitude increases.

In the workshops Les and Susan Fehmi offer, they teach the differences between the four attention styles as mentioned earlier. Narrow focus, as we have seen, is relevant and important under certain conditions and circumstances. Diffusing is an attention style in which the attention moves in the opposite direction, away from the narrow focus mode. The focus broadens or stretches like when one is focusing on a beautiful painting and then one diffuses one's attention to perceive the wall and the surrounding space as well. One can think of it as narrow becoming wide.

Objectifying and immersing as styles of attention are about one's relation with the aspect of reality one is attending to. When one objectifies, one goes into what I believe can be described as a witnessing awareness state or style of attention. One allows and observes, one does not engage. In guided meditation exercises I often encourage the person to look at or observe the thoughts that enter his/her mind almost as if he/she is witnessing leaves moving down a river. One does not engage with those leaves; one just observes them freely and allows them to move by calmly and lets them go. In this style of attention, one is not attached to the outcome and the self or the ego is separated from the occurrence or observation or aspect of reality.

Immersing as a style of attention is the opposite of objectifying. The ego engages or connects with something to the extent that the person loses its awareness of self. I would like to share a beautiful example of immersing that I experienced recently.

In the remote area of Namibia where I was on a sabbatical to complete the bulk of this book, I went on a tribal tour. The tour guide is also a waitress at the lodge. She is studying to become a teacher and works at the lodge during holidays to earn an income over and above the sponsored funds she receives for her studies from the lodge owners. While working at the lodge she stays with her grandmother in the little village of the Hambuku tribe where she grew up. I was a bit skeptical at first thinking that it would probably be a commercialized event and I also felt it may be invasive to the grandmother and other inhabitants of the village. This tour did however implicate a further contribution to Elizabeth's education so off we went. What a memorable, authentic, and enlightening experience it was!

After having walked some distance on a footpath (trodden by a few villagers and animals) through the bush, we arrived at Elizabeth's tribal home. There was her grandmother, sitting on the cleanly swept ground encircled by a few huts constructed from latte and mud. She was sitting beside a small fire which she had made. Apart from a few chickens and chicks, Elizabeth's grandmother and the tour party of four, there were no other living beings in the kraal. Elizabeth explained to us that her grandmother was going to prepare us a typical tribal meal. Elizabeth spoke to her grandmother in their native tongue, Thimbukushu which is one of many dialects spoken in the Kavango Region. The lady had a few flat baskets around her that each had a specific purpose. The one contained the harvested mahangu which is grain that gets pounded and processed in a certain way before it gets cooked on an open fire to prepare a porridge called "dimbombo dyo mahangu'. The grandmother started the pounding process in a cylinder shaped hollowed out part of a tree trunk with a long-rounded stick, the approximate length of a broomstick but considerably thicker in diameter. It was a beautiful ritualistic, rhythmic action accompanied by a chanting like sound. The grandmother tired after a while and our guide, Elizabeth, had to take over the pounding action. I could sense how she was conflicted, self- conscious and torn between two worlds – that of her heritage and the western civilization of which she has become a part by virtue of her studies and her work in the lodge. She was attending to the situation with an objective attention style – initially. Her emotional experience influenced her attention style as is often the case with all of us. Although she started pounding hesitantly and consciously initially, she became immersed and her reaction became instinctive, natural, and beautiful. She too succumbed to the need to chant rhythmically as if the sound was coming forth from the earth.

The objective attention style is not better or worse than the immersed style of attention, just as narrow focus is not better or worse than objectifying. A particular style of attention will serve us better than the other depending on the task or circumstances at hand. The goal is that we will be able to deploy all these styles of attention separately or concurrently at will.

Anxiety symptoms and even often depression symptoms, become less debilitating when clients engage in regular meditation practices. The person becomes more familiar with that space in which one can diffuse the focus slightly, a place where clinging on to the experience is no longer the only option. To start off with meditation suggestions at the onset of training a client suffering depression, will generally not be received well.

Crane and Soutar (2000), mention that many of the earlier protocols used in neurotherapy were designed to replicate many of the effects that are experienced during a meditative state. Meditation often leads to an increase in alpha and when this was identified, the alpha frequency band became the focus of much research and interest. In 1994, the bestselling author, spiritual teacher and medical practitioner, Deepak Chopra, published a paper with conclusive evidence that an increase in alpha power plays a role in both state and trait changes associated with meditation practice (Chopra, 1994).

It comes as no surprise that neurofeedback protocols that increase alpha power result in decreased anxiety levels and feelings of emotional wellbeing. To equate meditation practices to training that increases the alpha amplitude, is according to Dr Tarrant (2017) far too simplistic. The role of alpha in meditation appears to be related at least in part, to the degree of relaxation as well as to the degree of attention and focus. Most relaxation exercises also lead to an increase in alpha and reduced sensory intensity.

According to Basar et al. (1997), certain meditation exercises actually lead to a reduction in alpha activity.

Our current understanding of the associated neurobiology with different meditative states has grown much since the onset of neurofeedback, owing to the current brain imaging research. The type and style of meditation also have different effects on brain activity. Certain meditation styles and neuromeditation protocols are better suited to certain symptoms.

Three categories of meditation have been distinguished based on the effects on brainwave activity and attention. This categorization is not based on the different styles of meditation taught in eastern philosophies, yoga schools or other institutions of a spiritual nature. The three styles of meditation in question are Focused Attention referred to as FA from here on, Open Monitoring which will be referred to as OM, and automatic self-transcending, referred to as AST (Travis & Shear, 2010). There is another style of meditation called Loving Kindness/ Compassion meditation. This style of meditation may be familiar to readers who are familiar with the Dalai Lama's teachings. It is designed to produce a specific emotional state of empathy and compassion and is regarded to be a subcategory of FA by some authors and researchers. This style of meditation will be referred to as LK-C for the purpose of this discussion.

FA is probably the style of meditation that most readers will be most familiar with. It involves focusing the attention voluntarily on a chosen object such as the breath or a specific word or phrase often referred to as a mantra or affirmation. When the attention wanders off, the meditator is to observe and recognize this distraction and redirect the attention gently without judgment to the object of focus. The meditator engaged in FA shows an increase in frontal-parietal gamma power and coherence. Beta 2 (20–30 Hz) activity is also increased by FA (Travis & Shear, 2010). In a study, novice and experienced FA meditators' fMRI images indicated several areas of the brain involved in maintaining focused attention. The identified areas involved in FA, according to Petersen and Posner (2012) are the dorsolateral prefrontal cortex, the visual cortex, the superior frontal sulcus and intra parietal sulcus. A study that Lehmann et al. (2001) did on advanced meditators indicated increases in gamma activity that shifted to different regions of the brain depending on the type of processing involved. Visual centers were activated when the monks visualized the Buddha and the verbal centers were activated when mantras were the object of focus whereas the frontal areas were activated when the focus was on dissolution and reconstitution of the self.

Many studies have confirmed the involvement of the anterior cingulate cortex (ACC) in tasks pertaining to self-regulation of cognition and emotions. There appears to be a close correlation to the activation of the ACC during the sustained attention required during FA. Studies done on the effects of lesions in the ACC, confirm the importance of this region in self-regulation. According to Crottaz- Herbette and Menon (2006), the ACC is the major generator of attention-related activation regardless of the sensory modality involved.

The main challenge in focused attention meditation is to prevent the mind from wandering which is regarded as being a natural tendency of the mind. The Default Mode Network (DMN) has been implicated by many studies to be the main role player in mind wandering (Buckner et al., 2008). In FA, the focus becomes fixed on the object of meditation and inevitably drifts off to thought processes that involve the sense of self. This process is then observed through self-monitoring and thus the focus is returned to the object of focus. The ACC becomes activated in the process of becoming aware of the mind wandering (Craigmyle, 2013). It thus appears, according to Tarrant (2017), that FA meditation causes interplay between activation of the ACC and deactivation of the DMN. This process can be supported by a neurofeedback protocol designed to reward beta or gamma (fast brainwave activity) in the ACC and reward of alpha in the Posterior Cingulate Cortex (PCC) or the Precuneus. The mind set required to maintain activation of the ACC and deactivation of the Precuneus, is that of relaxed focus.

The following neurofeedback protocols have been suggested by Tarrant (2017) as helpful for focused attention (FA):

Standard protocol:

Reward beta2 (20–30 Hz) or gamma (30–40 Hz) at Fz
Reward alpha (8–12 or 8–10 Hz) at Pz

LORETA protocol:

Reward beta2 (20–30 Hz) or gamma (30–40 Hz) at the Anterior Cingulate Cortex
Reward alpha (8–12 or 8–10 Hz) at the Precuneus or Posterior Cingulate Cortex

Tarrant (2017) suggests that the proposed FA protocols ought to initially not include the fast brainwave (gamma or beta) and the alpha rewards, but only either the fast brainwave or the alpha reward.

Loving kindness/compassion meditation or LK-C is similar to AST meditation in that it involves the focus of attention on something specific. In the case of LK-C meditation, the focus is on unrestricted availability to help others. It differs from FA meditation in that the goal of LK-C meditation is to generate feelings of caring, love and compassion. This style of meditation results in the activation of areas of the brain involved in the perception of the emotional state of others. Two areas have been identified to be directly involved in experiencing empathy, namely the right anterior insula and the anterior cingulate cortex.

A lovingkindness/compassion surface training neuromeditation protocol involves rewarding alpha (8–12 Hz) at F4 with a simultaneous inhibit of 8–12 Hz at F3 or a 15–18 Hz reward at F3. The suggested LORETA protocol involves rewarding beta2 (20–30 Hz) or gamma (30–40 Hz) at the right insula and a beta 2 (20–30 Hz) reward or gamma (30–40 Hz) reward at ACC.

Open monitoring meditation (OM) is more commonly referred to as mindfulness meditation. Mindfulness meditation has become a very popular meditation style. There are various guided mindfulness meditations available online as well as many courses on offer that are readily accessible.

This style of meditation encourages a witnessing awareness rather than an attentional focus. In Buddhism, this style of meditation is referred to as Vipassana. In Tibetan Buddhism, the ideal meditation includes aspects of both FA and OM styles of meditation in a single practice. According to the Vajrayana teachings, the mind of the practitioner progressively gets transformed and frees itself from egocentric grasping and ignorance. Vajrayana is a system of Tibetan Buddhist meditation methods. These meditation methods are focused on freeing the mind from grasping which is considered to be the cause of confusion and suffering. Grasping traps us in the realm of delusion known as samsara. The opposite of samsara is referred to as nirvana or enlightened reality. The focused attention section of these meditations usually involves focusing on a deity such as Chenrezig which functions as a symbol of transformation. This then allows the enlightened self to surface after which the practitioner observes what is, free from projection, which is where the OM aspects of meditation then come into play. Many researchers and meditation teachers have likened Vajrayana teachings to the teachings of Jung.

In open monitoring meditation, the meditator does not attach to any object of attention. There is a non-judgmental monitoring of each thought, sensory experience, and emotion as they appear and drift by. The meditator releases each sensation, emotion or thought as it surfaces into consciousness.

The research studies done on the effects of OM meditation on the EEG, indicate an increase in theta power frontally as well as increased coherence in the theta band.

Although theta is mainly associated with deep states reached in meditation and sleep onset, a frontal midline theta rhythm has been identified to be involved in the performance of tasks (Aftanas & Golocheikine, 2001). According to Tarrant (2017), it has been established that the attentional networks of the anterior frontal lobes as well as the ACC are involved in generating this particular theta rhythm. Long term OM meditators appear to have different theta activation patterns compared to novice meditators. Experienced OM meditators demonstrate increases in theta over the frontal midline, whereas short-term meditators do not show an increase in anterior midline theta during meditation. This may be due to the fact that novice meditators are more anxious and frustrated at not reaching the required meditative state. OM meditation is more relaxed and inclusive than FA meditation which requires a narrower focus. OM meditation involves an ongoing monitoring of the self which implies involvement of the default mode network.

A neurofeedback protocol to utilize during an OM meditation would be a theta reward (4–8 Hz) at Fz or ACC (depending on whether it is power surface training) with or without an alpha inhibit at Pz or the Precuneus. Instead of the alpha inhibit in both cases, a beta 2 reward can be added at Pz for the standard protocol or at the Precuneus or PCC.

To a certain extent, automatic self-transcending can be likened to transcendental meditation. This meditation style is about moving beyond the procedures of the meditation (Tarrant, 2017). It entails moving through a state of sustained attention to mental silence. This meditation style has been studied extensively and it has been concurred that it leads to an increase in amplitude of low alpha (8–10 Hz) and alpha coherence (Travis & Shear, 2010). Increased low alpha power is associated with reduced external attention and expectation. The mind becomes more settled when low alpha power increases and does not grip onto or create concerns.

The neurofeedback protocol that leads to this state that is reached in AST meditation is the protocol that is discussed in chapter 5 under the alpha-theta training section. During this protocol, alpha is rewarded at Pz in the eyes closed condition. Alpha is rewarded with a gentle sound whenever it rises above a given threshold. This area is just anterior to the Precuneus which has been described as the most important region of the Default Mode Network (DMN). The Precuneus is involved in self- centered imagery and episodic memory retrieval as well as processes associated with identity. Reflective self-awareness is also an important function of this area of the brain. The Precuneus with the Posterior Cingulate Gyrus is involved in conscious information processing. In addition to surface training on Pz in LORETA training the Precuneus and/or the PCC can be trained directly.

The Medial Frontal Cortex is also part of the DMN and could be included in a neurofeedback protocol that is focused on the goals of AST which is quietening the mind.

The meditative state reached in AST meditation as well as the brainwave state, have much in common with Les Fehmi's alpha synchrony training (Fehmi & Robins, 2008). According to Fehmi, a multisensory experience of space results in large amplitudes of synchronous alpha activity. Alpha synchrony can be trained with neurofeedback protocols by training alpha in multiple regions.

A daily practice during which a multisensory experience of space is encouraged, can work wonders for clients that have high levels of anxiety and those who find it difficult to quieten their minds. This is best done early in the mornings in a calm environment – preferably outdoors – while lying on the back outstretched on a yoga mat. The senses are then systematically engaged one by one in the experience of the environment. The awareness of the environment can begin with the immediate environment and be systematically expanded to an awareness of the infinity of space.

Tarrant (2017) suggests that FA and OM meditation styles may be beneficial to ADHD sufferers seeing that both these styles train aspects of attention. OM may possibly also be helpful for those who wish to improve their self-monitoring and executive skills associated with self-awareness. Open monitoring may also be of particular significance in the treatment of anxiety. There is clear evidence that people with more theta activity have lower trait and state anxiety scores (Inanaga, 1988). A comparison study in which the EEG characteristics of the EEG of FA meditators and OM meditators were compared, found that OM meditators displayed higher frontal theta amplitudes (Dunn et al., 1999).

Most of the current brain imaging-studies pertaining to the effects of meditation are focused on stress reduction as a result of mindfulness or open- monitoring meditation.

AST protocols are suggested to be potentially beneficial to those suffering psychological disorders pertaining to the sense of self. There are neurofeedback practitioners that are already using the protocol that can be regarded as a form of AST training (rewarding alpha at the Precuneus) with personality disorders and addictions (Tarrant, 2017). According to Tarrant, Mark Smith has mentioned that this protocol appears to instill a calm sense of integrity in these patients. Quieting the distorted sense of self, may lead to the development of a healthy ego. The same process may then quieten the self-involved stories of the ego and allow the person to move on to a sense of spirituality and a broader form of consciousness (Jones & Bhattacharya, 2014).

Neurofeedback practitioners will be better able to determine which neuromeditation protocol would be best suited to their clients' needs if they practiced the different meditation styles to experience the influences of these meditation styles and by implication understand the influence the associated neurofeedback protocols on the EEG and more importantly, on the inner experience.

7.3 A Brief Summary of Three Styles and Benefits of Meditation

A brief summary of the styles and advantages of meditation based on the article Mind of the Meditator that was published in Scientific American (2014), authored by Matthieu Ricard, Antoine Lutz and Richard J. Davidson, follows.

The article is a result of extended studies on meditation by researchers over a period of fifteen years. The author is not going to focus on the measurable changes in function and structure in the brain in this section as a result of meditation, but on the potential benefits to enhance physical and emotional well-being. The goal of this section is to provide the novice meditator and the practitioner that considers integrating meditation into their practice, with a starting point. The three styles of meditation that are summarized here are the three main forms of Buddhist meditation namely focused attention, mindfulness, and compassion/ loving kindness meditation.

In focused attention meditation the meditator concentrates on the in-and-out-cycle of breathing. The mind has a natural tendency to wander – even in experienced meditators. The goal of the meditator is to refocus on the rhythm of the inhalations and exhalations as soon as there is an awareness of the distraction. Systematically, with daily practice, it becomes easier to sustain focus for longer periods of time. With the practice of focused-attention meditation the mind becomes centered and adept at being aware of distractions. A focused state can eventually be achieved with less effort.

Mindfulness or open-monitoring meditation involves observing all sensory sensations, bodily sensations, and thoughts as they appear. This observation of the different sensations, thoughts and feelings has to be from a neutral perspective which can be described as a non-reactive awareness. When the mind becomes preoccupied with any thought or perception, the meditator should return to a detached focus. In mindfulness meditation the meditator does not resist, judge, interpret or change any perception. The different sensations, thoughts and feelings are allowed without engaging with any of the perceptions. One's awareness of one's surroundings grows with systematic daily practice and with it a sense of psychological well-being develops as one becomes progressively less reactive. The practitioner develops the ability to regulate mental states and experience a sense of calm. Mindfulness meditation can contribute to a more stable and clear mind and emotional balance. The meditator acquires the ability to master the mind and to liberate it from inner confusion and dysfunctional conditioned patterns of inner chatter.

Compassion/loving kindness meditation cultivates an attitude of compassion towards other people. This style of meditation generally involves the repetition of a phrase or mantra that expresses unconditional love for others. In this practice the intent of the meditator is to alleviate the suffering of others. This form of meditation has proven to be beneficial to health care workers that are at risk for emotional burnout. It contributes to inner balance, strength of mind and courage in the same way that traditional prayer does.

The analysis of neuroscience research studies on meditation, clearly indicates the effects on both brain functioning and the physical structures of the brain. The reader that wishes to acquire more detail on the findings that lead to the acclaimed benefits of meditation referred to in this summary section, would be able to access the article referred to.

The author is privileged to have received relevant information on a number of people that went on a ten day silent retreat in 2018. A noted expert in the field of applied neuroscience from the States concurred that a comparison of the pre and post retreat QEEG recording of an individual on the retreat, indicated an increased calm state of mind. There were also indications of increased perceptiveness and stabilization of the temporal lobes. Increased alpha coherence was visible which is often observed with experienced meditators.

The neurofeedback practitioner that wishes to integrate meditation into their practice ought to be very sensitive to the needs and convictions of the client and ought not attempt to convince the client of adding a meditation practice or including a neuromeditation protocol in his/her training should that individual not be comfortable with the suggestion.

Chapter **8**

Neurofeedback and Attention Deficit Hyperactivity Disorder (ADHD)

8.1 Background and Introduction

I believe that most of the neurofeedback practitioners that introduced neurofeedback as an additional therapy to their practices in the 1990's and the first decade of the new millennium, did so mainly to have an additional treatment option for the ADHD population. There are, of course, also the specialist therapists that work mainly with PTSD or with Bipolar Disorder or Traumatic Brain Injury or a host of other disorders that added the therapy for different purposes. Most health care practitioners, however, get to work with a substantial number of ADHD sufferers. The prevalence of ADHD amongst adults in most cultures is estimated by the DSM- 5 (APA, 2013) to be 2, 5%. There are many sources that indicate the incidence of ADHD on a regular basis. In children, ADHD is the most commonly diagnosed pediatric psychiatric disorder and some sources indicate the incidence as being between 5 and 10% amongst children. The perception that the ADHD population is growing, is a common perception amongst researchers and therapists. The relevance of these facts and speculations to this book is that all neurofeedback practitioners come across individuals with full blown ADHD and individuals who have some attention and focus related difficulties. Neurofeedback has probably been used and is being used to address ADHD more commonly than any other disorder. Consequently, there are very many research studies with large sample sizes and also comparative studies on the efficacy of neurofeedback as an intervention for ADHD. In the book *Evidence-Based Practice in Biofeedback and Neurofeedback* (Tan et al., 2016), neurofeedback has been indicated as having a level 5 efficacy rating. This means that neurofeedback is both efficacious and specific. (The reader is referred to chapter 2 for a description and explanation of the different levels of statistical efficacy).

Before some of the studies are discussed, let us take a fresh look at ADHD. ADHD, when not understood or treated, can cause devastation. The divorce rate of ADHD sufferers is much higher than that of the normative group. Life partners often find it too demanding and stressful to continue in a relationship with the ADHD sufferer. Research has revealed that 80% of ADHD learners are underachievers. A recent study showed that between 60 and 80% of ADHD sufferers don't complete their schooling in South Africa. These children are more prone to drug abuse, to teenage pregnancies (40% of the teenage pregnancies in South Africa are due to ADHD) and to drifting from one job to the next. ADHD teenagers and adults are more often involved in motor vehicle accidents than the rest of the population. They often cause a lot of tension in the household due to their lack of a developed sense of responsibility and to recklessness. Not only their household but also their social lives, career lives and personal relationships are affected negatively by their lack of responsibility (Bester, 2014). Their social behavior often appears to be immature.

Clearly, the ADHD individual is at risk of not leading an actualized life and of both experiencing and causing a lot of discomfort. Fortunately, we live in an era where stimulant medication is no longer the only intervention option. Despite the fact that the largest mental health research organization, the American National Institute of Mental Health (NIMH) announced in May 2013 that they would no longer be basing their research on the DSM-5 (APA, 2013) categories of disorders, but rather on the cognitive and neurological components and despite the fact that the DSM- 5 was going to contain criteria including EEG-data for the diagnosis of ADHD, the diagnosis is still based on a list of diagnostic criteria. The good news is that there is more funding available for brain-based therapies than ever before since the shift away from the funding for the DSM-5 based categories has occurred. The three main groups of ADHD symptoms pertain to inattentiveness, hyperactivity, and impulsivity.

8.2 Criteria for Diagnosis

The symptoms specified in the DSM-5 are the following:

Inattentiveness

(a) The person often fails to pay close attention to detail and makes careless mistakes in school work, work or other activities (details are overlooked or omitted, for example, or the work is inaccurate).

(b) The person often has difficulty sustaining attention in tasks and play activities (finds it difficult to remain focused during lectures, conversations, or long reading sessions, for example).

(c) The person does not seem to listen when spoken to directly (the person's thoughts seem to be elsewhere, for instance, even in the absence of any obvious distraction).

(d) The person does not follow through on instructions and fails to finish school work, chores or duties in the work place (starts tasks but quickly loses focus and is easily distracted, for example).

(e) The person often finds it difficult to organize tasks or activities (for example, difficulty managing sequential tasks; difficulty keeping materials and belongings in order; messy, disorganized work; has poor time management; fails to meet deadlines).

(f) The person often avoids or is reluctant to engage in tasks that require sustained mental effort (school work or homework, for example; and in older adolescents or adults the preparation of reports, completion of forms and completion of lengthy papers).

(g) Items essential to the performance of tasks or activities are often lost (for example, school materials, pencils, books, tools, wallets, keys, paperwork, spectacles, cell phones).

(h) The person is easily distracted by extraneous stimuli (among adolescents and adults this may include thoughts about unrelated matters).

(i) Frequently forgetful in daily activities (doing chores, running errands, for example; among older adolescents and adults, the answering of calls, paying of accounts and keeping of appointments).

Hyperactivity and impulsivity

(j) The person often fidgets or taps hands or squirms in his or her seat.

(k) The person often leaves his/ her seat when remaining seated is expected (leaving their seat in the classroom or office, other workplace or in other situations where they are expected to remain in one place).

(l) The person runs around or climbs in situations where it is inappropriate (in adolescents or adults this behavior may be limited to feelings of restlessness).

(m) The person often has difficulty playing or engaging in leisure activities quietly.

(n) The person is often "on the go" or behaves as if he/she is" driven by a motor" (for example, is unable or finds it difficult to remain still for long periods, such as in a restaurant or during meetings; others may experience this as restlessness or an inability to keep up).

(o) He/ she often talks excessively.

(p) The person often blurts out questions before the questions have been completely formulated. He/she finishes others' sentences for them and finds it difficult to wait his or her turn to speak or contribute.

(q) The person often finds it difficult to wait his/her turn (difficulty waiting in a queue, for instance).

(r) He/she often interrupts others or intrudes on them (for example, interrupts conversations, games, and activities, or uses others' belongings without permission; adolescents and adults may intrude into or take over what others are doing).

8.3 Conditions for Diagnosis

Certain conditions are prerequisites for diagnosis, namely that the symptoms must be present continuously for six months; the symptoms must be inconsistent with the person's developmental level; at least some of the symptoms must have started presenting before the age of twelve; there must be clear evidence that the symptoms interfere with or reduce the quality of social, academic, or occupational functioning. The symptoms must also not be the result of schizophrenia or any other psychotic disorder and should not be better explained by another mental disorder, for example anxiety disorder, dissociative disorder, personality disorder or substance intoxication or withdrawal.

Several inattentive or hyperactive-impulsive symptoms must be present in at least two environments (for example, at school or place of work, among friends and family, or during other activities).

At least six symptoms under number one or six symptoms under number two must be present in children younger than 17. In older adolescents and adults, at least five symptoms under number one or five symptoms under number two must be present.

The symptoms must not be due to oppositional behavior only or due to defiance exclusively or be a result only of hostility or failure to understand tasks or instructions.

There are three types of ADHD which, according to the DSM-5 (APA, 2013), need to be referred to as presentations and not types any longer.

8.4 ADHD Predominantly Inattentive Presentation

This sub-group is also referred to as the inattentive group. ADHD sufferers from this group have a tendency to be very dreamy and get distracted by their own thoughts. They must present with at least six symptoms from group one of the DSM-5 (APA, 2013) criteria in two different environments if they are younger than 17 years old and at least five of the symptoms from number one of the DSM-5 criteria if they are older than 17 years. Some of the ADHD sufferers with the diagnosis of inattentive presentation have a few symptoms from group two as well – symptoms pertaining to hyperactivity and impulsivity. The number of symptoms from group two has to be less than five for adolescents and adults over 17 years and less than six for children younger than 17 or else they would be diagnosed with the combined presentation.

ADHD sufferers with the mainly inattentive presentation mostly have symptoms associated with low arousal levels (The reader is referred to chapter 5 for a reminder of the symptoms associated with under-arousal). When the neurofeedback practitioner uses a power training protocol, it would typically involve a high frequency reward (between 15 and 20 Hz) on C3 on the left hemisphere or on Cz. The inhibit bands would either be based on symptoms or guided by a QEEG. To use an inhibit of slow brain wave activity (between 2 Hz and 7 or 8 Hz) is common. This population often has an excess of slow brain wave activity.

Most of the research pertaining to neurofeedback as an intervention for ADHD is based on the theta-beta ratio, one channel amplitude training and ISF training protocols. Although we do not have enough research results from multichannel protocols yet, anecdotal evidence looks promising regarding the effects of live Z-score training for ADHD.

8.5 ADHD Predominantly Hyperactive-Impulsive Presentation

ADHD sufferers with the predominantly hyperactive-impulsive presentation are seldom overlooked. In fact, they appear to be everywhere. When the teacher drifts off to sleep at night she may well have visions of the hyperactive learner popping up in her alpha or theta state as well since he has been rather in his/her face all day. These children, and adults even, do not seem to have a sense of personal space and often disregard other boundaries as well. They can, for instance, be very direct, often untactfully direct that cause people to feel offended. Most people find ADHD sufferers from this group, quite invasive.

Lower arousal level types and more introverted people often find their talkativeness and restlessness exhausting. Due to their general lack of or poor impulse control, they are often judged and misunderstood.

ADHD sufferers with the predominantly hyperactive-impulsive presentation must have at least six symptoms from the second group of the DSM-5 criteria when they are younger than 17 years and at least five symptoms from the group when they are older than 17. They normally have a few (fewer than six for the sufferers younger than17 and fewer than five for the sufferers older than 17) of the symptoms from group one as well.

The predominantly hyperactive-impulsive subgroup of the ADHD population often present with many over-arousal symptoms. Symptoms associated with over- arousal are indicated in chapter 5. Single channel power or amplitude training protocols mostly involve enhancing SMR (sensory motor rhythm or 12–15 Hz activity) on C4 on the right hemisphere or on Cz. Inhibits are usually based on symptoms and often involve inhibiting very fast beta activity (22–36 Hz) and theta activity (4–7 Hz) Coherence and multichannel training protocols are ordinarily based on QEEG findings.

8.6 ADHD Combined Presentation

This subgroup of the ADHD population is the biggest group. Approximately 85% of ADHD sufferers present with at least six symptoms from group one of the DSM-5 (APA, 2013) criteria if they are younger than 17 or at least five symptoms from group one if they are older than 17 years, plus at least six or five symptoms depending on the prerequisites for diagnosis of the matching age group, from group two.

The main presenting symptoms of this subgroup in terms of arousal-level related symptoms generally include symptoms associated with both over-arousal and under- arousal as well as symptoms associated with unstable arousal.

Training protocols often involve training on both the left and right hemispheres over the sensory motor strip separately. On C3 higher frequencies are rewarded between 15 and 20 Hz (frequency bands mostly span over at least 4 Hz bandwidths, for example 15–18 Hz) whereas lower frequencies on C4 (12–15 Hz) are rewarded. Inhibit bands may be the same on both sides or may differ based on symptoms or QEEG findings.

A bipolar hook-up during which an active electrode is placed at C3, a reference electrode at C4 and a clip on ground electrode on A1, used to be a popular protocol before two and more channel training became readily available. The frequency to be rewarded would then mostly be 12–15 Hz.

With two channel training the two placement areas can be trained simultaneously at different frequencies. Both, enhance and inhibit bands can be set independently for the two sites.

8.7 ADHD and QEEG Findings

Over and above considering ADHD in terms of DSM-5 based criteria and merging the most prominent symptoms with arousal based symptoms and making training protocol decisions accordingly, the accessibility of QEEG's offers another possibility.

One research study quoted often, is the study done by Dr Robert Chabot from New York University (Chabot & Serfontein, 1996). This study indicated that ADHD sufferers can be divided into different subgroups based on EEG findings. It appears, according to this study, that 47% of the ADHD population have an excess of theta activity in the resting brain, 31% of the ADHD population demonstrate an excess of alpha activity in the resting brain whereas 7% have an excess of beta activity. Fifteen percent of the ADHD population show no deviances in terms of their EEG from the mean scores. The 7% with the excessive beta activity, are possibly the group that does not respond well to stimulant medication such as methylphenidate. More and more pediatricians and psychiatrists are beginning to show an interest in QEEG findings for this reason. This biological marker can enable physicians to make a differential diagnosis and select an appropriate treatment and prevent abreactions.

The small sub-group with an excess of beta activity, found mainly in the frontal regions, appear to be more prone to emotional outbursts and temper tantrums which may, according to Di Michele et al. (2005), be associated with frontal lobe self-regulation and inhibition control.

In terms of neurofeedback protocols, the training protocol will be focused on inhibiting the excess activity and frequencies to be rewarded will be adapted according to the findings of the QEEG.

8.8 ADHD Research Studies that Confirm the Sustained Effects of Neurofeedback

Theoretical models have been developed for the theta/beta ratio (TBR) protocol, the sensorimotor rhythm (SMR) protocol and the slow cortical potential (SCP) protocol. These three protocols are based on EEG research and have been very well investigated. They have well established efficacy in the treatment of ADHD. Randomized controlled trials as well as meta- analysis findings that support the conclusion that neurofeedback in the treatment for ADHD is efficacious and specific (level 5 efficacy) are referenced and some of those studies are discussed in this section.

The most recent meta-analysis conducted to date was performed by an international group of researchers that looked at all available studies involving the clinical benefit of neurofeedback on ADHD symptoms. It was published in the scientific journal *European Child & Adolescent Psychiatry*. The study is titled: "Sustained effects of neurofeedback in ADHD: A systematic review and meta- analysis" (Van Doren et al., 2019).

The researchers from The Netherlands, Germany and the United States associated with numerous universities, conducted a systematic review and meta- analysis to investigate the long-term effects of neurofeedback and different control groups, including medication. The researchers were selected to represent differing and opposing views on neurofeedback in order to ensure impartial, balanced and critical evaluation of the data. Data was compiled of more than 500 children with ADHD from 10 randomized controlled studies. The results of neurofeedback, active and non-active control conditions were compared. The active control conditions included medication. The clinical benefits were assessed after a follow-up period of on average six months after the treatment was concluded. Neurofeedback had a large effect on inattention and a medium effect on hyperactivity-impulsivity in the six-month follow-up analysis. At the six month follow-up period, there were no differences between the clinical effects of neurofeedback and the active control groups (including medication). For the non-active controls, there was a small effect on inattentiveness that disappeared at follow-up. The benefits of neurofeedback improved from outtake to follow-up which was not the case with the other treatments in the active control groups. In the medication control group, medication was used uninterruptedly and was not terminated during the six-month follow-up period. No additional neurofeedback sessions were administered in the six-month follow-up period.

The results of this study apply to the SCP, TBR and SMR protocols.

Another systematic review and meta-analysis was conducted by Sonuga-Barke and colleagues (Sonuga-Barke et al., 2013) on randomized controlled trials in the treatment of ADHD which included neurofeedback. The ratings demonstrated comparable effect sizes to the meta-analysis done by Arns and colleagues in 2009. In the teacher ratings there was a tendency towards significance (p=.07). The procedure and criteria of the meta-analysis was critically assessed by Arns et al. (2014) and it was concluded that the weaknesses of the study included that the changes in medication status were not considered, the selection of control conditions was not administered correctly and all studies did not involve the standard training protocols, namely SMR, TBR and SCP. When the data was reprocessed correctly, a significant effect was also obtained from the teacher ratings. The randomized controlled trials that had follow-up to six months and to two years, indicated that the clinical effects of neurofeedback did not disappear and indicated a tendency of further improvement of hyperactivity and impulsivity symptoms over time (Gevensleben et al., 2010).

The best known and most often quoted meta-analysis is probably the meta-analysis conducted by Arns et al. (2009). This meta-analysis was done on neurofeedback studies that have been conducted up to 2009. It was found that the results of the studies were mostly coherent. Non-randomized studies were included in this meta- analysis.

The meta-analysis conducted by Arns included 15 studies including 1 194 ADHD subjects. Five of the studies included in the meta-analysis were randomized controlled trials (RCTs) that included pre and post trials. It was concluded that neurofeedback resulted in large and clinically significant effect sizes for inattention and impulsivity and a medium effect size for hyperactivity. Based on the criteria accepted by the International Society of Neurofeedback and the Association of Applied Psychology based on the research criteria specified by the American Psychological Association (APA), neurofeedback treatment for ADHD can be considered efficacious and specific, meeting the criteria for level 5 treatments.

The meta-analysis conducted by Arns et al. (2009) included SMR training during which SMR is increased and theta (4–7 Hz) is decreased, theta/beta ratio protocols (TBR) during which beta activity at higher frequencies is increased and theta amplitudes are decreased, and operant conditioning of slow cortical potentials. SCP and SMR protocols have been successful in treating epilepsy mainly due to the fact that these protocols teach the individual to regulate cortical excitability more efficiently. Controlled studies comparing SCP and TBR protocols show similar effects on the core symptoms of ADHD.

In *Evidence-Based Practice in Biofeedback & Neurofeedback* (Tan et al., 2016), it is specified that the effect size for neurofeedback on symptoms of inattention are comparable to the effect size reported for methylphenidate. This conclusion is concurred by Arns et al. (2009), Faraone and Buitelaar (2009), Sherlin et al. (2010), in their respective studies. These results are on par with earlier referenced studies in which the effects of neurofeedback were compared with the effects of methylphenidate.

A brief overview of some of the initial studies that lead to the publication of the recent meta-analysis studies on the efficacy of neurofeedback in ADHD will be considered.

The first research done in terms of the SMR training protocol was based on the widely known animal research study conducted by Barry Sterman in the early 1960's that indicated that when 12–16 Hz activity is increased over the sensorimotor strip it results in a decrease in motor activity (Sterman et al., 1969ab). These findings instigated pioneering studies with humans that indicated that humans can learn to modify many aspects of the brains' activity through non-invasive EEG measurement in a combination of operant conditioning and neuroscience. The Sterman study was developed into training protocols for the hyperactive-impulsive ADHD subgroup. Enhancing the amplitude of SMR activity slowed the motor system down and SMR became known as the resting rhythm of the motor system. The counterconditioning or reversal phase study done by Lubar and Shouse (1976) had far reaching implications for neurofeedback and resulted in widespread interest from the scientific fraternity. That study would not be approved by a review board today, but it is the inclusion of the counterconditioning phase that gives strong support to the hypothesis that increased SMR was responsible for the positive changes in core ADHD changes in the study. The main findings were that the two neurofeedback protocols, increasing SMR and decreasing SMR had clear differential effects on the subjects. When neurofeedback was used to increase 12–14 Hz and decrease 4–7 Hz over the sensory motor cortex, the core ADHD symptoms decreased. When neurofeedback was used to increase 4–7 Hz activity and decrease SMR (12–14 Hz activity) ADHD symptoms increased. The improvement in core ADHD symptoms returned when SMR training was reintroduced and these changes were maintained when methylphenidate was withdrawn in the final phase of the study.

Maurice Sterman and Joel Lubar have over 50 peer-reviewed journal articles to date in which the effectiveness of neurofeedback in the treatment of the core symptoms of ADHD are documented.

For the purpose of compiling *The Evidence-Base for Neurofeedback as a Reimbursable Healthcare Service to Treat Attention Deficit/Hyperactivity Disorder,* Pigott and colleagues reviewed the controlled studies during the past decade that evaluated the effectiveness of neurofeedback in treating children with neurofeedback (Pigott et al., 2013). The studies included 701 children and adolescents.

According to that review not all children learned to regulate their EEG. Those that learned to regulate their EEG's best, showed the greatest improvement in symptoms associated with ADHD.

Neurofeedback, when compared to control groups, resulted in significant improvements in parent-rated core symptoms; teacher-rated core symptoms; continuous performance tests of core ADHD symptoms; neuropsychological measures of response inhibition, reaction time and concentration. Neurophysiologic measures relevant to ADHD including QEEG Attention index, Event-Related Potential (P300) during continuous performance testing and activation of regions in the brain related to attention and executive functioning using fMRI improved.

Neurofeedback proved to be significantly superior to sham neurofeedback in the review as well as significantly superior to EMG biofeedback, computerized cognitive training, cognitive behavioral training and waitlist control in improving outcome measures of ADHD core symptoms.

Neurofeedback training resulted in improvements equivalent to improvements achieved by stimulant medication. In a large randomized controlled trial, neurofeedback resulted in improvements equivalent to improvements by stimulant medication alone as well as medication in combination with neurofeedback.

Neurofeedback resulted in EEG changes consistent with the training protocol and these changes persisted in a follow-up assessment after six months as well as after two years. In follow-up studies neurofeedback resulted in significant improvements in core ADHD symptoms that were sustained after six month and two-year follow-up assessments after termination of treatment.

(The studies that were analyzed in the review of which the conclusions were presented can be accessed in the document mentioned above that is available on the ISNR website and elsewhere).

In addition to the review conducted by Pigott et al. (2013), a meta-analysis published online in *Journal of Attention Disorders* in 2012 (see Hodgson et al., 2014; Pigott et al., 2013) indicated that neurofeedback was found to be more than twice as effective in the treatment of ADHD core symptoms than the six other treatments it was compared to namely working memory training, behavior modification, school- based behavior therapy, behaviorally based parent training and behavioral self- monitoring treatments. The five commonly suggested treatments showed negative effect sizes compared to the control group conditions. Four neurofeedback studies involving 301 ADHD child and adolescent subjects finding neurofeedback highly effective were not even included in this meta-analysis due to the cut- off date for study inclusions.

Another breakthrough for neurofeedback in terms of making it more accessible and known as a viable alternative to medication in the treatment of ADHD also occurred in 2012. *Practice Wise* is the company that maintains the ranking of research support for child and adolescent psychosocial treatments of the American Academy of Pediatrics (Practice Wise, n.d.). *Practice Wise* awarded biofeedback/ neurofeedback the highest level of evidence-based support for the treatment of ADHD. The ranking methodology (similar to the ranking system of the APA, ISNR and AAPB) was applied to over 600 randomized controlled trials of psychosocial treatments in support of mental health. The neurofeedback studies were coded by three independent raters. The coding was based on variables pertaining to the quality and relevance of the research including the number of RCTs and resulting effect size of the biofeedback/neurofeedback treatments compared to the experimental control group conditions. The bulk of the studies were on the efficacy of EEG neurofeedback.

The conclusion that can be safely drawn, based on the research to date on the efficacy of neurofeedback in the treatment of ADHD core symptoms involving SCP, TBR and SMR protocols, is that neurofeedback is an efficacious and specific treatment for ADHD.

Chapter 9

Neurofeedback and Anxiety

A chapter on anxiety is included in this book for various reasons. Symptoms and discomfort pertaining to anxiety disorders may arguably be the second most common reason why people seek neurofeedback intervention and all neurofeedback practitioners may consequently be experienced or seeking to become more knowledgeable in dealing with anxiety. Another reason for focusing on anxiety specifically is because of the efficacy and high success rate of general biofeedback and neurofeedback in the treatment of anxiety and anxiety disorders. In the third edition of *Evidence-Based Practice in Biofeedback & Neurofeedback*, Tan et al. (2016) general biofeedback and neurofeedback has, based on the research done to date of the publication, been rated a level 4 treatment (which means that is efficacious based on the research guidelines for efficacy levels as described in chapter 2).

Anxiety disorders are referred to as biopsychosocial disorders. Although we will be taking a fresh look at anxiety and considering all the known components that are involved in anxiety, it is probably the biological component and in particular the involvement of the central nervous system in the presentation of symptoms relating to anxiety, that make general biofeedback and neurofeedback potential main role players in treatment or training plans for those who suffer anxiety to a debilitating extent. Cognitive behavior therapy (CBT) is regarded by many as the golden standard in treating anxiety disorders but possibly bio-and neurofeedback are catching up. The reader may want to refer to chapter 6 again for the discussion of the physiological stress response. We will however consider the involvement of different physiological systems afresh in this chapter albeit from a less technical perspective. This chapter is meant to bring an improved understanding of the anxiety phenomenon to practitioners and lay readers alike.

Anxiety is in essence an emotion and all human emotions are normal. It is however a secondary emotion and is mainly based on fear which is a primary emotion. Anxiety can thus be considered to be normal in a moderate degree. Anxiety is necessary and often protects us in that it causes us to strive and grow. Think of the anticipated threat you perceive when you see a falling tree or a driver that has lost control. You fear the potential consequences and avoid an accident. The student that fears that he/she will fail at his/her tests, studies harder and succeeds. Our concern is with symptoms of anxiety that negatively influence the quality of the individual's life on any level and not with the normal stress response that is functional. To better understand anxiety, we will, however, consider the dynamic of the normal response.

David Barlow, well known for his pioneering work on anxiety, defined anxiety as a future-oriented mood state that is focused on the anticipation of negative events (Barlow, 2002). If we define normal as being usual, ordinary, regular, or common, we would not be able to consider anxiety as being abnormal. Most, if not all, humans experience anxiety regularly and probably more than usual during times of transition and challenge and often anxiety serves us as mentioned before. It would be a matter of concern if an individual would not experience anxiety during trying times. That could in fact be indicative of psychopathology.

Low to moderate levels of anxiety can be beneficial. It heightens our arousal levels in situations where it may be necessary. It can make us more task- orientated, focused, alert and motivated. Certain chemicals such as adrenaline and noradrenaline are released, but beyond a certain point too much of these and other chemicals (to be discussed further on) have a very negative effect on our performance and on our health. Our focus then moves away from the task and zooms in on the physical discomfort we feel which becomes a vicious cycle. We attempt to deal with the distressing thoughts about the discomfort by worrying, which is counterproductive.

Anxiety is considered pathological when it interferes with a person's functioning and overall well-being. According to Jacofsky et al., (2013) the three factors to be considered in the gauging of whether the anxiety in question is normal or adaptive or pathological, are duration, intensity and frequency. Abnormal anxiety is disproportionate to the situation or circumstances that triggered the response. When the duration, intensity or frequency becomes chronic or impairs an individual's quality of life, it becomes pathological. There are different anxiety disorders that are variant forms of abnormal or pathological anxiety. The different anxiety disorders are characterized by different symptoms. The main considerations by which adaptive or normal anxiety are distinguished from abnormal anxiety, are the same however. When the anxiety causes significant distress or when it impairs social functioning, occupational functioning or functioning in any other important area of the individual's life, it can be considered abnormal anxiety. From the perspective of the neurofeedback practitioner, the only important consideration is whether the person's functioning is affected negatively, in which case the person will be experiencing discomfort.

The National Institute of Mental Health indicated in 2008 that forty million Americans suffered an anxiety disorder each year. That percentage indicated a prevalence rate of 18, 1%. The first episode of anxiety is indicated by the same study to occur before the age of twenty-two. Whether or not this prevalence rate is representative of different countries and cultures or not, it is reasonable to assume that anxiety symptoms are very common and cause discomfort to millions of people. Should we accept these statistics as being roughly representative of most groups of people, that would mean that anxiety affects the lives of roughly one out of five individuals.

The symptoms of anxiety can be divided into physical, emotional, cognitive, and behavioral symptoms. The physical symptoms include a feeling of restlessness, shortness of breath, sweaty palms, racing heart, chest pain or discomfort, muscle tension, trembling, feeling shaky, nausea or diarrhea, butterflies in the stomach, dizziness or feeling faint, hot flashes, chills, numbness or tingling sensations, an exaggerated startle response and sleep disturbances or fatigue.

The physiological symptoms are based on the changes that occur in the body when the fight or flight response is triggered. The body cannot distinguish between a real threat, in which case a fear response would be appropriate, and an imagined or anticipated threat or danger, which is what anxiety is.

The emotional symptoms include feelings of apprehension, distress, dread, nervousness, feeling overwhelmed, panic, uneasiness, worry, fear or terror and jumpiness or edginess.

The thoughts people experience when having anxiety are often described as worry (Bourne, 2000). Common themes according to Jacofsky et al. (2013) are concerns about specific things that may happen, for example "what if . . .' -thoughts. Another common cognitive symptom is that the anxiety sufferer needs to be certain about something in particular so they will feel the need to reaffirm repeatedly. This is often something insignificant. The thought may be something like "I must have certainty". They will, for instance, have obsessive thoughts about the significance of the anxiety symptoms. They could also get stuck on the thought that people may laugh at them. Some people with phobias for enclosed spaces will repeatedly think that they will not be able to escape. Another common obsessive thought is that the person has concerns about going crazy. The anxiety sufferer may also get stuck on a thought like "Oh my God, what's happening to me?".

Behavioral symptoms include avoidance behaviors such as, for instance, avoiding elevators or social situations or any anxiety provoking situation. The person suffering anxiety may present with escaping behavior in that they run out of a church or crowded shopping mall. They may engage in unhealthy or risky behavior in an attempt to get relief from anxiety by drinking too much or using addictive substances. They may attempt to reduce anxiety by remaining in their restricted safe space which results in limiting their daily activities. They may become overly attached to a person or safety object and resist being separated from the person or object.

People with anxiety disorders often have problems with concentration, memory, appetite, and mood.

In the biopsychosocial model of anxiety, the causes of anxiety are categorized in three groups, namely biological causes, psychological causes and environmental or social causes.

The biological component of anxiety includes the body's physiological or adaptive response to fear as well as genetic traits which we inherit. Bourne, (2000), speaks of a personality type that we can inherit that is more sensitive and reactive to stress. Despite the fact that we may have inherited a heightened receptivity to stress, that alone cannot cause an anxiety disorder. Psychological factors such as our thoughts and beliefs about our experiences and our perceived sense of control over our lives all influence whether we regard something as being a threat or not. Our thoughts about ourselves and our environment play an important role in the development of an anxiety disorder. Anxiety develops from the perceived gap between one's estimated ability to cope with a challenge and the perceived or estimated difficulty of the task or challenge (Jacofsky et al., 2013). The bigger the gap, the bigger the risk of developing an anxiety disorder. A person with a lack of confidence will necessarily estimate the challenge or goal to be achieved as beyond his/her ability.

The third component that has an influence in the development of an anxiety disorder, is the environment. According to Barlow (2002), the social component of the biopsychosocial model implies that environmental factors may trigger, shape and strengthen the biological and psychological weaknesses. These factors may include tragic events, financial problems, or loss. Role models can also have a significant influence on the development of an anxiety disorder. Peer pressure groups may have an influence in that the individual becomes preoccupied with the evaluations of the peers which may lead to excessive worrying, avoidance behavior and feelings of anxiety.

According to the social learning theory (SLT) of Albert Bandura (1977), individuals learn new ways of thinking and behaving by observing others, unlike the more traditional view of behaviorism which teaches that we learn behavior as a result of a direct experience. According to SLT a person may have learned to become anxious based on contact with other people. The social environment also influences our development of beliefs about ourselves. In CBT a healthy environment is created in which the therapist becomes a new role model that expresses confidence in the individual's abilities. Social learning according to the social learning theory, may thus not only contribute to the development of an anxiety disorder but may also facilitate recovery from an anxiety disorder.

The biological component of the biopsychosocial model of anxiety is of special interest to the neurofeedback practitioners and those anxiety sufferers who wish to consider general biofeedback or neurofeedback as an intervention.

The main area of focus in the rest of this chapter will be the role of six of the interrelated systems in the body, including the central nervous system in their influence on anxiety experiences, rather than the genetic component of the biological factors. According to Jacofsky et al. (2013), genetic predisposition has been implicated in panic disorder and phobias). The systems involved are the nervous system, the cardiovascular system, the respiratory system, the digestive system, the excretory system and the endocrine system. These systems are responsible for the electrical, chemical, and physiological changes that affect the presentation and the experience of anxiety symptoms.

We can think of the command center of the body as being the brain that coordinates the other systems and dictates their actions. It is consequently important for us to consider what happens in the brain when it perceives danger or anticipates a threat. The important distinction between fear and anxiety is that fear is a reaction to the presence of danger whereas anxiety is the reaction to anticipated danger. It is essential to note that the mind cannot distinguish between the two. When the individual is busy with thoughts about an anticipated threat in the future the mind responds in the same way as when the threat is present. At the thought of danger, the body gets messages from the brain to prepare itself. Chemical and electrical messages are sent from the brain to prepare the body for protecting itself (the fight response) or to escape the danger (the flee response). Two important structures in the brain involved in activating the chemical changes are the hippocampus and the amygdala which are both part of the limbic system. The limbic system represents the emotional center of the brain. The hippocampus is mainly responsible for memory functions. When the body goes into a higher state of arousal due to a perceived threat, the hippocampus becomes activated and checks for memories of previous similar experiences which then heightens the symptoms of fear and/or anxiety. The amygdala is responsible for regulating emotions such as fear (Jacofsky et al., 2013) but also for scanning the environment for signs of danger and sending the alarm signal when dangers are detected.

The amygdala communicates with the hypothalamus (amongst other structures and regions of interest) which has a very important function with respect to anxiety. The hypothalamus controls the autonomic nervous system including chemical and hormonal neurotransmitters. The autonomic nervous system and the chemical substances involved have important roles in the production of anxiety symptoms as the body prepares itself for dealing with the threat. When the body senses danger, the amygdala thus sends a message via the hypothalamus to the autonomic nervous system to prepare for fight or flight.

The autonomic nervous system (ANS) has two sub-systems that have opposing effects. These sub-systems are the sympathetic nervous system (SNS) and the parasympathetic nervous system (PNS). Although the working of the SNS and PNS have been discussed in chapter 6 in terms of the stress response, it is discussed in this chapter as well so that this chapter on anxiety can function as a standalone chapter for different applications.

Only one of the sub-systems of the ANS can be active at any given time. The SNS has been compared to the "on" position of a light switch and the PNS to the "off" position (Jacofsky et al., 2013). The SNS is thus responsible for preparing the body for the fight or flight response whereas the PNS initiates the rest and digest response. It is important to understand that the "on" and "off" positions in our analogy implicate an all or nothing response. Once the sympathetic nervous system has been triggered it has a chain of reactions. It has been said that it takes 90 seconds to reverse this reaction when circumstances are optimal in terms of the absence of the threat and ideal actions in terms of thought processes and other factors. As mentioned earlier, when the stress response is appropriate, it is functional and can save our lives. When we experience an inappropriate and extended or chronic stress response however, it can be very debilitating. Other than that, the chemicals hormones and neurotransmitters, associated with activation, may become depleted when anxiety symptoms do not abate.

Back to the snowball effect once the SNS has been triggered: The adrenal glands get the message to release adrenaline and noradrenaline, also known as epinephrine and norepinephrine. These chemicals act as fuel to the body. Some of the readers may be aware of the extreme lethargy associated with hypo activity of the adrenal gland. When the threat has passed and the person stops anticipating a further danger or threat, the PNS kicks in and activates relaxation. The anxious feelings and physical sensations, until the PNS restores a state of relaxation, include feelings and sensations of dizziness, light-headedness, chest pain, racing heart, tingling sensations, breathing difficulties, nausea, upset stomach, stomach pain, dry mouth, constipation and perspiration. These symptoms are created by the activation of the sympathetic nervous system in order to activate other parts of the body that may be needed to function optimally during fighting or fleeing.

These physiological symptoms involve the cardiovascular system, the respiratory system, the excretory system and the digestive system. A better understanding of these symptoms can be very helpful during the extreme discomfort of the experience of the symptoms. We tend to cope much better with discomfort of which we understand the origin and dynamic than symptoms that we fear the origin of. The spiral of anxiety is such that it feeds itself. The more uncertainty exists about what is happening, the more the cognitive, emotional, and psychological associated symptoms get exacerbated. A closer look at the involvement of the cardiovascular system in the sympathetic nervous system (when the fight and flight response is activated) shows us that the heart beats faster in order to pump more blood because of the additional oxygen required by the muscles to be able to function optimally.

The faster heartbeat can cause extreme discomfort to the extent that a person can fear that they are having a heart attack. This is not an uncommon perception. A further complicating factor is that the body restricts the blood flow to areas that do not need it as much as the large muscles in the arms and legs may need it in a crisis. The blood flow will, for instance, be restricted to the fingertips and toes. Skin temperature is a marker of anxiety that is addressed in general biofeedback and is also often added to neurofeedback. Hand warming visualization exercises are also recommended as a stress management tool and are described elsewhere in this book.

The blood flow to the brain is also restricted temporarily which often causes the most uncomfortable anxiety related symptoms. Feelings of dizziness, light- headedness and a sense of unreality are not uncommon. This temporary restriction of the blood flow to the brain happens because the fight and flight response is more focused on the ability of the body to fight or flee than on improving cognitive clarity. Temporary memory problems and concentration problems can also ensue. No long lasting harmful effects are caused during this process other than the discomfort and the impact that it has on the individual psychologically.

The respiratory system is affected immediately when the heart starts beating faster in order to increase the availability of the amount of oxygen. The additional oxygen provides more energy to the muscles immediately. The person experiencing this chain of events will feel out of breath or as if they cannot get enough air which in turn contributes to the feeling of light- headedness. Tightness in the chest can also be experienced. (The importance of breathing is central to general biofeedback and has been discussed elaborately in chapter 6).

The SNS also affects the excretory system in that it causes the body to perspire. Perspiration controls the temperature of the body and prevents it from overheating in a crisis situation. When the muscles and the heart work very hard, heat is generated. Perspiration also makes a person more slippery which serves the function of making it difficult for the attacker to hold on to the individual.

The digestive system gets shut down during anxiety because in a crisis situation – the ability to digest food is not regarded as important. The body does not lose any energy or fuel so to speak to what is not of crucial importance during the anticipated crisis. Many gastrointestinal symptoms result from the shutting down of the digestive system by the sympathetic nervous system. Nausea and stomach pains and dry mouth are not uncommon. There has been a lot of focus on the relation between the brain and the gut during the past decade.

The activation of the SNS causes the entire body to work harder which often results in exhaustion and fatigue.

The nervous system communicates with the rest of the body, excluding the endocrine system, with electrical signals. The communication of the endocrine system occurs via chemical messengers. The two types of chemical messengers involved are hormones that travel throughout the entire body through the bloodstream and neurotransmitters that are operational in the brain. Two hormones, adrenaline and noradrenaline are released by the adrenal glands when the sympathetic nervous system is activated. The adrenal glands are part of the endocrine system. These two chemicals are found in the brain as well and are therefore neurotransmitters as well. Adrenaline and noradrenaline are activating and cause the heart rate to accelerate and the blood pressure to rise.

Corticotropin releasing hormone (CRH) is another stress related hormone which plays its part in activating the body. According to Jacofsky et al. (2013), research indicates that high levels of CRH are hypothesized to be associated with anxiety related symptoms in humans. This hormone is also involved in the activation of the hypothalamic-pituitary-adrenocortical (HPA) axis. The HPA, a part of the neuroendocrine system, is also involved in the stress response and has been associated with anxiety and depression.

The chemical substances in the brain involved in relaying messages between neurons are called neurotransmitters. The neurotransmitter most commonly associated with anxiety symptoms is serotonin. Selective serotonin inhibitors (SSRI's) are often prescribed for anxiety disorders because individuals suffering anxiety generally have a deficit of serotonin. The use of SSRIs, increase the availability of serotonin. Serotonin also affects mood, appetite, and sleep.

Gamma-aminobutyric acid (GABA) is another neurotransmitter that is involved in anxiety. GABA is an inhibiting neurotransmitter that slows the neural transmission down and calms the brain. Individuals with deficiencies of GABA are believed to be more anxious because of the fact that their bodies will always be with heightened arousal and readiness for any eventuality. Benzodiazepines (a group of medication) are believed to increase the release of GABA which then slows the body down.

Let's remind ourselves again that the stress response in the body is a normal and necessary response designed to protect us and help us to survive. The normal stress response is activated in the face of a perceived threat or dangerous situation and dissipates when the threat is over. Ledoux (1998) discussed the simple example of fearing a stick until we register that it is not a snake. He described the process by which the autonomic nervous system and the limbic areas of the brain react before the cortex gets involved. In this description the fight/flight response which was discussed earlier in this chapter gets activated. This process explains the fight/flight mechanism from a physiological perspective.

Porges (1995) describes the freeze mechanism that can replace the fight/flight response. Porges argues that the unmyelinated vagal nerve (not the myelinated vagal nerve) which is the tenth cranial nerve can trigger an alternative to fight/ flight that represents a freeze action and presents as immobilization, passive avoidance, PTSD, and the inability to move forward.

There ought to be a healthy dance between the activation of the sympathetic nervous system, the deactivation of the sympathetic nervous system and the activation of the parasympathetic nervous system. When we need to flee from a lion or fight off an attacker, the process of the activation of the sympathetic nervous system serves a protective function and does not cause long lasting and lingering discomfort. (I am not referring to the potential psychological trauma involved in facing a lion!). When all the above mentioned physiological and neurochemical processes occur and the added available energy is not applied in a fight or flight action, it causes immense discomfort. What makes it worse is that seldom or ever is that energy appropriate to the sufferer of an anxiety disorder because the perceived threats are anticipated and the circumstances in which they are perceived, do not allow for jumping, running, fighting, shouting or any type of release.

The reader will now understand that certain biological and neurochemical processes can put an individual at a heightened risk of developing anxiety symptoms. A biological or neurochemical predisposition on its own is not believed to be able to cause an anxiety disorder. Individuals with a biological predisposition to anxiety in conjunction with a psychological vulnerability are more likely to develop an anxiety disorder (Jacofsky et al., 2013).

The psychological components relevant to the development of an anxiety disorder have been indicated by research to be perceived control, cognitive appraisals, cognitive beliefs, and cognitive distortions. An elaborate discussion of these components is beyond the scope of this book and will therefore be discussed very briefly for the sake of those readers that may want to do further research on these components.

According to Dr David Barlow (2002), psychological vulnerability to anxiety may be developed because of an early life experience of a lack of perceived control over stressful life circumstances. Children who regularly have the perception that they have no control over the events of their lives may develop a tendency to expect negative outcomes and develop a sense of helplessness. Both over- protective and under-protective parenting styles can lead to the development of the perception that the world is a dangerous place. Ongoing childhood trauma can also cause a psychological vulnerability that may lead to the development of an anxiety disorder.

Lazarus and Folkman (1984) have distinguished between different categories of cognitive appraisals. A cognitive appraisal is the way in which an individual evaluates an occurrence or situation. Some types of appraisals lead to positive beliefs whereas a stress appraisal leads to a belief that harm will occur. Such a belief will lead to an experience of anxiety. The secondary appraisal, pertaining to the individual's perceived ability to control the event or circumstance, is also a determining factor in whether the individual will experience anxiety or not.

Ellis (1997) is of the belief that stressors in the environment are not what determine behavior or emotional responses, but that the belief of the individual about his or ability to cope with the stressor is what determines behavior. The core beliefs of the individual about himself and the world are the organizing principles by which any situation is interpreted or understood. These core beliefs are often not conscious beliefs. One of the goals of cognitive therapy is to bring these core beliefs into awareness (Jacofsky et al., 2013).

According to Beck et al. (1985), people are likely to make errors in their thinking in their appraisals of situations. These errors are called cognitive distortions. Two common cognitive distortions pertaining to anxiety involve the overestimation of the threat and the under-estimation of the individual's ability to cope with the threat.

In cognitive behavior therapy (CBT) the individual is taught to change problematic beliefs and thinking patterns and to engage in adaptive behaviors. As mentioned earlier, CBT has been considered the "gold standard" of treatments for anxiety disorders.

That anxiety will be treated is advisable because it has the potential to affect quality of life considerably. It can affect academic performance, cause an individual to resist important medical examinations and result in an individual avoiding normal, healthy activities and social interaction. According to the DSM-5 (APA, 2013), anxiety qualifies as an anxiety disorder when it becomes habitual, relatively chronic, impairs everyday life significantly and meets the diagnostic criteria of panic disorder, agoraphobia, specific phobia, generalized anxiety disorder, social anxiety disorder, separation anxiety disorder or selective mutism. Many heart rate variability (HRV) studies, biofeedback-assisted relaxation training studies, skin conductance studies, electro-myographic biofeedback studies (EMG) and neurofeedback studies have been conducted with generalized anxiety disorder, alcohol abuse with comorbid anxiety, anxiety accompanying eating disorders, anxiety in gifted children and panic disorder, to mention but a few, with varying results. According to Tan et al. (2016), thirty years of research have shown therapeutic benefits of general biofeedback for students' anxiety, anxiety accompanying medical disorders, and conditions and anxiety disorders. There is adequate evidence to support that general biofeedback meets the Level 4: Efficacious standard of clinical efficacy for student anxiety, anxiety accompanying medical disorders and anxiety disorders. There is a growing body of evidence that proves the efficacy of neurofeedback specifically as a modality of biofeedback, for anxiety. Of the many available research studies, a few have been selected to be included in this chapter.

A randomized controlled study of 45 individuals with a diagnosis of generalized anxiety disorder (GAD) was published by Rice, Blanchard and Purcell (1993). The individuals were treated with frontal electro-myographic (EMG) biofeedback, neurofeedback to increase alpha, neurofeedback to decrease alpha activity or were treated with a pseudo- medication control condition. The participants completed eight training sessions at a frequency of two per week.

All participants completed the STAI (State Trait Anxiety Index), the Welsch-A Scale and the Psychosomatic Symptom Checklist. These anxiety checklists were completed at baseline before treatment, two weeks post treatment and six weeks post treatment. The participants were also monitored with HR (heart rate) in a relaxation trial and also in two stress conditions.

The results showed significant decreases on the STAI in all four treatment conditions and not in the control group. The alpha-increase training groups showed significant improvements on the Welsch-A Scale and so did the EMG groups. In the post- intervention assessment it was only the alpha-increase group that showed reduced reactivity of HR. The authors suggested that alpha-increase training in neurofeedback and EMG training in general biofeedback, seemed the most promising modalities in the treatment of anxiety.

In another study of 45 individuals with GAD conducted by Agnihotry et al. (2007), the 45 participants were randomly assigned to a surface EMG relaxation group, an increase alpha-EEG group and a control group. The participants received training for twelve consecutive days. Post treatment, the alpha-increase group as well as the EMG relaxation group showed significant improvements on the State and Trait Anxiety Index. Galvanic skin resistance was measured as a physiologic index of relaxation and improved post treatment with both groups.

According to H. Corydon Hammond in an article published in *Journal of Adult Development* (2005), Moore reviewed eight studies of training GAD with neurofeedback, and although according to Hammond there were problems with the training periods, seven of the studies still showed clear positive clinical outcomes. In this article Hammond mentions many more research studies in which alpha- enhancement neurofeedback had positive clinical outcomes with anxious alcoholics, PTSD sufferers and OCD sufferers.

According to Cynthia Kerson (2017), anxiety is often the symptom of underlying dysregulations. In her opinion, adolescents and young adults tend to be very interested in their health and often experience that medication and other alternative treatments do not render success. Adolescents and young adults appear to be the age group that is at high risk of developing anxiety. According to a study conducted by Blanco et al. (2008), the diagnoses of anxiety and depression are on the rise across the lifespan, with the largest effected age group being teenagers and young adults.

In her chapter titled "Neurofeedback as a Treatment for Anxiety in Adolescents and Young Adults" in the book *Handbook of Clinical EEG and Neurotherapy*, Cynthia Kerson (2017) mentions that the neurofeedback protocol and assessment options have increased making it a more effective treatment modality than ten years ago. She suggests that the neurofeedback practitioner ought to be attentive to excessive beta amplitude (which may include spindling) alpha asymmetry in the frontal lobes and non- attenuating posterior alpha with eyes open based on an eyes- closed assessment. These three brainwave patterns in the assessment are shown to be specific to anxiety. Kerson suggests that one training protocol may not be enough and that she has had more success with training posterior pathologies first. Protocol importance ought to, according to Kerson, be based on symptoms and goals after a QEEG recording. When considering training the excessive beta, 20–24 Hz excessive activity is often representative of worry and rumination while excessive 25–30 Hz activity often represents muscle artefact.

Alpha/Theta training (discussed in chapter 5) is considered a helpful protocol for anxiety by many practitioners and researchers.

In their chapter entitled "sLORETA Neurofeedback as a Treatment for PTSD", in the book *Handbook of Clinical EEG and Neurotherapy* (Collura & Frederick, 2017), Getter et al. indicate that information from neuroimaging studies suggests that a specific network involving the amygdala, the vmPFC and the hippocampus is very significant in PTSD. Fear is attributed to hyper-activation of the amygdala and to the exaggerated sensitivity of PTSD-individuals to threatening signals. Intervention in the activity of one of the structures involved in the relevant network, can affect the entire network which results in a reduction of symptoms of PTSD (Getter et al., 2017). The same authors recognize the efficacy of enhancing alpha as suggested by many researchers in the treatment of PTSD disorder but also to consider the efficacy of low resolution tomography (LORETA) neurofeedback for the treatment of PTSD. Although the authors of the mentioned chapter indicate that their suggested LORETA neurofeedback protocol for PTSD sufferers still needs to be evaluated, they report anecdotal evidence of the efficacy of increasing theta activity in vmPFC.

Based on anecdotal evidence from my own practice as well as the anecdotal evidence reported in clinical discussion groups and mentoring programs in South Africa, it appears that the success rate of general biofeedback training as well as neurofeedback training involving alpha-enhancing protocols is very high.

In 2019 one of our own neurofeedback practitioners in South Africa, Karlien Balt, did a presentation at the ISNR conference on the efficacy of ISF (Infra Slow Frequency) neurofeedback training on adults suffering anxiety.

It is safe to conclude that not only has neurofeedback become a viable and responsible choice of treatment for anxiety disorder, but that the rapidly expanding body of evidence of the efficacy of different sub modalities of neurofeedback in the treatment of anxiety disorders, makes individualized customized protocols possible that may well bring relief to those individuals who do not respond well to medication.

Chapter 10

Neurofeedback and Depression

Depressive Disorders are undoubtedly and predictably among the disorders that have been researched most frequently on the premise of the high and it appears, ever increasing, prevalence and incidence of depression among different age groups.

All health care workers from different disciplines work with clients and patients suffering symptoms of depression regularly. The two main reasons for the inclusion of this chapter in the book is to provide knowledge to the reader suffering depression with which to illuminate the darkness depression exudes and to better equip neurofeedback practitioners who work with depressive clients to change the experience of the sufferers of depression. An additional reason is that referring clinicians will take note of the efficacy of neurofeedback as a treatment for depression in order to be able to make better informed and responsible referrals especially for those patients who are resistant to medication, whether it be for physiological or emotional reasons.

In the current *Diagnostic and Statistical Manual of Mental Disorders* (DSM-5) (APA, 2013) different kinds of depressive disorders are listed, distinguished by duration and the link to various causes. It is stated in the DSM-5 that the common feature in all of the depressive disorders is the presence of a sad, empty or irritable mood, accompanied by somatic and cognitive changes that significantly affect the individual's capacity to function. The difference between depressive disorder due to another medical condition, substance or medication induced depressive disorder and major depressive disorder is the duration, the timing or the presumed etiology. Exclusion and inclusion criteria of depressive disorders specified in the DSM-5 are contentious matters which lead to the inclusion of a footnote, and will be discussed briefly further on. For the purpose of this book, we will be focusing mainly on major depressive disorder.

The persistent feeling of sadness or loss of pleasure or interest, characterizes major depression. Major depression is a mood disorder that affects the way you feel about life in general. Having a helpless or hopeless outlook on life is the most common symptom of depression. Other feelings may include feelings of worthlessness, self-hate, and inappropriate guilt. When there are persistent feelings of sadness and loss of pleasure for at least two weeks and the presence of five or more depressive symptoms are prevalent, the criteria of major depressive disorder as specified in the DSM-5 are met. The symptoms are: *sleeping too much or too little; psychomotor retardation or agitation; change in weight or appetite; loss of energy; feelings of being worthless or guilty; a perception of poor concentration* and *an inability to think or make decisions and repeated thoughts of death and/or suicide* (Beidel et al., 2014).

In terms of mood, the person suffering depression may experience *anxiety, apathy, general discontent, guilt, loss of interest in pleasurable activities, mood swings* or *sadness*. Sleep patterns are generally affected negatively and depression may either cause *early awakening, insomnia, restless sleep* or *wanting to sleep too much*. The behavior of the individual suffering depression may be affected in terms of being more *agitated, crying excessively, being irritable and isolating him-/herself* and *avoiding social interaction*. The depressed person will often withdraw from activities he/she used to enjoy or looked forward to doing. He/she will no longer have an interest in his/her hobbies or sports he/she used to love and avoid going out with friends. Symptoms of major depression include *decreased sex drive* and *even impotence*. A *feeling of constant fatigue* which leads to *excessive sleeping* is not uncommon. Sleeping too much may, of course, lead to insomnia which in turn feeds the feelings of fatigue. The lack of sleep may cause or exacerbate anxiety. Depression and anxiety often occur together. Anxiety, discussed at length in the previous chapter, is characterized by nervousness, feeling tense, feelings of dread or danger, rapid heart rate, trembling or muscle twitching, difficulty with focusing and worrying.

According to Timothy Legg (n.d.), depression often affects men and women differently. Men with depression often present with symptoms such as irritability, risky behavior, escapism, misplaced anger and substance abuse. Both men and women can present with mood swings which can range from an outburst of anger to crying uncontrollably without any external trigger.

Suicide is always a real threat in the presence of major depression. In 2013 more than 42,000 people committed suicide in the United States (Legg, n.d.). Usually people suffering depression will talk about suicide or make a first attempt at suicide before succeeding at it.

There is, according to Dr Corydon Hammond (2005), a robust body of evidence that suggests that there are biological predispositions that often exist for depression (and also for anxiety and obsessive-compulsive disorder) and that relatively new research has indicated that medication is often only mildly more effective than placebo (a substance or treatment of no intended therapeutic value). EEG biofeedback or neurofeedback offers a viable and non-invasive alternative to the treatment of depression. The efficacy of neurofeedback in the treatment of Depressive disorders has been ranked at level 4 in *Evidence-Based Practice in Biofeedback and Neurofeedback* (Tan et al., 2016). In other words it is considered to be efficacious after an analysis of the available research. Neurofeedback has been found to be statistically significantly superior or equivalent to control conditions.

Very often the biological aspects of mental disorders are neglected simply because the average psychologist and therapists from other disciplines are not trained in ways to modify the functioning of the brain. Davidson (1998) summarized and documented research information that clearly indicated a difference in activation levels of the left and right prefrontal cortex. Many EEG studies summarized by Davidson indicate that the left frontal area is associated with more positive affect and memories whereas the right hemisphere is more involved in negative emotion. Higher amplitudes of left frontal alpha in comparison to right frontal alpha which implies alpha asymmetry, indicates a biological predisposition to depression. The higher alpha amplitude in the left frontal cortex indicates that the left frontal area is less activated. These individuals may consequently be less in touch with positive emotions and more aware of negative emotions associated with the right hemisphere.

A study done by Henriques and Davidson (1991) also indicated that the left hemisphere is associated with approach motivation, whereas the right hemisphere is more associated with withdrawal behavior (Hammond, 2005). When the left hemisphere is in an idling state in an alpha rhythm, there will be more withdrawal behavior as well as an absence of positive affect.

A study done by Dawson et al. (1992) indicated that even infants of depressed mothers displayed reduced left frontal EEG activation. A study duplicated by Field et al. (1995) proved the reduced left frontal activation in 3–6 month old infants of depressed mothers. Baehr et al. (1997) as well as Askew (2001) indicated that frontal alpha asymmetry may be a state marker of depression and a trait marker of a vulnerability to depression. Askew (2001) found a strong correlation between frontal alpha asymmetry and scores on the Beck Depression Inventory (BDI).

Based on the vast body of research on the significance of frontal alpha asymmetry in depression, Rosenfeld (1997) developed a neurofeedback protocol for modifying frontal alpha asymmetry. His protocol is F4-F3/ F3+F4 with placement of a reference electrode at Cz. Rosenfeld reported on a series of case studies of depressed patients (Rosenfeld, 2000). Before the neurofeedback sessions, the patients were taught to breathe diaphragmatically for 15–30 minutes and to warm their hands to 95 degrees Fahrenheit. Active electrodes were placed at F3 and F4 and both referenced to Cz. Training sessions twice a week were divided into 50% neurofeedback and 50% psychotherapy. In some cases the BDI and Minnesota Multiphasic Personality Inventory (MMPI) scores declined as the alpha asymmetry improved.

Baehr et al. (2001) reported on one- and five-year follow-ups on three patients treated with a frontal alpha asymmetry neurofeedback protocol that there were substantial changes in symptoms as well as in frontal alpha asymmetry. The alpha asymmetry remained eliminated on the long-term follow-ups. This is very significant to the field of neurofeedback because there are numerous studies conducted by Allen et al. (1993, 2004), Gotlib et al. (1999), Kwon et al. (1996) that indicated that medication caused remission of the symptoms but that the frontal asymmetry remained, indicating a continued vulnerability to future depression.

Hammond (2000) reported a case study with his own protocol to address alpha asymmetry with an eight-and-a-half-month follow-up. The protocol he used involved electrodes on FP1 and F3 with an inhibit of slow alpha and theta and a reward of 15–18 Hz for 22 minutes after which time the reward frequency was changed to 12–15 Hz for eight to ten minutes. The severe depression of the patient was alleviated and the frontal alpha asymmetry was eliminated.

In *Journal of Adult Development* Hammond (2005) reports on another sample of nine patients with an average age of 43 years ranging from 34 to 50 years that met the criteria of alpha asymmetry of the Rosenfeld protocol and depression according to the MMPI. Eight subjects completed the treatment. After twenty thirty-minute sessions, seven out of the eight subjects showed significant improvements after a one year follow up with no psychotherapy or medication. Including the drop-out as failure, the results indicated that 77,8% showed significant improvements. The post treatment MMPI scores indicated a mean decrease of 28, 75 t-scores Peeters et al. (2014) reported a pilot study of nine subjects suffering depression receiving a maximum of thirty sessions of alpha asymmetry neurofeedback. Alpha asymmetry declined significantly and five showed significant reduction or complete remission of depressive symptoms as scored on the Quick Inventory of Depressive Symptoms. For treatment of alpha asymmetry in this study, active electrodes at F3 and F4 were referenced to A1 and A2.

An alternative neurofeedback protocol to treat depression, involves enhancing faster alpha in the occipital-parietal region. Although there is clear evidence that this protocol has successfully increased cognitive performance, there is limited evidence of the success of the protocol for the treatment of major depression.

Although the significance of biological markers has been established and renders it important that the responsible neurofeedback practitioner will establish whether there is indeed frontal alpha asymmetry, there is also research available that has indicated the significance of other biological factors. Certain structures of the brain have been indicated in their involvement in depression as well as certain neuronal pathways, specific neurotransmitters and also differences in neuroplasticity according to recent research studies. The influence of hormone levels in the bloodstream can also affect the entire body as well as the brain. The effect of cortisol on depression has been well researched. It is still not clear, however, whether higher cortisol levels are a cause or an effect of depression. As is the case with the development of anxiety disorders, there are also psychosocial factors that play a role in the predisposition to depression.

The structures of the brain that have mainly been implicated in the presence of depression are the frontal lobes, limbic structures, and the hypothalamus. We have already discussed the phenomenon of slowing in the left frontal lobe that can be addressed very efficiently with alpha asymmetry protocols.

Abnormalities in neuronal pathways that use certain neurotransmitters that communicate information may have an effect on the frontal lobes and the limbic structures. Collections of neurons that produce neurotransmitters have their somas or cell bodies in the brainstem, which is the structure below the cerebrum. Long axons get projected from these cell bodies to various areas of the cerebrum. One such a pathway starts in the raphe nuclei of the brainstem and is responsible for the secretion of serotonin. There are different groups of raphe nuclei at different levels of the brainstem that send many axon projections to different areas of the cerebrum, including the frontal lobes and to the limbic structures. The role of serotonin in depressive disorders is well known and is a main focus of a group of anti-depressants called serotonin reuptake inhibitors. The SSRIs make more serotonin available in the communication processes in the brain. Another pathway starts in the locus coeruleus which also sends long axons into the cerebrum and releases norepinephrine which also has a significant role in depression. Another pathway starts with the ventral tegmental area in the brainstem and communicates with different areas of the cerebrum, including the frontal lobes and limbic structures by means of projections of axons and in the process dopamine gets supplied to the brain.

The role of dopamine in depressive disorders has also been extensively researched. The disciplines involved mostly in addressing the neurotransmitter balances that have an influence on the development and enduring of depression are psychiatry and pharmacotherapy. Other influential factors in the focus on the role of the neurotransmitters in depression, is the funding available for research and marketing where the drug companies play a significant role.

The "new kid on the block" in terms of the role players in the etiology of depression, is neuroplasticity which is in essence the ability of the brain to form and reorganize synaptic connections especially in response to learning or experience. It is hypothesized that negative early childhood experiences and exposures may influence the neuroplasticity of the brain in a way that make it more vulnerable to depression. Neuroplasticity is a main premise of the success of neurofeedback. This concept was discussed at length in previous chapters.

Most neurofeedback practitioners and other clinicians will have experienced concern about a sudden diagnosis of major depressive disorder of a person that they have consulted for a period of time. They will possibly be aware of circumstances that have changed in the individual's life that equates to trying times, but they would never have suspected the individual to have major depressive disorder.

The diagnosis done by a psychiatrist will undoubtedly be correct according to the DSM-5 (APA, 2013). The author is guiding the reader in a roundabout way to think about depression from a wider perspective. A main reason for this tour if you wish, through the perspectives of the different lenses of the different disciplines with mostly honorable motives, is for the neurofeedback practitioner to think of other possible protocols that may be helpful for those sufferers of depression symptoms that do not necessarily have frontal alpha asymmetry.

According to Dr. Allan Horwitz from the Health Institute for Health, Care Policy and Aging Research at Rutgers University in New-Brunswick, who has dedicated most of his research to the DSM, said psychiatry was in a crisis in the 1970's and had little credibility (Horwitz, 2010, 2014). Their jurisdiction was threatened by other fields because of the fact that psychoanalysis had little relevance to medicine. Many researchers emerged and focused more on biological psychiatry. The third party insurance payments also had a role to play in this significant shift. Claims would not be honored that were based on a general and vague diagnosis that could not be substantiated by measurable evidence. At a presentation at the Penn Centre for Neuroscience and Society in 2017, Dr Horwitz explained that the criteria for the diagnosis of depression and other mental disorders in the DSM-I and DSM-II were very general and vague. Anxiety was regarded as an underlying component in all of the neuroses, not only of depression. Psychotic depression was regarded as a separate and severe condition. Depressive disorders were separated from ordinary sadness.

Robert Spitzer is described by Dr Horwitz as the key role player in the DSM- III which had very little in common with the DSM- I and DSM-II. Definitions had no causal explanations. It was a revolutionizing way of thinking about mental disorders. It was focused on symptoms and there were no vague referrals to conditions being controlled by subconscious processes or referral to any other causes of conditions. Psychiatry needed a medical model and needed specificity.

In the DSM- III normal and disordered conditions were conflated according to Dr Horwitz. The DSM-III has very specific rather than general criteria for diagnosis. From that point onward, anxiety was regarded as a specific separate problem and sub-divided into nine distinct conditions whereas depression then became the core mood disorder. The relevance of the brief walk through the history of the changes of the descriptions and perceptions of what depression is, is the spectacular growth in the prevalence of depression since the beginning of the DSM-III in the 1980's. Depression became the most common condition to be treated in the DSM-III. In fact in the United States 38% of all out patient diagnoses was depression despite the other 300 disorders specified in the DSM-III (Horwitz, 2010, 2014). Currently, the diagnosis of depression by far outweighs the diagnosis of anxiety.

According to Ronald Kessler's National Comorbidity Survey Replication (2005), which entailed a random sampling of the population of the United States of 9282 adults, indicated the prevalence of the eight most common mental disorders (excluding substance abuse) to be as follows:

• Major Depressive Disorder	16.6%
• Specific Phobia	12.5%
• Social Phobia	12.1%
• Conduct Disorder	9.5%

• Oppositional-Defiant Disorder	8.5%
• Attention Deficit/ Hyperactivity Disorder	8.1%
• Generalized Anxiety Disorder	5.7%
• Intermittent Explosive Disorder	5.2%

A rise in the prescriptions of SSRI-anti-depressants from 1988 at 20 million prescriptions to 120 million prescriptions in 1998, with a continuing increase into the twenty first century, is of significance (Horwitz, 2017). These prescriptions include prescriptions from the field of psychiatry and general medicine.

The question as to what has caused the extremely high growth in depression, is one that has been raised perhaps by the reader and other health care practitioners, but also by many researchers and experts analyzing this phenomenon from different vantage points. A well-known book among health care practitioners is *The Loss of Sadness: How Psychiatry Transformed Normal Sorrow into Depressive Disorder* by Horwitz and Wakefield (2007).

The DSM-5 which was published in 2013 does not contain most of the changes that were suggested. It is very similar to the DSM-IV (APA, 1994). Psychiatry is currently steeped in neuroscience and many of the suggested changes involved biomarkers identified by neuroscience for many disorders. This is a major point of contention. In terms of the diagnosis of depression, issues of contention are the criteria for exclusion and inclusion of the diagnosis as mentioned earlier in this chapter. Bereavement was the only exclusion until it was removed. When a person meets the criteria for MDD specified in the DSM-5 but they have a loved one that has died, then they were not diagnosed with DMM until very recently when the exclusion was removed. The question was if that should not have served as a model for exclusion for other losses or particular circumstances that have the inevitable result of depression symptoms. Should there thus not be a distinction made between ordinary distress and a disorder? Perhaps a person presents with depression symptoms because they have lost their home or their job or because circumstances in their personal lives have changed in that they are suspecting a partner to have another secret relationship. The president of the American Psychiatric Association at the time, John Oldham, said that the bereavement exclusion is very limited (see Brooks, 2012; Frances, 2012). He asked how a strong reaction to having your entire home wiped out by a tsunami is different to a strong reaction after the death of a loved one or spouse. Perhaps the person needs to consider relocation because of the political situation in the country (this may have bearing on the fact that the author is a South African!). People go through periods of growth and change that are often associated with symptoms of depression. There are possibly as many potential causes for depression as there are people and different circumstances.

According to the DSM-5 (APA, 2013), it is normal to present with any number of depressive symptoms for less than two weeks. With the anxiety disorders the periods that are stipulated are three months and in some cases six months which is possibly a more realistic time frame during which to obtain some degree of objective perspective. Studies have followed by Wakefield, Schmitz and others that posed the question whether the bereavement exclusion for major depression disorder ought to be extended to other losses and that resulted in a footnote to be added to the DSM-5 regarding exclusions that according to Horwitz, is confusing. The other matter that was raised in research is whether a distinction ought to be made between uncomplicated and complicated responses to bereavement and other losses in an attempt to separate neurosis from psychosis once again.

The result of the studies and responses by relevant parties was that the bereavement exclusion was removed and an advisory note was added stating the following: "The normal and expected response to an event involving significant loss (e.g. bereavement, financial ruin, natural disaster), including feelings of intense sadness, rumination about the loss, insomnia, poor appetite and weight loss, may resemble a depressive episode. The presence of symptoms such as feelings of worthlessness, suicidal ideas, psychomotor retard, and severe overall impairment suggest the presence of a MDE in addition to the normal response to loss."

According to Horwitz at al. (2017), the advisory note added to the DSM-5 for MDD is so vague that it has no communicative or research value. He also states that it conflicts with the diagnostic criteria, that it abandons the longer duration for grief, and worsens the confusion between normal sadness and depressive disorder.

The combination of normal and pathological reactions to situations in a diagnosis has implications on different levels. There are for instance different treatment implications for sadness and pathology.

In my practice, as I believe in the practices of many other practitioners, individuals with questionable diagnoses show up in search of an alternative to a cocktail of medications that renders them desperate and to an extent dysfunctional. Perhaps this is more evident in the diagnosis of major depressive disorder because of the mere numbers involved. It is definitely not in the scope of practice of most neurofeedback practitioners at this point in time to suggest changes in medication, unless of course the neurofeedback practitioner is a psychiatrist. In the United States and possibly elsewhere, there are progressively more psychiatrists adding neurofeedback to their practices. In South Africa that is not yet the case. It is, however, within our scope of practice to relieve discomfort. The better informed we are and the more aware we are of different perspectives and possible mistakes – many based on poor self-reporting skills – the better equipped we are to assist in improving the quality of life of the individuals we work with. The responsible neurofeedback practitioner, unless he/ she is a psychiatrist, will not suggest changes in medication. Communication with the prescribing psychiatrist is essential because there will also be changes in responses to medication during the neurofeedback training process.

The neurofeedback practitioner can often assist even when the person suffering symptoms associated with depression does not present with frontal alpha asymmetry. The accurate tracking of symptoms by means of questionnaires and other measurements is essential. Often when depression symptoms are present that would have been categorized as normal sadness by a different set of criteria, normal high frequency power training protocols and other multiple channel protocols that are focused on other relevant aspects of dysregulation other than alpha asymmetry, relieve discomfort.

Chapter 11

Neurofeedback for PTSD and Developmental Trauma

11.1 Introduction

It is time to think differently about the treatment of emotional suffering and mental illness: This is the opening statement of the foreword of this book by Sebern Fisher. In the treatment of no other disorder or cause for emotional suffering than for that of the consequences of trauma, is it clearer that neurofeedback is not only a viable option but the best available option to date. Neurofeedback is currently the only intervention through which the brain learns to regulate itself. The person entangled in fear, anger (or even rage) and shame in the horrific aftermath of trauma, remains a victim of the brain's desperate maneuvers of dedication to its own survival. The often extreme, socially- unacceptable and complicated symptoms trauma survivors present with, make it difficult for partners, family, friends and even therapists to deal with. The symptoms differ in severity depending on the insults suffered. The symptoms stem from fundamental differences in brain regions and brain networks of the victims of trauma clearly indicated by fMRI studies and related neuroscience research studies. When the fear circuitry and the arousal levels are calmed down and when the Default Mode Network is restored or activated, the symptoms dissipate or become less intense as the brain of the person with a history of trauma begins to regulate itself. Symptoms resulting from a history of trauma, reflect a brain problem as opposed to a personality, mental or behavior problem. A symptom- based diagnosis for the population of people with a debilitating history of trauma mostly leads to ineffective treatment plans. Emerging neuroscience research disambiguates that initial intervention for trauma-related symptoms ought to happen at the level of the brain. Once the brain is calmer and there is access to the verbal and inhibitory structures, psychotherapy ought to follow.

The inclusion of this chapter in the second edition of this book, is not only relevant and significant, but also urgent. The neurofeedback practitioner and other readers will get exposure to latest and relevant neuroscience research and hopefully gain insight into what Sebern Fisher calls the "cascade of terror" (2020) that unfolds in the brains of trauma survivors and washes through their lives over and over again leaving devastation in its wake. Neurofeedback, as a modality of applied neuroscience, can change this destructive pattern.

Two decades ago, we as neurofeedback practitioners, were whispering to one another about the anecdotal evidence we had of miraculous transformations of trauma cases we witnessed in our private practices, not yet fully understanding the dynamics involved and fearful of judgement by mainstream practitioners. And here we are today, understanding, because of scientific evidence based on neuroimaging and electroencephalogram studies exactly why the traumatized brain responds better to certain neurofeedback protocols than to any other indicated therapy.

Although the approach in neurofeedback in dealing with trauma ought to always be that of calming the brain, irrespective of whether the intervention is for post- traumatic stress disorder (PTSD) or for developmental trauma disorder (DTD)-a distinction will be made between the two in the interest of clarity.

11.2 Post-Traumatic Stress Disorder (PTSD)

The increased awareness of the effects of trauma was kindled after the American Psychiatric Association (APA) added PTSD as an official diagnosis to the DSM-III in 1980 (APA, 1980). The focus of PTSD was initially mainly on the effects of war but evolved to an understanding that a much wider population than war veterans are affected by trauma.

People who suffer PTSD have generally either experienced or witnessed a traumatic event such as war, a tsunami or any other natural disaster, an accident that resulted in emotional or physical shock or injury or any violent personal assault such as rape, torture, armed robbery or motor vehicle hijacking. The sufferer may have been witness to any of the above-mentioned or other atrocities or even to murder. The examples are intended to remind therapists that traumatic events are often culture and time specific and that the screening for trauma ought to be done accordingly.

Some other conditions and disorders related to PTSD in mainstream approaches, are acute stress disorder (which is not fundamentally different from PTSD), adjustment disorder (where the stressor is not severe or outside the parameters of the average human experience) and reactive attachment disorder which is a disorder found in children who have been neglected and cannot form an attachment with their caregivers. Disinhibited social engagement disorder is also an attachment disorder that can develop when a child does not receive appropriate nurturing and affection. Such a child is then not closely bonded to the parents and therefore bonds very easily when meeting strangers and is overly friendly with them. The attachment disorders, however, are better understood when looking through the lens of developmental disorder which follows further on in this chapter.

Having experienced or witnessed traumatic events can result in the prevalence of numerous symptoms or combinations of symptoms. Symptoms can include flashbacks, nightmares, panic attacks, eating disorders, verbal memory deficits, substance abuse, cognitive delays, emotional numbness and avoidance of places people and activities that are reminders of the trauma. PTSD sufferers often experience symptoms involving fear, anxiety, and sadness. The various combinations of symptoms can simulate different disorders or conditions in different individuals often resulting in futile treatment efforts.

It is beyond the scope of this book to discuss the diagnosis of PTSD and other related disorders in terms of the symptoms specified in the DSM-5 (APA, 2013), but it is relevant however to consider fear, unstable arousal levels and dysregulated nervous systems as common denominators to all trauma related diagnoses.

As mentioned, previously PTSD was typically associated with soldiers and war veterans who had had traumatic experiences during battle. The incidence of PTSD proves to be significantly higher and the unfurling much wider. According to an article entitled "Adjustment Disorder: Current Status" (Patra & Sarkar, 2013) indicate that PTSD affects approximately 3,5% of U. S. adults and that the incidence amongst women is twice as high as the incidence amongst men.

In the article entitled "Regulating posttraumatic stress disorder symptoms with neurofeedback: Regaining control of the mind" (Nicholson et al., 2020) Dr Ruth Lanius and her understudies indicate the incidence of PTSD to be 10% amongst public safety workers internationally. In the same article the result of a survey done by the World Health Organization in 11 countries on the incidence of PTSD is referred to. The survey indicated that PTSD was associated with 20,2% of sexual assault cases. A cross-national systematic review of 10 neurofeedback studies also quoted in the above-mentioned article, pertaining to the success of neurofeedback for PTSD patients, indicated positive improvements on at least one PTSD-symptom in all 10 studies (Nicholson et al., 2020).

Neurofeedback is considered a more personalized approach than other mainstream approaches to which a significant percentage of PTSD patients are resistant. The many different protocols that are deployed to target the different circuits and brain regions involved in PTSD, makes it a flexible treatment that enables improved self-regulation which has a marked effect on most presenting symptoms of PTSD. Recommended protocols will be discussed towards the end of this chapter.

The brain dynamics associated with PTSD will be discussed alongside the discussion of the brain dynamics involved in DTD.

11.3 Developmental Trauma

In Allan Schore's book, *Affect Regulation and the Origin of Self: The Neurobiology of Emotional Development* (1994), he indicated that the maturing brain structures of the infant are influenced by early adverse circumstances and influence socioemotional development and the development of the self. This work lead to increased focus on the effects of early trauma. In 2005, psychiatrist and professor of Psychiatry at the Boston University School of Medicine, Dr Bessel van der Kolk, suggested the diagnosis of developmental trauma disorder (DTD). Developmental trauma used to be referred to as "complex PTSD" or "early trauma". In an article by Tori DeAngelis (2007) Dr van der Kolk is quoted as follows: "While PTSD is a good definition for acute trauma in adults, it doesn't apply well to children, who are often traumatized in the context of relationships. Because children's brains are still developing trauma has a much more pervasive and long-range influence on their self-concept, on their sense of the world and on their ability to regulate themselves" (DeAngelis, 2007). From a neurofeedback perspective- based on neuroscience findings- developmental trauma like PTSD, is proven to be an arousal related disorder.

Developmental trauma can occur from the moment of conception prior to the onset of conscious verbal thought. The incidents, insults or period of trauma or neglect will not be recalled consciously by the child or the adult if it occurred during a pre-cognitive and pre-verbal developmental stage of the brain. The survivor will however live in a state wherein the mind and the body are constantly aroused, just like the PTSD survivor.

The term developmental trauma is used to describe childhood trauma and neglect characterized by chronic abuse and harsh adverse experiences and circumstances before birth and during childhood. Attachment disruption is an inevitable result of DT.

The ACE study, better known as the *Adverse Child Experiences Study* (see Anda & Felitti, 2003; initial surveys began in 1995) provided a rough guideline that is widely accepted as an indication of the existence of different types of abuse and neglect during childhood that predict future health problems. More importantly from an intervention point of view when we consider the results of many ACE -based research studies, we begin to understand the magnitude of the implications. The incidence of individuals with high ACE scores, reflects the incidence of brains of survivors of developmental trauma that cannot regulate, and consequently cannot quiet fear. These brains have embedded in their very fabric, probably locked in in certain frequencies (to be clarified in the following section) the original fear: the fear of survival. When DT goes untreated the consequences as projected by the ACE are dire.

The ACE score is determined by ascertaining the number of affirmative responses to the existence of ten different circumstances describing ten different types of trauma. The higher the ACE score the higher the risk for chronic disease as well as of emotional and social problems. An ACE score of 4 or higher for instance, is indicative of an increased risk of pulmonary lung disease by 390% and an increase of 1 220 % in the risk of attempted suicide. The outcome of the study that included 17,000 subjects, indicated that childhood trauma was very common and that there is a direct link between childhood trauma and the adult onset of chronic disease, depression, suicide and violence (either as the perpetrator or as the victim). If the circumstances specified in the ACE study were prevalent in the life of the child younger than 18, it would be a fair assumption to make that traumatic circumstances were also present when the child's brain was still in pre-cognitive and pre-verbal state. A further indication of the study was that a combination of different types of trauma increased the risk of health, social and emotional problems. The ACE study also indicated that people rarely experience one type of trauma only and that sexual abuse and verbal abuse are ordinarily coupled with other adverse events.

To obtain an ACE score, a person needs to add the positive responses to exposure to the following ten conditions prior to the person's 18th birthday that reflect five personal and five indirect experiences of adverse events *(The categories as specified by US Centre of Disease Control. The reader can find the specified questions and the prediction rates of specific lifelong negative emotional and physical outcomes in the original study as mentioned above. The findings have since been confirmed by numerous studies across the world).*

- emotional abuse
- physical abuse
- sexual abuse
- mother treated violently
- household substance abuse
- household mental illness
- parental separation or divorce
- incarcerated household member
- emotional neglect
- physical neglect

A meta-analysis of all the ACE studies done across the world in 2017 funded by the Welsh Government, may also be of interest to the reader and is easily accessible should the reader wish to do further research and verification.

The prevalence of developmental trauma is clearly high. By considering the indicators of the ACE study every reader will have seen a few (at least) familiar reflections in that mirror. Many or most healthcare practitioners drawn to trauma work have a deep understanding of the effects of trauma that lies beyond reason born from experience. It was not until recently that I truly realized that not everybody is driven, propelled, impelled, goaded even, by what Sebern Fisher so aptly refers to as a "pulse of fear" in her book (2014). Those who have suffered development trauma are driven by fear. The concept of developmental trauma disorder (DTD) offers an explanation and understanding of the symptoms from an array of other diagnoses. The most valuable compass that I am aware of regarding gaining insight into and an understanding of developmental trauma, is Sebern Fisher's book mentioned above.

Neuroscience illuminates the daunting reality of the existence of millions of fear- driven brains with clarity and insight. The areas and networks of the brain affected by trauma are discussed and illustrated in the next section. The "fear- driven brain" needs to be guided to improve its regulation in order to calm the arousal and the fear. All neurofeedback protocols (to be discussed towards the end of this chapter) ought to serve this goal.

The adults, teenagers and even younger children that suffered adverse childhood experiences show up at our private practices with many different diagnoses. Those diagnoses include bipolar disorder, borderline personality disorder, (BPD), dissociative identity disorder (DID), reactive attachment disorder (RAD), PTSD, any of the depressive disorders, any of the anxiety disorders (characterized by feelings of anxiety and fear) attention deficit hyperactivity disorder (ADHD) or obsessive- compulsive disorder (OCD). DTD can also be masked as one of many other of the 297 disorders in the

DSM-5 (APA, 2013). Ruth Lanius (see Nicholson et al., 2020) indicated that there are more than 600,000 symptom combinations with which those with trauma histories can present. These clients often show up for assistance after having explored many mainstream and alternative interventions. They are often resistant to both medication and talk therapy. Many healthcare practitioners with good intentions feel hopeless after futile attempts to stabilize the survivors of developmental trauma. They are often resistant to most mainstream therapies because of their dysregulated nervous systems, irrespective of their diagnosis. In Sebern Fisher's book (2014) as well as in her webinars and mentoring sessions, she teaches that the dysregulated brains of this population render them unsusceptible to talk therapy and that a DSM-diagnosis is not helpful. She no longer regards these and related disorders as distinct but as manifestations of dysregulated nervous systems. According to Sebern Fisher (2014), irrespective of how the sense of motherlessness is felt or expressed by the DT population, it is best understood from a central nervous system perspective.

The highly reactive nervous systems of the survivors of trauma can be trained to calm down, to activate brain structures that inhibit the fear response and to influence networks involved in affect regulation to come online. Once the brain has acquired the ability to regulate emotion, psychotherapy and possibly other indicated therapies ought to be phased in.

11.4 The Traumatized Brain-Reaction

Although brain structures and networks have been described in chapter 3, areas, structures, and networks affected most by trauma are described and discussed in this chapter as well but from a different perspective. This chapter can consequently be read as a standalone chapter. An understanding of the arousal model is most relevant to the interpretation of this chapter. Those clinicians that do not work from the perspective of the arousal model on a regular basis, are recommended to read chapter 5 again. Due to space restrictions the arousal model will just be referred to in this chapter and not elaborated on.

A discussion of regions and networks in the brain that are affected by trauma and neglect follows and is based mainly on Sebern Fisher's webinar series on The Nature of Forgetting (2020).

Permission has been granted by Sebern Fisher and by Ruth Lanius to use content and illustrations from the webinar series. Some quoted research studies and illustrations will pertain mainly to DTD, others to PTSD and often the illustrations and studies will be relevant to both PTSD and DTD.

Every major system of the brain (developing and developed) from the brainstem to the cortex, is affected by early childhood abuse and neglect. The fetus of the abused pregnant mother is already affected by the mother's fear responses. The amygdala that helps in the modulation of stress reactivity and is involved in the vulnerability to mood disorders develops at an early embryonic stage and the development is altered by high levels of cortisol which is the body's main stress hormone (Buss et al., 2012). Research has revealed that physical abuse during pregnancy is a significant predictor of attachment problems.

The key structures involved in emotional regulation that are impacted by developmental trauma and mostly by PTSD as well, are indicated to below.

DEVELOPMENTAL TRAUMA IMPACTS KEY STRUCTURES
UNDERLYING EMOTIONAL REGULATION

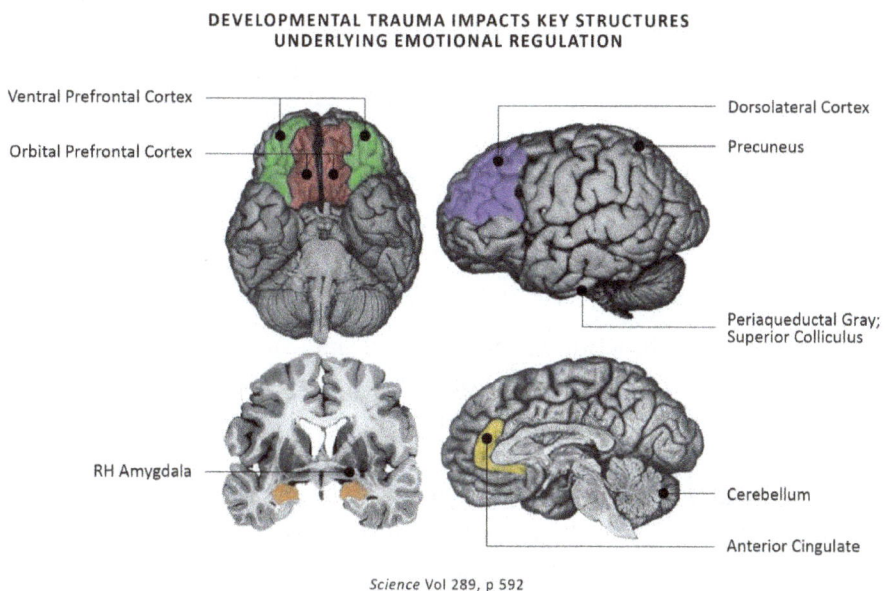

Ventral Prefrontal Cortex
Orbital Prefrontal Cortex
Dorsolateral Cortex
Precuneus
Periaqueductal Gray; Superior Colliculus
RH Amygdala
Cerebellum
Anterior Cingulate

Science Vol 289, p 592

Figure 11.1: Key structures impacted by DT. Adapted from Davidson, R. J., Putnam, K. M., & Larson, C. L. (2000). Dysfunction in the neural circuitry of emotion regulation--a possible prelude to violence. Science, 289(5479), 591-594. doi:10.1126/science.289.5479.591

- The *precuneus*, located at the back of the brain, relates to our sense of being - to our very sense of existing. It can be described as the seat of self-awareness. It provides the individual with a sense of self in time in space. The precuneus is a core region in the default mode network (DMN) and is also involved in episodic memory retrieval. Reduction in DMN connectivity is normal in aging and a prominent problem in Alzheimer's Disease. Studies have shown significant reduction in connectivity in victims of trauma that is not age related. Brain networks and how they are affected by trauma, is discussed and illustrated below. A sensor placed at Pz in the 10/20 Placement System (see figure 2.1 in chapter 2) will target the precuneus.

- Another brain region crucially important to emotional regulation, namely the *ventral medial pre-frontal cortex (vmPFC)* is also affected by trauma. This area of the brain plays a vital role in the inhibition of the amygdala which is a key role player in the fear response. This area, when activated, gives access to mindfulness during certain stages of meditation practices and provides a sense of coming into the body.

- The *dorsal medial pre-frontal cortex*, implicated in theory of mind, the narrative of self and the sense of me, is also impacted by trauma. In meditation practice, the meditator initially draws the focus away from words and inner chatter, out of the dorsal medial pre-frontal cortex and into the ventral medial pre-frontal cortex to be mindfully present in the body. With dissociative patients these structures do not come online at all when needed and also show severely impaired connectivity to the amygdala in less severely debilitated cases of PTSD and DT.

- The normal functioning of the *pre-frontal cortex* in its entirety is impaired by a trauma history. The normal functioning of the pre-frontal cortex enables an individual to perform executive tasks, to make logical decisions, to pause before reacting and to evaluate and integrate information obtained from the brain, from the body and the environment. This area of the brain plays a major role in the inhibition of the amygdala. Connectivity and communication between the deeper structures involved in fear detection and response and the prefrontal cortex is essential in the process of neutralizing and calming fear. (The work of Bessel van der Kolk and Ruth Lanius pertaining to the malfunctioning of the prefrontal cortex in patients with a history of trauma, is discussed below). If the fear circuitry is not inhibited by the frontal areas of the cortex, the fear goes unchecked and the trauma victim is subject to its relentless onslaught.

- The *amygdala* has been known for some time to hold center stage in the fear system and the fight/flight or freeze response. (These responses of the autonomic nervous system have been described in chapter 6 and will be illustrated and summarized in this chapter as well). It has become evident however from the

252

latest related neuroscience research, that some responses that have been assigned to the amygdala, originate from the brain stem.

The following illustration shows the results of a study by Ruth Lanius (Nicholson et al., 2020) that indicates that none of the patients screened for early childhood trauma and neglect had connectivity between the pre-frontal cortex and the amygdala.

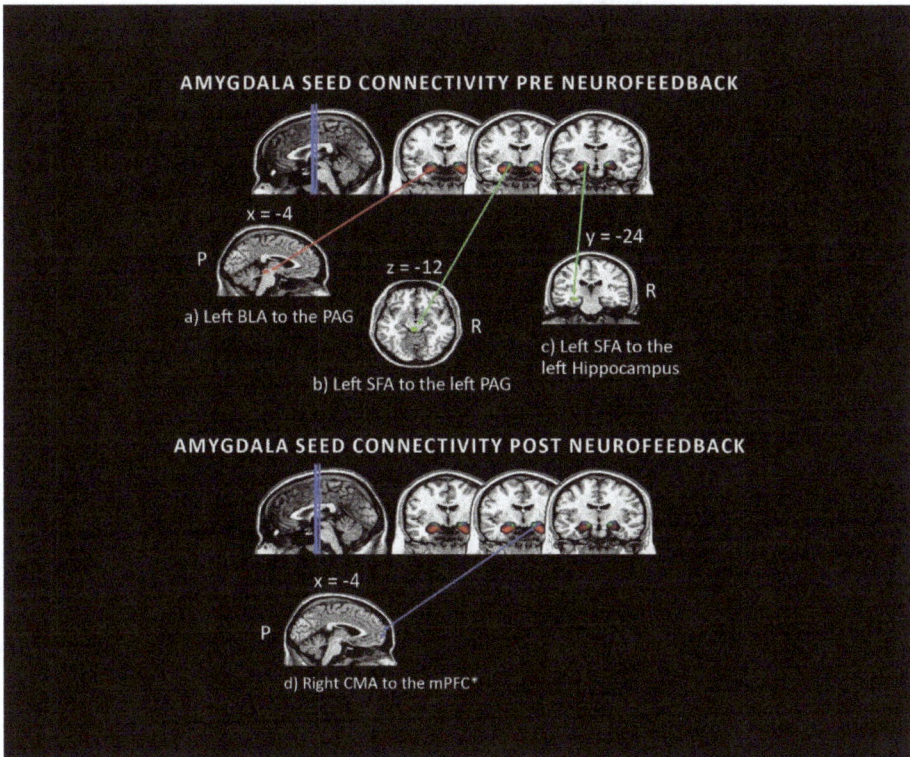

Figure 11.2: Amygdala connectivity with the vmPFC pre and post neurofeedback. Reprinted with permission from Ruth Lanius.

All of the participants with DT showed connectivity between the periaqueductal gray, the superior colliculus and the amygdala.

After one session of neurofeedback involving alpha training, the fMRI's of 80% of the subjects indicated the beginning of connectivity between the amygdala and the pre-frontal cortex and reduced connectivity between the amygdala and the periaqueductal gray (PAG).

A change in the connectivity of the amygdala involving reduced communication with the periaqueductal gray and the superior colliculus and increased connectivity with the vmPFC is associated with reduced arousal and reduction in PTSD symptoms.

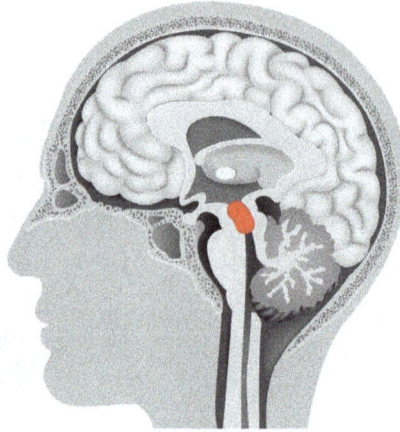

PERIAQUEDUCTAL GRAY

Figure 11.3: Periaqueductal gray- lateral view. Redesigned by Alesha Otto.

- The *periaqueductal gray* plays an important role in the autonomic response and consequently in the behavioral response to threatening stimuli. The PAG is described as the brain's threat detector that activates the amygdala in the presence of perceived danger (Fisher, 2020). It is also the primary control center for descending pain. The PAG contains enkephalin producing cells that suppress pain. Enkephalin has the same properties as morphine opiates.

- The *superior colliculus* is also involved in detecting and registering threat signals through the senses. It is a layered multi-sensory structure and lies on the roof of the midbrain.

- The significance of the *cerebellum* of the individual with a history of early childhood trauma, has been the focus of many recent research studies. Treatment protocols in neurofeedback involving the placement of the electrodes closer to the inion ridge in accordance with the findings of the significance of the cerebellum in the presence of a history of trauma, are being investigated by trauma specialists and neurofeedback practitioners.

254

The cerebellum is the first structure to inhibit the temporal lobes and is activated mainly through holding and rocking according to Sebern Fisher (2020). Many individuals with early childhood trauma and neglect have no recollection of ever being held or rocked and many probably never have been.

There is a body of research indicating that the cerebellum is not only important in physical balance and rhythm but also in emotional balance. Lesions in the central cerebellum, called the vermis or limbic cerebellum and in the lateral hemisphere of the posterior cerebellum can result in the cerebellar cognitive affective syndrome (CCAS). This syndrome includes deficits in executive abilities, visual-spatial problems linguistic impairments and severe affective disturbance ranging from emotional blunting to disinhibition and psychosis (Schmahmann, 2004).

Considering the close proximity of the cranial nerves and the vestibular system to the more primitive parts of the brain that are affected in trauma, presenting symptoms can be interpreted and protocols adapted accordingly.

Problems with physical balance, posture, clumsiness, and rhythm are very typical symptoms associated with developmental trauma in the presence of which protocols closer to the inion ridge to target the brain structures involved would be appropriate. According to Sebern Fisher (2020), these children, teenagers or adults never had a caretaker to orient them to the world.

We can thus conclude that neuroscience has made it increasingly clear that there are multiple regions in the brain involved in trauma and in fear reactions. It is not just the amygdala responsible for the flight/flight or freeze response that is overactive in the person with a history of trauma. Many other structures, including structures from the reptilian or lower mid-brain (PAG and the superior colliculus) and the mammalian brain (limbic or midbrain) are involved as well. These primitive structures are dedicated to survival and cannot be shut down by the pre-frontal cortex. Studies in fact show that there are no connections between the pre-frontal cortex and the subcortical structures involved in threat detection in the severely traumatized population. In this regard the work of Ruth Lanius (Nicholson et al., 2020), Bessel van der Kolk (2005, 2016), Rob Coben et al. (2014), Allan Schore (1994, 2003ab) and other neuroscience researchers is invaluable. These structures cannot be reasoned with, are not accessible through words and therefore it is clear that talk therapy will not be able to regulate these pre-verbal structures in and reactions from the brain.

When the fear detection in the brain is not contextualized or inhibited by structures and networks functioning optimally, the CNS creates what Sebern Fisher describes as a "cascade of terror".

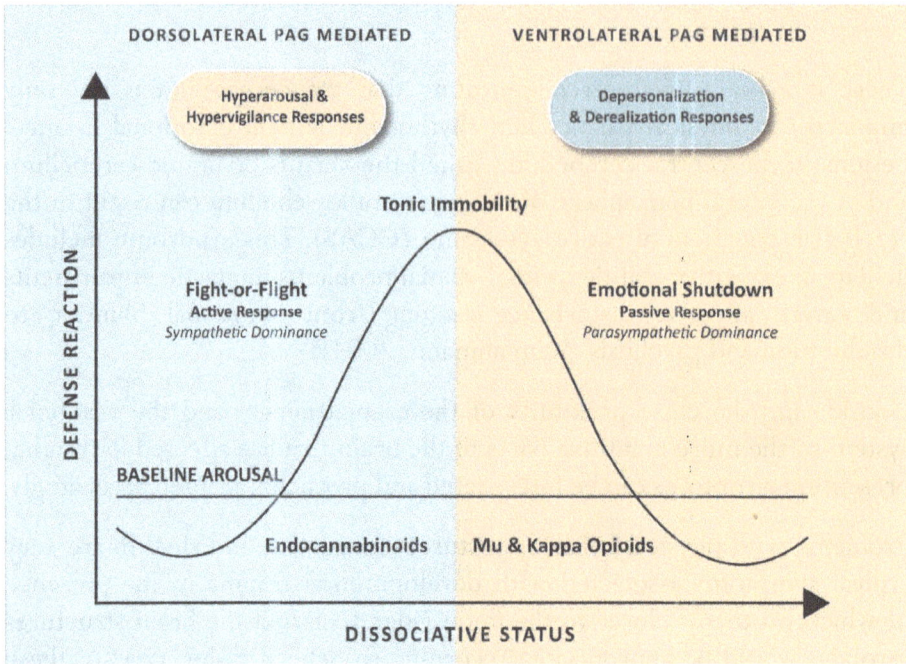

Figure 11.4: Fight/flight and freeze response. Redesigned by Alesha Otto and printed with permission from Ruth Lanius.

When a fear signal is registered in the reptilian and midbrain structures dedicated to fear detection, prior to it becoming conscious, there are significant measurable events that occur at millisecond intervals. Already in that pre- conscious cortical timing of evoked potentials there is a discordant unfolding of electrical activity in the hypervigilant brains of those with a history of trauma. At 200 milliseconds after a stimulus there is a non-conscious measurable response and at 300 milliseconds there is the first conscious recognition of whatever caused the alert. An organized response throughout the brain follows that then contextualizes the stimulus. In the PTSD- brain there is disorganized reactivity without accurate interpretation of for instance the sound of a car backfiring.

The traumatized as well as the non-traumatized brains go through a period of gathering information after a potentially startling stimulus. That period is represented by the initial upward curve of the bell curve in the illustration, toward the arousal baseline horizontal line. What is of significance is how the rest of the process unfolds after the defensive reaction has commenced. The dorsolateral PAG activates toward a fight/flight response that results in the release of endocannabinoids. The sympathetic tone of the autonomic nervous system is dominant at this point and the arousal level goes higher. The sympathetic activation causes a fight or flight, hyper-aroused, hypervigilant response. Porges (2011) refers to this activating response orchestrated by the sympathetic nervous system as the "first line of defense". Certain physiological reactions are associated with this response (See chapter 6 *Physiological responses to Stress and Tension*). The trajectory can go further if the terror provoking stimulus is intense enough- into tonic immobility -when both the para-sympathetic and sympathetic systems become equally activated.

The tonic immobility can be understood as a fight/flight response put on hold through the activation of a braking mechanism. During the tonic immobility or emotional shutdown phase of the trajectory, opioid analgesics are released. When, according to the individual's neuroception, the fight/flight response is not going to be able to ensure survival and the sympathetic nervous system is too aroused, the dorsal vagal (the unmyelinated vagal nerve) has the ability to shut down the entire system and cause the freeze response. The "second level of defense" as Porges (2011) refers to it, is the freeze response which can involve dissociating, physiological immobilization, depersonalization, derealization and even the loss of consciousness. It also presents as passive avoidance in some and is often associated with PTSD. Tonic immobility associated with a defense reaction has also been described as "feigning death" or "playing dead" which is not uncommon in the animal kingdom. (The expression "playing opossum" which means to play dead, is derived from the opossum which is a marsupial from North America. The heart rate and breathing of opossums slow down when they are under threat and they become unconscious).

The healthy and normal activation of the parasympathetic nervous system through increased vagal tone is associated with the regulation of stress responses and causes the individual to pendulate appropriately between relaxation and arousal. The freeze response does not involve healthy and normal activation of the parasympathetic nervous system. In neurofeedback terms it is important to remember that the freeze response is often mistaken as depressive-like symptoms and then treated incorrectly on the left hemisphere by rewarding high frequency brainwave activity.

Before we discuss specific neurofeedback protocols to address the indicated areas and regions affected by trauma, it is important that we will consider how some neural networks are affected by a history of trauma as well and ascertain the role of those networks in regulation and arousal. In this process we remain focused on the main goal which is to lower the arousal of the traumatized brain ever on high alert to respond to any perceived threat, as well as on the goal of improving emotional regulation.

Intrinsic Connectivity Networks and Trauma

Functional connectivity of different brain regions, referred to as networks, is now understood to be important in cognitive tasks and behavior. Disruption in any of the networks have dire consequences on multiple levels of functioning. Research has shown that developmental trauma impacts negatively on the three major networks in the brain. The most debilitating consequences probably stem from the clear disruptions in the default mode network (DMN).

Below is an illustration of some of the identified networks in the brain to illustrate the complexity and the sensitivity of the communication pathways. There are millions more that have not yet been identified.

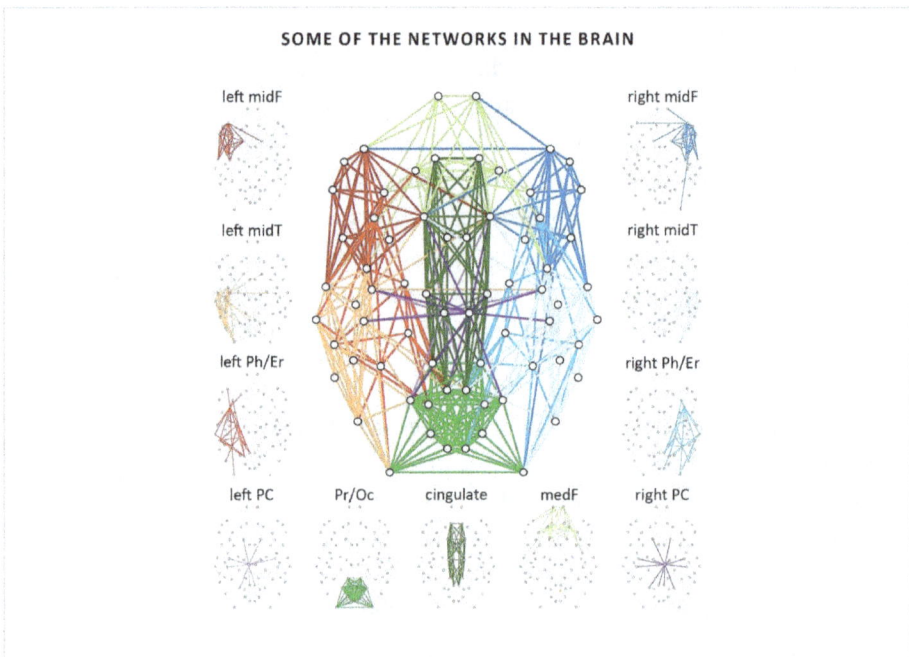

Figure 11.5: Some known networks in the brain. Reprinted with permission from Sebern Fisher. De Reus, M. A., Saenger, V. M., Kahn, R. S., & Van den Heuvel, M. P. (2014). An edge-centric perspective on the human connectome: Link communities in the brain. https://royalsocietypublishing.org/doi/pdf/10.1098/rstb.2013.0527

The three intrinsic connectivity networks in the brain that are affected by trauma are the *salience network (SN), the central executive network (CEN)*, and the *default mode network (DMN)*. Dysfunction in these three networks are often associated with psychopathology (Nicholson et al., 2020).

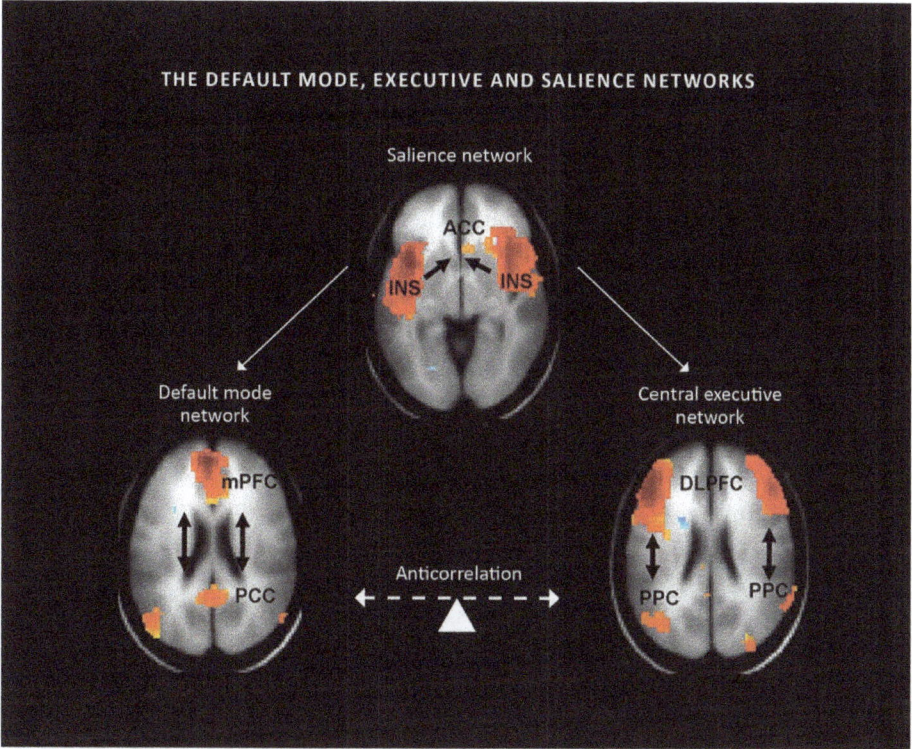

Figure 11.6: The three intrinsic networks affected by trauma. Reprinted with permission from Sebern Fisher. Nekovarova, T., Fajnerova, I., Horacek, J., & Spaniel, F. (2014, April 22). Bridging disparate symptoms of schizophrenia: A triple network dysfunction theory. http://www.frontiersin.org/articles/10.3389/fnbeh.2014.00171/full

The *salience network* is regarded to be a large- scale brain network in humans comprising primarily the insula and the dorsal anterior cingulate cortex. The insula provides information to the brain from the body. The raw data is received at the posterior insula (T6) and then gets interpreted at the anterior insula which corresponds to the F6/F8 placement in the 10/10 International Placement System. The insula is thus involved in what Stephen Porges (2011) refers to as interoception which is the perception of the internal physiological state of the body. Eating disorders are often associated with DTD and are possibly related to disruption in the salience network. The substantia nigra, ventral striatum, amygdala, dorsomedial thalamus, and the hypothalamus also form a part of this network. It's primary function, as the name suggests, is in detecting and filtering stimuli and distinguishing between significant, important, conspicuous and non-important stimuli. The SN then also recruits other relevant networks. This network has an important role in integrating sensory, emotional, and cognitive information to derive a sense of self or self-awareness. It is also involved in social behavior and communication. Neuroimaging studies of PTSD sufferers have shown an increased connectivity between the limbic circuitry and the SN at rest. (Fisher, 2020). This hyper-connectivity will result in an exaggerated fear of danger or hypervigilance - an extreme alertness that undermines the quality of life.

The *central executive network* is crucial to the cognitive control of behavior. The CEN connects areas of the dorsolateral prefrontal cortex and the posterior parietal cortex. The CEN is crucial to the cognitive control and regulation of behavior, emotion and thought. When this network is healthy and functions well, we can generally control our behavior by thinking before we act. In the brain with trauma history, this network does not function optimally. A study by van der Kolk (2016) indicated that neurofeedback improved the executive function in formerly untreated adults with early childhood trauma, significantly (Fisher, 2020).

The *default mode network* is the largest network in the brain. The concept of the DMN is a relatively new one and is not without controversy. Researchers and neuroscientists don't all agree on which structures should be included in this network. Most agree that this network includes the following brain regions: the medial prefrontal cortex (mPFC), the posterior cingulate gyrus and the inferior parietal lobule. The other brain regions that are also regarded to be part of the DMN are the temporal cortex, the hippocampal formation and the precuneus.

The DMN is a network of interacting brain regions that is active when a person is not focused on the outside world or busy with a specific task. There are many recent research studies focusing on the intrinsic activity of the brain during resting-states. Increased activity is noted in the DMN during tasks involving autobiographical, episodic, and semantic memory, mind wandering, perspective taking and future thinking. The DMN has been described as the "self-other-network".

When this network does not function optimally, there is an impaired awareness and perception of the self and of the other. A main goal of neurofeedback as an intervention for victims of early childhood trauma ought to be to normalize the functioning of the DMN. The DMN is considered the backbone of cortical integration (Alves et al., 2019).

Neuroscience research abounds in imaging and EEG studies indicating irregular activity in DMN's of individuals with histories of trauma.

A study on the alterations in the DMN connectivity in PTSD related to early-life trauma was conducted by Bluhm et al. (2009). The result of that study is illustrated on below.

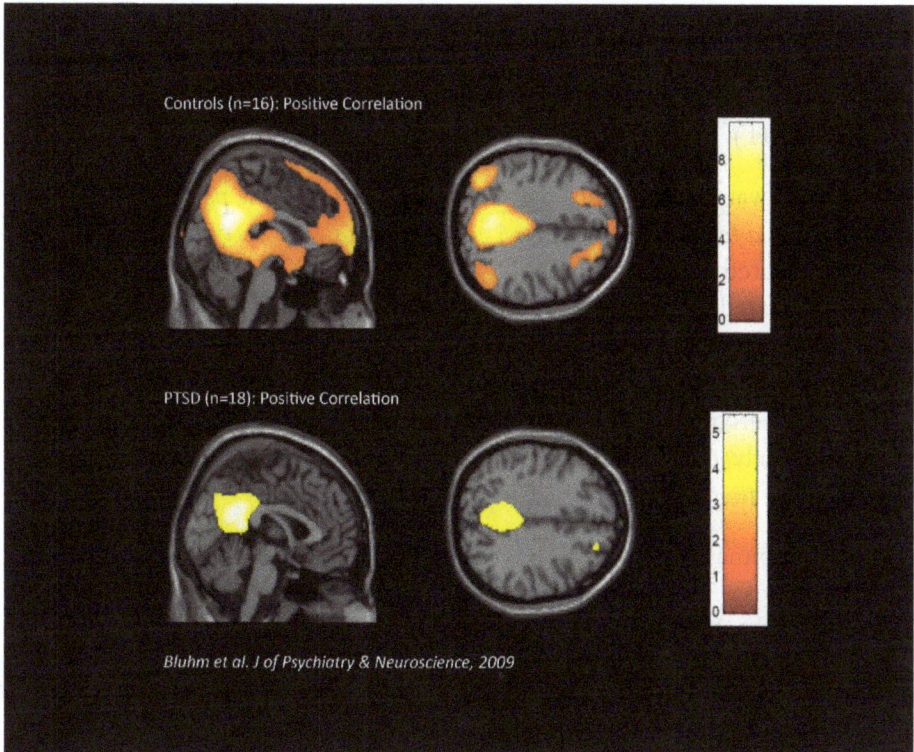

Figure 11.7: DMN activity at rest, Controls vs PTSD. This slide is printed with permission from Ruth Lanius.

Adult female patients with a primary diagnosis of PTSD as a result of childhood abuse and healthy controls were recruited for inclusion in the study. The subjects were allowed time to acclimatize to the scanner environment and a high- resolution anatomic scan was taken before the resting state scan. Several steps were taken to minimize conditions that would make it difficult to enter a relaxing state. The subjects were then requested to close their eyes, to relax and to allow their minds to wander during the five and a half minute scanning procedure. Functional images were acquired to obtain whole-brain coverage. None of the subjects from the healthy controls or from the PTSD reported any anxiety during the procedure.

Direct comparison of the healthy controls and those with histories of early childhood abuse revealed that patients with chronic PTSD - related to early-life trauma show significantly reduced connectivity within the DMN during a resting state. These brain regions including the PCC, precuneus and mPFC have been associated with self-referential processing during the resting-state and are consistent with the notion of altered self-perception and consciousness as a result of early-childhood trauma (Bluhm et al., 2009). The findings of this study are consistent with other studies- a few of which are mentioned below-showing abnormal functional connectivity within many of the DMN regions in participants with histories of trauma (both PTSD and DT).

Another relevant study entitled *Default mode alterations in post-traumatic stress disorder related to early-life trauma: A developmental perspective* (Daniels et al., 2011) indicated that altered DMN connectivity in individuals with PTSD has been related to prolonged childhood maltreatment. In the same article it is suggested that the deficient DMN connectivity in adults who have suffered early childhood trauma and neglect, appears to be similar to the DMN connectivity of healthy children aged seven to nine years. It appears thus that early childhood trauma may interfere with the developmental trajectory of the DMN.

Other neuroimaging studies (referred to in the same article) suggest that dissociative experiences also involve brain regions implicated in the DMN (Daniels et al., 2011).

According to Ruth Lanius (Nicholson et al., 2020), it is stated that there is decreased connectivity at rest in key hubs of the DMN of PTSD patients.

A prerequisite for the DMN to develop is the presence of a 'good enough' parent. Without a sense of safety and protection and guiding constraints, this network develops poorly if at all. When the PTSD patients in one of the above- mentioned and illustrated studies were off task, their fMRI's involving regions of the DMN showed severely disrupted activity representing a lack of a sense of self as well as the absence of the ability to inhibit fear (which is a core function of the mPFC proven to be inactive with the PTSD and DT patients during resting states). This is a most significant finding with major implications. Sebern Fisher emphasizes repeatedly in her mentoring and from other teaching platforms that attempts at restoring the functionality of the DMN through neurofeedback is of paramount importance.

In our clinical practices it may be difficult to observe the behavior of DT patients when they are not engaged in any task although we acquire related information. The readers I am certain will have noticed the extreme discomfort from anecdotes from some patients and from observations of friends and acquaintances with a history of trauma when they are not engaged in an activity or task. Without the inhibition of fear from the mPFC in the presence of triggers or threats the fear goes unchecked. Bearing in mind that the DT brain is always scanning for threats and the fear response is constantly triggered, it implicates extreme discomfort. The person with developmental trauma is not only exposed to the stimuli that cause natural startle responses (which are generally significantly amplified in this population) to sudden noises, but also to thousands of sensory perceptions and experiences associated with the original insults that can trigger fear reactions.

Margaret is a 31-year old multi-talented and creative individual. She had suffered quite severe early childhood neglect and abuse and has had no contact with her divorced parents since she was eighteen. She saved money while working as an au pair in Holland and could afford to pay for her own studies when she returned to South Africa. She arrived at my practice with a diagnosis of ADHD and comorbid anxiety. She was concerned that she may lose her job at a corporate firm due to her lack of focus. Margaret did indeed present with attention related problems as well as impulsivity and what appeared to be fluctuating bouts of severe anxiety. She defined herself as being hyperactive. Her perception or her account of her behavior was based mainly on the feedback from others. She reported that she was perceived as being reactive, controlling, argumentative, impulsive and there were many other negative renditions of her traits each of which she insisted on justifying. Margaret described herself as not being able to sit still or to rest. She planned projects ahead of time and often did not follow through. I had difficulty to attain an authentic grasp of the essence of her or of the core of her discomfort. My sense was she was not in the room with me or that she had compiled a presentation that she delivered to me- notes and all! She was hasty, impatient and a core part of her was absent. It was a challenge to relate to her initially. When we started investigating her experience during resting states, it became evident that she avoided being idle to great lengths and that we were not dealing with straightforward ADHD and resulting anxiety. She simply could not retreat to her inner thoughts when she was idle. She experienced extreme discomfort and heightened anxiety when she was not actively engaged in an activity. While on task, when the task was challenging or pleasant enough, she could "rest in it and escape into it". She did not enjoy her work at all because there was no challenge. Her mind would start wandering and then she would become extremely anxious and panicky which resulted in intense headaches and other physical symptoms which implicated instability of arousal.

Interpreting her behavior in terms of probable malfunctioning of the DMN provided insight into why previous attempts at therapy that did not include brain training, were futile. The discomfort she experienced when idle and the difficulty I experienced in trying to locate her amidst all that she related, was probably related to the absence of a sense of self resulting from her dorsal medial prefrontal cortex (where the sense of "me-ness" resides (Fisher, \2020) being offline. When the DMN is supposed to come online during idle states, another important area that proves to have impaired connectivity with the population of individuals with histories of adverse childhood experiences is, as we have seen from research studies, the ventral medial prefrontal cortex that is vital in its function of inhibiting the amygdala. The client's heightened anxiety when not actively engaged in a task that requires focus, could probably be related to the absence of the inhibition of the amygdala implicated by the absence of the activation of the ventral medial prefrontal cortex. The consequences of a malfunctioning DMN are vast and potentially devastating.

The necessity of prioritizing the restoration of the DMN in patients with a history of trauma is self-evident.

Initially her training involved improving her attention, but it soon became evident that fear was at the core of her discomfort. The executive functions of the frontal cortex are mainly inaccessible when the PAG detects danger and activates the amygdala to initiate a fear response. We abandoned the attention-based protocols quite soon and proceeded with different approaches to lower the arousal, quieten the fear and restore a sense of self. She responded very well to right sided training at T4-P4, C4 and P4 as well as to C5- C6 . When her fear-driven behavior and anxiety became less, we commenced with 4Channel Z-score training that included the major hubs of the DMN with placements at F3, F4, P3, P4 and Fz, Pz, T3, T4. The Z-score training was alternated with amplitude training with decisions based on tracking the symptoms carefully. The young woman's life changed quite dramatically. She finally stopped sabotaging her relationships and even chose to locate her estranged mother. Panic attacks were something from the past. By the time I left Cape Town, she had plans to become engaged and her career as a professional photographer had taken off. Anxiety surfaced again shortly after my emigration, but she is currently responding very well to arousal protocols.

In unspoiled places in countries in Southern Africa one often finds swarms of flying ants after a summer rain shower in the late afternoon. They have fairy-like delicate wings and a short lifecycle. While camping on the banks of the Orange River close to the Namibian border, I found one in a puddle of rainwater. There in the water, it had lost its magnificence and could not be its natural self. It could dedicate itself only to futile attempts to survive-unless it would be thrown a lifeline. It reminds me of how vulnerable we are when our environment changes- when we are subject to an altered milieu. If we think of the evolved brain with all its circuitries intact as the landscape that has adapted to our needs to be fully functional human beings and liken it to the African sky in which the flying ant can thrive for a short period of time, it conveys a sense of our vulnerability. The time of day, the quality of the light and all aspects of the climate have to be in a particular perfect balance for it to be an actualized flying ant for a while. When the brain that presents the individual with the potential of an optimized human experience like the African sky to the flying ant, loses its balance, the experience of the individual changes. When the more advanced and modern circuitries are not functioning as they should, when there is no inhibition of the fear circuitries, when the brain is on high alert and dedicated to survival, we find ourselves weighted down in an ocean of fear. Neurofeedback is the lifeline that can restore the environment to one in which the trauma survivor can reach for the sky again instead of desperately struggling to stay afloat.

11.5 Common Symptoms Often Simplified and Mistaken

I have included this section because I believe that all of us have a tendency at some point at least to view symptoms through a lens. We develop tunnel vision zoomed in on whatever it is that we are coming to terms with cognitively or emotionally. Because of the books that I have written on ADHD for instance, I saw ADHD symptoms everywhere and the danger is that those and most other symptoms boxed in by a diagnosis can simulate almost any condition or disorder. The diagnosis is not what matters, we have established that. The diagnosis is mostly a hindrance and places a restriction on how we think about symptoms. The symptoms on the other hand are important. It gives us information about the discomfort that we are dedicated to alleviate, but we need to think about the origin of that symptom in terms of the brain. When there is impulsivity for instance, we need to consider whether it is simply an ADHD related problem or is it trauma related and therefore fear driven.

All neurofeedback practitioners work with people with DT. The symptoms they present with can match the symptoms of many diagnoses as we have seen. This section serves as a further reminder to look beyond the diagnosis to the history of the individual and to the brain.

The healthcare practitioner ought to be able to recognize the consequences of trauma for adequate referrals. The neurofeedback practitioners who have their basic training in other disciplines without a background in psychology, ought to be able to recognize the often confusing cluster of symptoms as the threads interwoven   in the shroud of trauma, in order to make informed protocol decisions and once the regulation of the brain has improved, to make referrals to trauma psychotherapists.

"A good deal of what we see as mental illness or as behavioral disorder has its roots in the density of developmental trauma" (Fisher, 2014). The challenge to the therapist is to pick up on the underlying fear through the layers of diagnoses and treatments with which the trauma victims mostly show up with on the doorstep of the neurotherapist to try yet another approach to rid themselves of the shackles from the aftermath of trauma. Mostly they do not show up with a diagnosis of PTSD or DT and they are not aware that the reason for their hyper- aroused nervous system is rooted in trauma or neglect. They do not understand the concept of an over-aroused or unstable central nervous system that keeps them alert to any possible threat either - until they do! When the underlying fear is explained in terms of neuroscience and arousal, there is relief.

Entwined in the fabric of the shroud of trauma with the threads of fear, shame and guilt, there is often the thread of abuse. The DTD sufferer often engages in abusive relationships or in codependent relationships. Their lack of self-worth and desperate need for recognition, acceptance, approval, and validation, often lead to bad choices pertaining to partners. Once in the spiral of abuse it is difficult to find the way out - especially when you are mostly functioning in survival mode from a state of fear as trauma victims do. Neurofeedback practitioners often witness how, when the higher cortical regions are accessed due to the calming of the fear circuitry, the trainee no longer desperately clings to the boat of a dysfunctional relationship as if his/ her life depended on it. The trauma survivors become able to make sound and rational choices that are beneficial to their wellbeing once fear is no longer the driving force.

It remains such a privilege to witness the transformation that occurs when a person finds his/her voice. *As it is in Heaven* is a Swedish film directed by Kay Pollak which I believe most readers will still remember mainly for the theme song "Gabriella's song" by Stefan Nillson with lyrics by Py Bäckman. In the movie, a renowned international conductor retires in the North of Sweden where he buys the old elementary school in a little village at which he endured bullying as a little boy. He then starts helping the local choir grow and develop and literally guides them to finding their voices. Their personal stories unfold and as they find their voices, their choices and their journeys change. They become liberated from their submissiveness to abuse and become empowered. The neurofeedback practitioners often witness these awe - inspiring transformations when the trauma victims get liberated from the shackles of fear.

Some of the effects of neglect and trauma are more predictable than others according to Sebern Fisher (2020).

Poor emotional regulation is one of the predictable symptoms of DT due to inaccessibility to the frontal structures involved in emotional regulation and the inhibition of fear reactions. It is probably also one of the most debilitating consequences that impacts on the victim's relationships, his/her work performance and basically every area of life. The survivors of trauma can be very fearful, volatile, intense, manic, unpredictable, impulsive or have anger outbursts after which they often experience shame. These types of symptoms are often perceived as being part of a bipolar disorder profile and not understood as being fear-driven from a hyper aroused nervous system in the wake of early childhood adversity. When improving the regulation of the arousal levels through neurofeedback, these incidents become less frequent and less intense.

Life for the victim of early-life trauma is generally complicated and difficult. "Going with the flow" is very seldom if ever a possibility. Whereas the average person generally looks forward to new experiences, holidays, engaging with new people and other pleasures life brings across our paths, the trauma victim dreads new experiences, anticipates potential danger and at the most endures each new day while yearning for the possibility of returning to a safe place. Mostly they don't participate in life- they are onlookers imprisoned by their fear. They find difficulty in being mindfully present in the moment and enjoying even the simplest of pleasures like a walk on the beach There are of course, different degrees of debilitation suffered by DT victims depending on varying factors, but it is important that the core concept of being imprisoned and debilitated by fear, be understood.

The DT victim always has attachment problems varying in degree based mostly on the severity of the trauma. It is important that any trauma disorder be perceived as a spectrum disorder. Symptoms associated with dissociation, depersonalization and derealization that are often a result of early-life trauma, can also vary in degree and are best understood in terms of the autonomic nervous system response illustrated in figure 11.4.

Cognitive development and learning ability can be impaired due to early childhood trauma and neglect. In areas that are impoverished and where substance abuse is rampant, one is more likely to come across children with learning difficulties due to trauma and neglect than due to ADHD or TBI.

Hyper- as well as hypo-sexuality can often be assigned to a history of trauma. When sexual abuse is part of the trauma history, sexual behavior of the victim is generally affected.

People that have suffered trauma, generally have problems with not only emotional regulation, but also with physical regulation. Relatively common physical conditions in the face of trauma history are an impaired immune system, chronic inflammation, and disease. The ACE-study clearly indicates that trauma victims often present with physical symptoms as well and predict the dire consequences if DT goes untreated.

Trauma victims often have a high pain threshold. If we consider the fact that we perceive by means of contrast, it is logical to assume that most wounds and typical pain sensations one comes across in daily life due to minor accidents, pales in comparison to the insults suffered by trauma victims. Self-harm (which is not an uncommon occurrence in this population) although more complicated than that, can be a part of this dynamic. Poor interoception (sense of the internal state of the body) controlled mainly by the orbito-frontal cortex which is often offline in the brains of the trauma population, is implicated in the high pain threshold as a common symptom in DT.

Impulsivity is often one of the common presenting symptoms of the traumatized brain. Impulsive reactions when the fear response has been triggered is inevitable if the stimulus that caused the fear response is not contextualized. The areas of the brain that neutralize fear responses and make sense of stimuli that activated the fear centers are often not available to the DT patient. The "cascade of terror" (Fisher, 2020) then unfolds as illustrated in figure 11.4. The option of thinking before acting is often not available to this population - but for a different reason than what is the case with young children and the ADHD-sufferers. In young children the right prefrontal cortex that is involved in inhibiting impulses is not yet fully developed. In the ADHD population impulsivity is associated with frontal cortical slowing. The impulsive responses of the DT patient are more explosive and harsh in nature because it arises as a defensive reaction. The unchecked responses often present as anger and are fueled by fear.

Other typical symptoms with which the traumatized brain acts out that can also very easily be mistaken for ADHD, pertains to feelings of being overwhelmed, difficulty with organizing and decision making. They can be overwhelmed by the simplest of decisions like for instance having to choose something off a menu. This is possibly best understood if you attempt to think what it would feel like if you had just received a phone call informing you of your child that had fallen ill suddenly and it is then expected of you to choose what to eat. The brain of the person with unprocessed trauma history is not in a relaxed dominant alpha state while sitting at a restaurant by the beach. The urgency of the alert state that you can recall when you imagine a crisis, is the same urgency the trauma survivor attempts to push to the background all the time in order to appear normal.

It is likely that the trauma survivor will find the loud voices and all the other sensory experiences in the restaurant very invasive, threatening, and disturbing. The person may either then act out in an inappropriate way by aggressively indicating that all the people are too loud or that the music is too loud or the person may internalize the discomfort with a whole host of potential symptoms including a panic attack or freeze response. The trauma survivor that was triggered by the sensory overload in the restaurant may also experience different physical symptoms including light headedness, heart palpitations, discomfort in the stomach or any part of the digestive system. Sweaty palms, dryness in the mouth or any other physical symptom associated with the sympathetic tone of the autonomic nervous system (see chapter 6 on the physiological responses to stress and tension) may arise. Should you think of this behavior in terms of a social anxiety disorder rather than interpreting it in terms of brain function, it may limit your consideration of protocol options.

Validation also goes to the core of early childhood neglect or abuse. The initial validation of the child's existence comes from the primary caregivers. Other than the attachment symptoms that can stem from a lack of a sense of self, the absence of recognition and approval in the life of the child that suffers neglect, it results in profound deep-seated lack of self-worth. It leaves the child with a constant background yearning for recognition and mostly remains a theme in the wake of the individual's journey through life. Should the origin of this behavior not be investigated, the neurofeedback practitioner could very easily make the mistake of wanting to lift the mood, the energy, and the confidence of this individual by doing left sided high frequency training. At the core of the presenting symptoms in DT there is fear that always needs to be calmed.

In her book *Emotional Alchemy: How the Mind Can Heal the Heart*, Tara Bennett-Goleman (2002) writes with great insight and compassion about how the lenses through which individuals view the world are shaped by past experiences. She describes fear and panic to often be the signature emotions of a history of abandonment, while sadness and feelings of hopelessness are often indicative of a history of deprivation. Dominant emotions of resentment and anger can often be traced to subjugation due to domineering parents. Rage is according to Bennet-Goleman (2002) frequently a result of mistrust born from betrayal and abuse whereas the emotions of shame and humiliation are associated with a conviction of unlovability. This book is, in my opinion, a helpful aid in developing a deeper understanding of and sensitivity to the many masks of the aftermath of trauma and neglect.

Many DT victims manage to have functional and meaningful lives. They design their lives skillfully with activities, routines, rituals, and safe places to which they can retreat and escape. The daily responsibilities, the expectations of others and exposure to new situations cause more stress and discomfort to those with developmental trauma histories than what is caused by the demands of daily living to the average population. Regular daily living, even during holidays, adds to their allostatic load.

McEwen and Steller, (1993) write comprehensively about the allostatic load in *Stress and the Individual. Mechanisms Leading to Disease* which is essentially the wear and tear on the body that accumulates when an individual is exposed to repeated or chronic stress. The underlying dynamic involves elevated or fluctuating endocrine responses due to exposure to challenges that the individual experiences as stressful. Many factors have been identified that contribute to allostatic load including genetic factors, diet, exercise, and other lifestyle factors to name but a few. The relevance of allostatic load to PTSD and DT is obvious.

Fisher (2014, p.184) sums up the ongoing effects of the aftermath of trauma eloquently as follows: "Beneath everything else, patients with developmental trauma suffer exhaustion at the core, from holding themselves together and from falling apart. When the allostatic load is too great, stress topples the patient into feeling exhausted, far beyond tired".

11.6 Neurofeedback Treatment Protocols for PTSD and DTD

Sebern Fisher suggests (2020) that the two main components on which neurofeedback protocol decisions ought to be based are the history of the patient and neuroscience. The two main goals to obtain are to quiet the fear by lowering the arousal and to restore the connectivity between the main hubs of the DMN.

Ruth Lanius states (see Nicholson et al., 2020) that common targets in neurofeedback ought to be based on the observed altered patterns of neural functioning in the patients with a history of trauma. Both large-scale neural oscillations as well as localized brain regions are implicated in research findings.

Neurofeedback protocols for trauma victims are mostly aimed at regulating alpha oscillations related to intrinsic connectivity networks and also at regulating amygdala activation including control from the mPFC.

In their study Ros et al. (2014) have found that people with a history of trauma often show drastically reduced alpha oscillations which is regarded a global index for chronic hyper-arousal.

The Peniston and Kulkosky research (1991) was in fact the first one to prove that the regulation of alpha brain waves reduced the PTSD symptoms in veterans. Not only was it evident that the protocol reduced hyperarousal symptoms , but also that the reward of alpha and theta brain wave activity, resulted in changes in the DMN and the SN which are intrinsic connectivity networks known to be directly involved in PTSD (Nicholson et al., 2020).

The treatment protocols discussed in this section are based on protocols being used for DT-related symptoms successfully internationally. The latest understanding of the significance of training closer to the inion ridge in the face of trauma, is still in the experimental stages and won't be discussed in detail in this edition.

Sensory Motor Strip and Parietal Placements

Sebern Fisher (2020) indicated that she mostly inhibits the frequency band of 1-6 Hz when working with DT patients. One mostly sees high amplitudes of delta and theta brainwave activity in this population. Sebern Fisher believes that the memories of trauma, neglect and abuse may be locked in into those frequencies which were the dominant frequencies of the developing mind when the insults occurred.

The upper inhibit band, when one works with two inhibit bands, is suggested to be 22-36 Hz unless differently indicated by the EEG, the QEEG or the reaction of the client.

Many neurofeedback practitioners (especially those trained in the arousal model) still to this day begin treatment with one channel amplitude training. Many of those practitioners prefer to begin treatment over the sensory motor strip. In the section on the arousal model in chapter 5, it was indicated that right sided training generally has a calming effect. The most common frequency to reward on C4 is 12-15 Hz. To start off with this protocol for trauma victims is a viable option and the patient's response will provide the neurofeedback practitioner with valuable information. This frequency may be too high for some. The neurofeedback practitioner will be guided by the reaction to the treatment protocol. C4 is a safe and well-researched placement from which to determine ideal frequencies.

There are those practitioners who prefer to begin the calming of the central nervous system by training the right parietal lobe at P4 or the posterior cingulate at Pz directly over the precuneus which is implicated in trauma as we have seen. The initial reward frequency is often alpha 8-11 Hz. It is generally safe to train here and seldom leads to any abreaction. Tracking the symptoms of the client carefully is paramount in finding optimal responses to treatment. There is also anecdotal evidence that alpha down training may be helpful. Research studies implicating the significance of the alpha oscillations in trauma have been quoted. Alpha down training over the precuneus has also shown significant reduction in DT-symptoms.

Some clients respond well to training on Cz at 12-15. Those experiencing discomfort due to ongoing inner chatter and those having difficulty in switching states, often experience relief with this protocol. It can also be helpful to those whose brains have resorted to OCD-type symptoms in dysfunctional attempts to improve regulation. Although it is the anterior cingulate (Fz) that is overactivated in OCD and is directly involved in regulation of emotion, most practitioners avoid starting off with frontal training. It appears that Cz training often does have a positive effect on OCD -related symptoms. If one considers the connectivity networks (see figure 11.5) it becomes clear that entire networks can be affected from different regions.

Inter- and Intra- Hemispheric Placements

In chapter 5 the reader will have noticed that trauma survivors often present with symptoms associated with instability of the central nervous system or unstable arousal. Some of the more common symptoms of unstable arousal with which the trauma survivors often present are manic-depressive cycles, mood swings, panic attacks, phobias, oppositional and defiant behavior, attachment symptoms, migraine, attention problems, seizures or seizure-like symptoms, a variety of pain symptoms, neurological, immune and autonomic symptoms. (See section 5.2.4.1 for a complete list of symptoms associated with instability of the CNS).

T3-T4 is considered to generally have a stabilizing effect on those with instability of arousal. Many practitioners start training at 12-15 Hz on the temporal lobes. For some this frequency is too high. The step-down temporal lobe protocol is also known to contribute to stability. I was first introduced to this protocol by Dr Roger DeBeus during a training workshop he presented in South Africa in 2006. Training commences at 12-15 Hz for three minutes followed by 11-14 Hz for three minutes and then training continues by stepping down at 1 Hz increments every three minutes all the way down to 8-11 Hz. Training at 8-11 Hz continues for approximately 12 minutes. I have witnessed much success with this protocol for children with DT presenting with conduct disorder symptoms.

In Sebern Fisher's book on DT (2014) she warns practitioners to be mindful of rigidity when training at T3-T4. She reminds the reader that it is not always easy to distinguish between stability and rigidity and training on the temporal lobes for too long, holds the risk of losing fluidity.

T4-P4, often starting with rewarding 10-13 Hz remains a popular protocol for bringing relief for emotional instability that is so often found in the wake of trauma. This protocol targets the fear circuitry and structures situated in the temporal lobe and accesses the DMN as well. This protocol mostly results in significant calming.

Training at C4-P4 especially when there are digestive issues or other prominent physical symptoms which is often the case with trauma victims is recommended. The goal remains to ascertain which frequency calms the CNS and increases the parasympathetic tone.

I have come across abreactions from T4 placements. The dedicated neurotherapist eventually develops an enhanced ability to tune in, so to speak, to the client's brain. With the trauma population there are often so many comorbidities that it is not possible to remain focused on the theory or on the client's QEEG. Some of the comorbidities will theoretically require opposing protocols, but it serves to remember that the brain has probably adapted and compensated in ways beyond what we can measure or make sense of. If we remain focused on the experience of the client, we will find frequencies and placements that calm the fear that sometimes defies reason.

There is significant anecdotal evidence that C5-C6 is a protocol that can be used with success in the trauma population as well. Ed Hamlin has had much success with this protocol for those with a diagnosis of bipolar disorder. It was mentioned earlier that it is not unusual that patients with DTD present with symptoms of bipolar disorder.

In Sebern Fisher's book (2014) on neurofeedback in the treatment of DT, as well as in her webinars and mentoring sessions she repeatedly reminds the neurofeedback practitioners that the goal with DT is to lower arousal and that the reward frequency needs to go as low as it needs to go to make that possible. She reminds that there is a wide spectrum of 0-45 Hz to consider.

Most practitioners that have been in the field for decades have been trained to mainly consider the reward frequency to be a bandwidth in the range of roughly between 8 and 18 Hz. Sebern reminds us that some need to train at reward frequencies as low as 0-3 Hz. Rewarding such low frequencies, does not, according to Fisher (2014) increase the amplitudes of slow brainwave activity. The arousal level is rather being "leveraged" while the slow brainwave activity is being lowered by inhibiting the slow frequencies. Having the same reward and inhibit band is sometimes necessary. Starting off at very low reward frequencies, however, is not recommended.

Training on or just above the inion ridge has been proven to be justifiable by the latest research in neuroscience indicating the significance of areas in the brainstem involved in trauma history. Protocols involving these areas are still in infancy and neurofeedback practitioners are advised to stay abreast of the research and anecdotal evidence in this regard.

FPO2

According to Fisher (2014), the work of Allan Schore (1994, 2003ab) that indicated the significance of the role of impaired development of the prefrontal cortex in affect regulation, lead to consideration of training at FPO2 for those with a history of developmental trauma. Fisher warns that caution ought to be exercised in this regard. It is suggested that if there is severe reactivity, that T4-FT8 be considered as an alternative to "reach" the insula which is another structure involved in inhibiting the amygdala.

Although FPO2 is not specified in the 10-10 system, it is indicated in the EEGer software. The active electrode is placed to the left and slightly above the left corner of the right eye in the little notch at the top end of the nose just below the right brow bone. The client ought to be lying back with closed eyes for practical reasons.

The neurofeedback practitioners that received their didactical training close to the turn of the century, will know that most practitioners remained hesitant to train at FPO2. Due to growing evidence of the significance of the targeted area in relation to the effects of trauma on the brain as well as to the anecdotal evidence of the positive effects of the application of this protocol trailing trauma, it is currently used more frequently.

Fisher (2014) suggests starting off with a reward frequency of 4-7 Hz while inhibiting 0-6 Hz and beta3. The goal remains the same: find the frequency that quiets the fear for the specific individual. The treatment time per session on FPO2 is typically between 1 and 5 minutes. Although the result is mostly positive and very calming and often induces a feeling of improved self-control, fear memories can be activated. This protocol is currently still contraindicated for those with a seizure disorder unless much improved stability is evident in which case extreme caution still needs to be exercised.

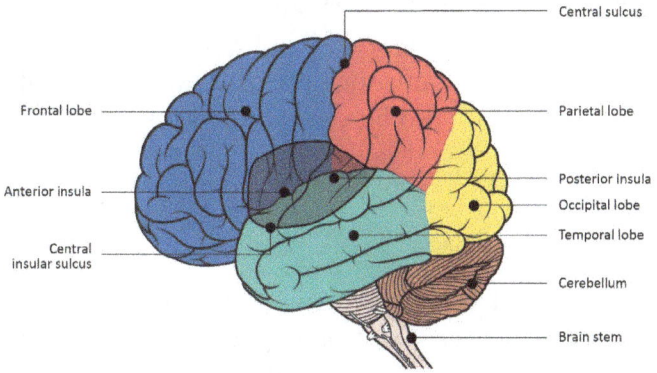

Figure 11.8: The position of the insula and other regions. Redesigned by Alesha Otto.

Z-score-, sLORETA- and ISF-protocols

Neuroscience research findings pertaining to the areas of the brain that are significant in brains of the victims and survivors of trauma are abundant. The involved regions and networks have been discussed. Whether regions or networks are being targeted that are under-developed or those that are over-activated or over-aroused, the protocol decisions ought to be substantiated by significant research results and a sound foundation in neuroanatomy and neurophysiology. The neurofeedback practitioner ought to not only have knowledge of the anatomical structures of the nervous system but also understand how the structures of the nervous system work together. The default mode network or any other relevant region or network can for instance be trained by various Z-score multi-channel placements (the reader is referred to section 5.4 that specifies the functional interpretation of 4 Channel training positions and section 3.5 specifying the location and function of the Brodmann areas).

sLORETA- training where the region of interest can be specified (see section 5.3) as well as the combination of LORETA and Z-score training can be used in scientifically based protocol decisions in the treatment of the results of trauma.

Protocol decisions for Z-score and LORETA training are often if not mostly guided by QEEG-reports.

Research results in ISF training on autists have indicated improvements in the networks associated with the sense of self (see section 5.7) which is a very relevant factor for the trauma population. A study conducted in South Africa has also shown the positive effects of ISF training for anxiety-related symptoms. According to Mark Smith (2017) ISF training leads to improved autonomic functioning which implies a healthier sway between the parasympathetic and sympathetic tone which is evidently significant to the trauma population. ISF can also be combined with sLORETA in infraslow sLORETA training.

11.7 In Closing

Intervention for the DT population has to commence at the level of the brain. Neuroscience suggests that initial intervention from any other perspective will have limited if any success. Psychotherapy, however important after improved regulation of the brain, cannot be successful when the patient does not have a developed sense of self or of other. The impaired connectivity of key structures in the DMN with those who have a history of early childhood neglect and abuse, implies inaccessibility of brain functions that are prerequisites to the success of talk therapy.

The following information from the *Association for Child and Adolescent Mental Health* on the effects of traumatic life experiences during childhood and adolescence published in 2016, in the *Child and Adolescent Mental Health Journal*, reveal disturbing facts and confirm the irrefutable fact that intervention ought to commence at the level of the brain: The centers for Disease Control and Prevention estimate that child maltreatment may be the most costly public health issue in the United States. Eradicating child abuse in America, would reduce the depression rate by more than 50%, alcoholism by more than 66%, suicide, drug abuse and domestic violence by 75%. "The current practice of applying multiple distinct comorbid diagnoses to traumatized children prevents a comprehensive treatment approach. Approaching their problems from a framework of memories of discreet traumatic events ignores the fact that the damage affects the brain's neural circuitry and goes well beyond dealing with discrete painful events. Our great challenge is to learn to utilize the brain's neuroplasticity to reorganize defective brain circuits" (Van der Kolk, 2016).

The statistics on the incidence of depressive disorders, suicide (see chapter and anxiety disorders (see chapter 9) are alarming. Many of those suffering in the aftermath of DT as well as PTSD are interwoven in the statistics of depression and anxiety and other diagnoses that receive less attention, but more are not factored into those statistics. Many are silent prisoners of fear, shame and rage and are tossed around helplessly in what feels like a flimsy, vulnerable boat on the tumultuous ocean of life, desperately trying to survive. Life remains for those under the burden of trauma only a quest for survival- just that- until someone throws them a lifeline of the possibility of quieting the fear and consequently improved self-regulation. Only then does the option of thriving, not only surviving, appear on the horizon.

Irrespective of the approach of the neurofeedback practitioner or the software and the hardware deployed, the goals remain clear: the reduction of arousal and fear, improved affect regulation and the restoration of undeveloped or malfunctioning networks affected by trauma.

As neurofeedback practitioners we currently have the most appropriate skills and equipment to address this pandemic of a different nature than the one we are in the wake of, but equally or more devastating, that has infiltrated most societies of the human race. With knowledge and access to resources comes responsibility and privilege. It is the responsibility as it is the privilege of all neurofeedback practitioners to be able to recognize the many faces of trauma, to stay abreast of the relevant research and the valuable shared knowledge and insights of experienced trauma neurofeedback practitioners. Based on this rich pool of knowledge and experience, appropriate protocol decisions can be made responsibly.

With this intervention at the level of the brain we don't only have access to an intervention that can transform the trauma victim's life from being a survivor to being one who thrives, we can literally save thousands of lives.

Chapter **12**

Case Studies

Introduction

The case studies presented in this book include case studies of clients from different age groups with different disorders and varying levels of discomfort. A few trusted and experienced neurofeedback practitioners from South Africa have been requested to make contributions to this book in this regard. The case studies were selected on the basis of being representative of a broad spectrum of clinical profiles that the average neurofeedback practitioner in South Africa gets exposed to. I believe that the selection of case studies ought to be fairly representative of the case load and also not foreign to the neurofeedback practitioners in the international arena. In the United States, it is possible for neurofeedback practitioners to work with specific disorders only, which enable them to sub-specialize in particular areas of expertise so to speak. Although the body of neurofeedback practitioners in South Africa is growing significantly, we still need to work in very diverse fields. Some neurofeedback practitioners started working with substance abuse, for instance, which they hadn't necessarily done prior to when they added neurofeedback as a modality to their practice. We find the same with epilepsy, with trauma and traumatic brain injury to mention but a few. The ideal is, of course, that the neurofeedback practitioners will focus on disorders and problem areas that coincide with their original training and their areas of expertise. One of the purposes of a book such as this one is to promote the field of neurofeedback to the extent that sub specialty becomes a viable option. Currently, communication between the different specialists involved in a particular problem is essential as is appropriate referrals.

A few testimonials of clients are included in the following chapter. These two chapters are intended to be a rewarding and pleasant read to all of those people seeking an alternative option for a problem they are burdened with. For the therapists, it serves as reminder why it is that we have embarked on this neurofeedback journey. Hopefully, those healthcare practitioners that started researching the field of bio-/ neurofeedback with a skeptical attitude

278

may consider including neurofeedback in their practices instead.

The names and other biomarkers of the cases that are being presented have been changed in order to protect the privacy of the clients. The cases are true cases and true reports from the indicated therapist and/or clients themselves. The case studies are not presented in a particular format because approaches of neurofeedback practitioners differ. The different formats are also attempts to meet the needs and interests of a very heterogeneous target group. In some cases I have included the thinking processes of the therapists involved in the compilation of a treatment plan in order to bring added perspectives to all bio-/ neurofeedback practitioners.

Consent was obtained from all of the individuals whose cases are presented in this book.

12.1 Case Study: A 60-Year-Old Male with Blepharospasm, Anxiety and Related Discomfort.

This case study was contributed by Louise van der Westhuyzen, the previous president, and a founding member of the Biofeedback Association of South Africa (BFSA). Louise is an occupational therapist registered with the Health Professions Council of South Africa. Her practice is in Plumsted in the Western Cape, South Africa. She is a general biofeedback and neurofeedback practitioner with BCIA Board Certification. Louise has been incorporating neurofeedback and other biofeedback modalities into her practice for the past 16 years. Louise dedicates much of her time and effort to promoting biofeedback in the health care field in South Africa.

JC is a 60-year-old male with a diagnosis of many medical conditions, including blepharospasm and facial dystonia, possibly being the most debilitating at the onset of his journey with Louise. Blepharospasm refers to a condition during which uncontrolled contraction of the muscle of the eyelid or "blepharo" occurs. The diagnosis of blepharospasm is applicable to any abnormal blinking or twitching of the eyelids resulting from any cause ranging from dry eyes to Tourette's syndrome to tardive dyskinesia. Facial dystonia is characterized by forceful contractions of the jaw and/ or tongue which often results in difficulties in chewing and in speech. This excessive involuntary contracting of the eyelids and muscles in the left side of the face, impacted on JC's driving ability, his work performance, and his social functioning (WebMD, n. d.).

JC experienced a lot of anxiety in his work environment but also in his dysfunctional marriage. In an attempt to experience less discomfort, JC avoided situations with high sensory input. At the onset of his new journey,

279

he had already had a history of generalized social withdrawal and two episodes of major depression. He did not have the ability to read social cues and facial expressions which often left him feeling confused and overwhelmed in social situations. JC also presented with sleep difficulties pertaining to sleep onset as well as frequent awakenings.

At the age of 30, JC was diagnosed with hypertension and at 35 with hyperlipidemia (genetic or acquired disorder that results in a high level of lipids, including fats, cholesterol, and triglycerides, in the blood). At the age of 52 he was diagnosed with type II diabetes and hypothyroidism. At 52, JC had coronary artery bypass graft (CABG) surgery after which he developed depression.

Louise's evaluation included an intake interview during which she obtained relevant history, a stress assessment with Biofeedback-script, a sensory profile obtained from a standardized questionnaire, an indication of depression and anxiety related symptoms based on the Amen Depression Anxiety Checklist, a mini EEG and QEEG and a psychiatric evaluation of Asperger Syndrome.

Louise considered the neuroanatomical structures involved in some of the presenting symptoms to be the basal ganglia (benign essential blepharospasm is considered a basal ganglia dysfunction), the primary motor cortex, the anterior cingulate and the secondary motor areas.

The stress assessment results as well as the mini-EEG on the following homologous sites: F3 and F4; C3 and C4; P3 and P4 as well as Pz, Cz and Fz, are indicated to the right:

Stress Assessment

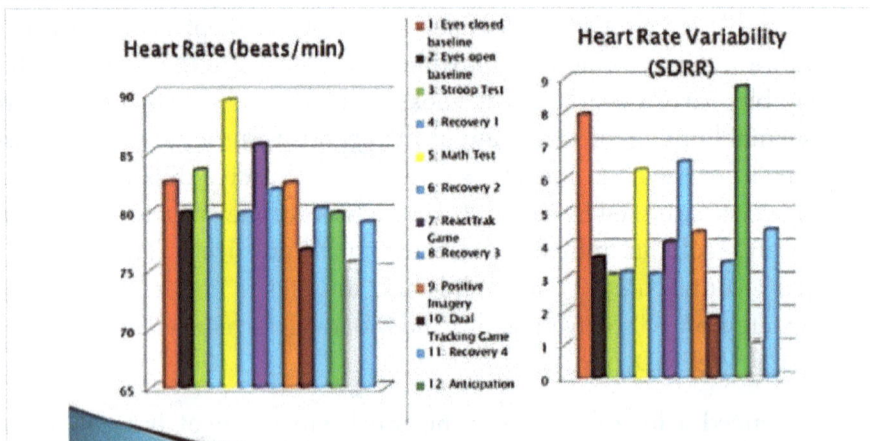

Figure 12.1: Stress assessment graphs of different biofeedback measurements (Reprinted with permission from the registered software user).

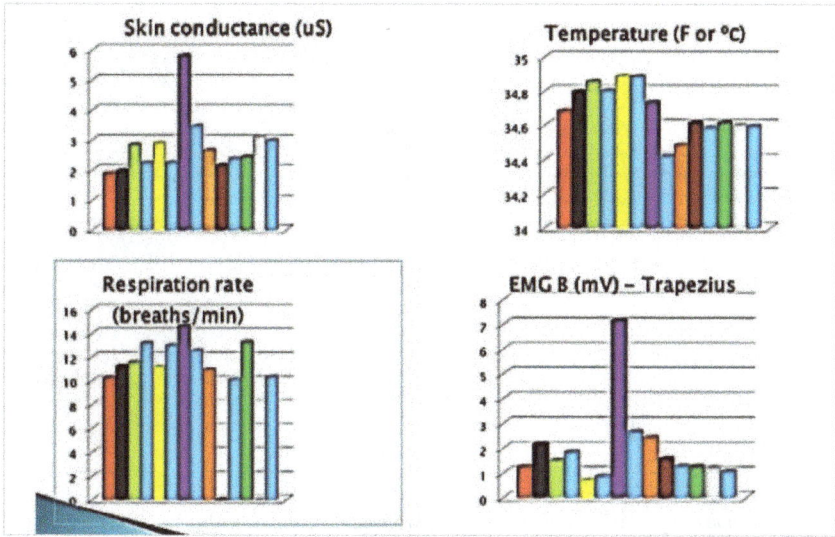

Figure 12.1: Stress assessment graphs of different biofeedback measurements (Reprinted with permission from the registered software user).

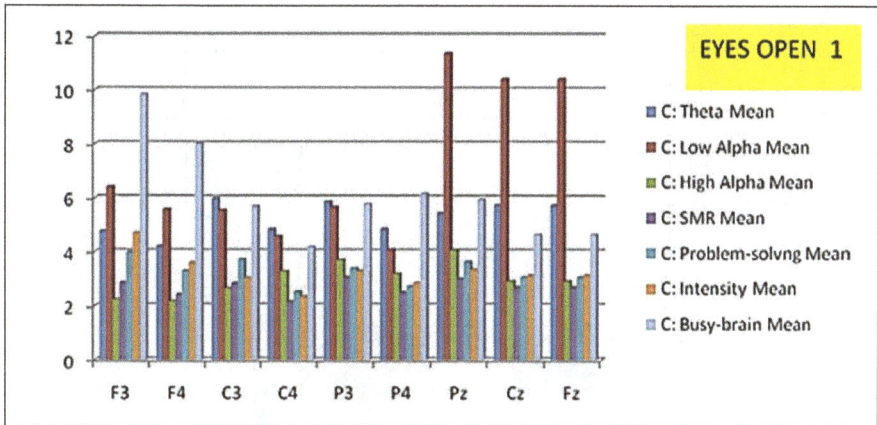

Figure 12.2: Stress assessment summary on homologous sites and central strip (Reprinted with permission by the registered software user).

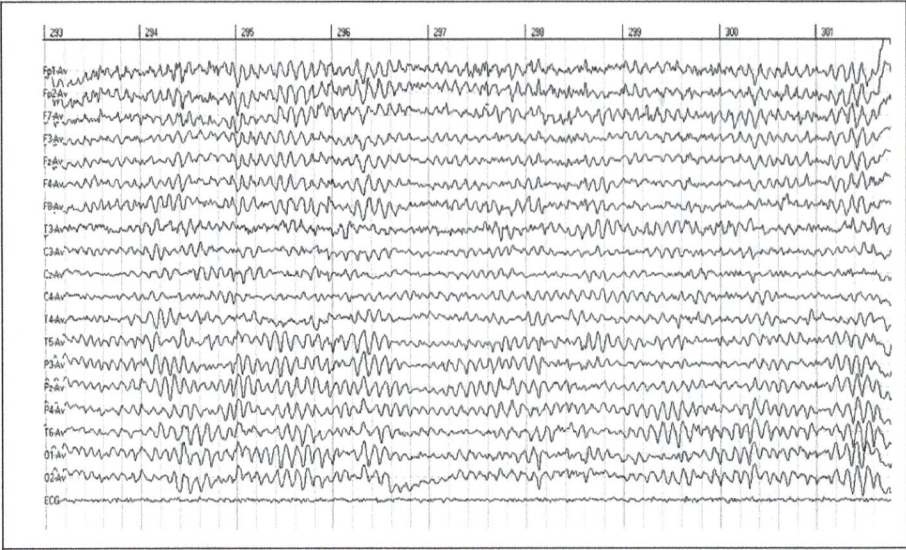

Figure 12.3: Section of raw EEG recording on 10/20 placements (Reprinted with permission by the registered software user).

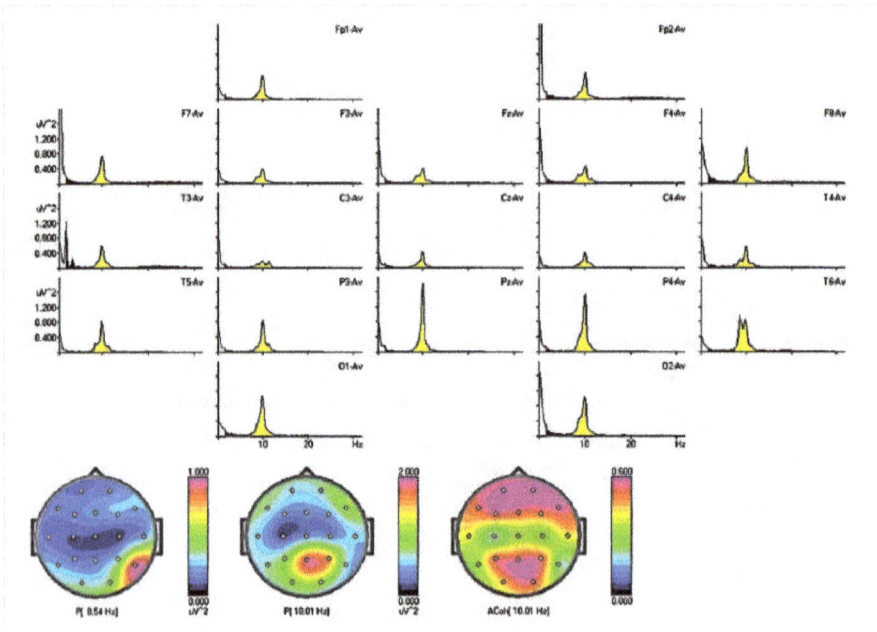

Figure 12.4: Alpha peak frequency distribution on the 10/20 placements (Reprinted with permission from the registered software user).

Louise indicates that the above profile is typically associated with affective regulatory issues resulting potentially in symptoms associated with depression as well as with symptoms associated with anxiety. She considers the problems the client has in terms of the lack of emotional insight and the absence of the ability to read social cues correctly to be linked to the right temporal slow peak frequency. The excessive frontal alpha may in her opinion, be associated with the blepharospasm because the muscles involved in eye movements are located in this area. The high alpha amplitude over the anterior cingulate area can lead to obsessive-like traits that may include an over focus or rumination on physical symptoms. Excessive alpha in this area is often associated with "stuckness".

Various interventions led to improved measurable outcomes as well as to dramatic changes in the client's life experience.

In terms of general biofeedback training, the following modalities were applied:

- Electromyography (EMG) training during which muscle tension is measured and addressed, was applied. The electromyogram sensors feed information back to the client about any changes in muscle tension. Second placement of an EMG sensor on the shoulder can not only assist the client in relaxing, but can also be useful in teaching diaphragmatic breathing. (See section 6.2.6 in chapter 6 for more information on electromyography).

- Peripheral skin temperature training and skin conductance measurements during which the client learns to control body temperature, skin conductance and relaxation was part of the general biofeedback training plan. Visualizing and focusing on increasing the skin temperature, assists the client with relaxation. When the client feels stressed there is a small rise in skin conduction and a small drop in skin temperature. Galvanic skin response is an indicator of skin conductance and increases linearly with a person's level of overall arousal (Nakasone et al., 2013). (See section 6.2.2 in chapter 6 for more information on peripheral skin temperature).

- Heart Rate Variability training is known to reduce anxiety and stress (Mikosch et al., 2010) and to improve cognitive functioning in stressful conditions (Prinsloo et al., 2011). HRV training has also been researched extensively in relation to mental processing and emotional stability (Thayer et al., 2009) as well in relation to certain physical conditions. Given the

283

multitude of conditions that can potentially improve when a person increases the variations in time between their heartbeats and the fact that many of the conditions are relevant to the client, it made good sense to include HRV in JC's treatment plan. (For more information on HRV training the reader is referred to chapter 6, section 6.2.5).

In terms of neurofeedback training, Louise used the following protocols:

- Alpha/theta training was done with an active electrode placement on Pz. Both alpha amplitudes and theta amplitudes were rewarded and beta activity was inhibited. This decision was guided by the QEEG as well as by the client's symptoms.

- At Cz down-training was done of frequency bands 6–10 Hz and 22–36 Hz.

- Down-training of frequency bands 4–10 Hz as well as of 22–36 Hz was done on Fcz.

- Two channel training was done on C4+T4 where the 12–15 Hz frequency bandwidth was enhanced while the 22–35 Hz frequency bandwidth was inhibited

The protocol decisions were based on a culmination of information attained through the QEEG, the symptoms of the client, all other collateral information as well as the ongoing tracking of symptoms.

Louise utilized the alpha/ theta protocol to induce calmness and improve the quality of sleep of the client. The protocol she used on the frontal lobes was meant to activate the frontal lobes by suppressing the alpha activity. This would have a noteworthy effect on the client's mood. The enhancing of the 12–15 Hz frequency band on the right hemisphere was to have a calming and stabilizing effect on the motor system.

The FCz protocol would address focus, attention, and anxiety components.

Louise's thinking about the training on FCz also included consideration of the fact that the training on that placement area could influence the activity of the anterior cingulate gyrus which could potentially in turn be affecting the mirror neuron activity through the connections of the cingulate to the frontal and parietal lobes. Should the effects on the mirror neuron system become clear, the client's sensory and motor aprosodia could be addressed without having to train on sites T6 and F6.

The heart rate variability training (HRV) could "do more than help". The connections of the brainstem nuclei to the striatum, diencephalons to the cortex and in particular to the anterior cingulate, may have a direct impact on the Asperger's symptoms with which JC presented.

The decisions on the number of sessions and the duration of the treatment were based on ascertaining the measurable outcomes and tracking the client's symptoms on an ongoing basis.

Louise emphasizes the relevance of the Systems Theory of Neural Synergy in her approach.

The neurofeedback training was focused on addressing the symptoms pertaining to the lack of the ability to read and mirror emotions, the client's poor self-regulatory skills, poor attention to his external world as well as his anxiety. Many researchers and authors have indicated the value of incorporating neurofeedback and general biofeedback modalities. The polyvagal theory of Porges (2007) describes the different roles of the unmyelinated vagus and the myelinated vagus. The unmyelinated vagus or the dorsal vagal complex responds to threats through immobilization, shutdown and passive avoidance and is activated during PTSD when a person believes that he will die. A different mechanism involves the sympathetic nervous system in response to threats. The response of the SNS together with the endocrine system results in mobilization, fight or flight or active avoidance. The SNS inhibits the unmyelinated vagus and mobilizes the individual for action. The third system in play which is considered to be the most recently developed system in terms of evolution is the myelinated vagus system. This system rapidly adjusts cardiac output and promotes social engagement (Thompson & Thompson, 2015). According to the same authors, daily stressors will result in a decrease in the myelinated vagal response and a corresponding increase in sympathetic drive in most people. Relaxing muscle tension, emptying the mind of negative ruminations and diaphragmatic breathing to increase HRV, can decrease the sympathetic drive and restore the myelinated vagal system that results in a state of calm. Louise states that this polyvagal theory often influences her approach to compiling a treatment plan: "Both neurofeedback and general biofeedback influence dynamic circuits and no matter from where we access the nervous system with an intervention, the nervous system will seek its own new balance and equilibrium."

JC's treatment also included CBT from a psychotherapist, prescribed medication from a psychiatrist, lifestyle changes, a biofeedback home program including mindfulness meditation and treatment of his eye with heat and massage by an optometrist.

Below are the changes in the mini-QEEG recording eight months after the onset of the client's bio-/neurofeedback training program in comparison to the initial recording:

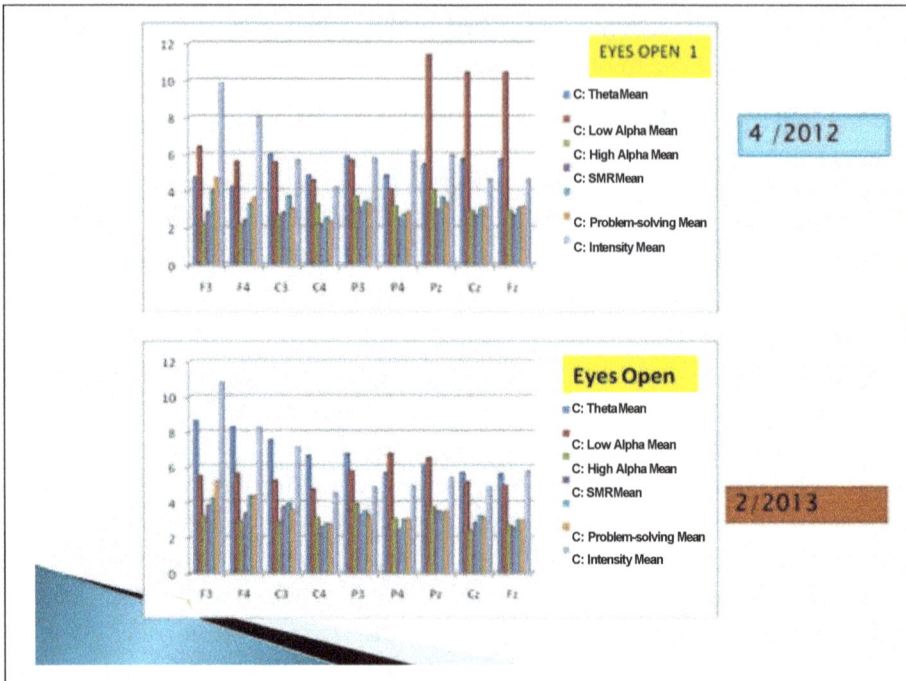

Figure 12.5: Pre- and post-treatment graphs.

The most dramatic changes involving the lowering of the low alpha bandwidth over the central strip (Pz; Cz and Fz) implies increased activation of the cingulate gyrus related to many of the client's prominent symptoms.

JC reported dramatic changes in his lifestyle and significant relief of his symptoms. Once the blepharospasm was under control, he felt liberated and was able to drive without fear of his eyes wanting to close. As lecturer to MBA students, he felt less overwhelmed and better regulated and focused.

JC's personal and social life was also affected positively. He could muster up the courage to end an abusive relationship without fear of being alone. He also no longer needed to isolate himself and could meet with friends in coffee shops and attend other social events. His sensory sensitivity became significantly less. After he had abstained from off-roading for a long period of time, he once again took to remote off road destinations in his 4x4 vehicle from where he could pursue his passion for photography.

In the process of his training, JC got to know, understand, accept and respect himself much better and he is currently assisting families with getting to grips with children that have been diagnosed to suffer an autism spectrum disorder.

12.2 Case Study: An 18-Year-Old Female Presenting with Headaches and Migraines

This case study is a contribution by Louise van der Westhuyzen.

Zoë is an 18-year-old grade 12 student. She is a very diligent and high performing student. Next year, she wants to go to university and is concerned that she may not be accepted despite her good academic performance and achievements. In South Africa, the allowance criteria for all degree courses offered at universities have become exceedingly higher. Those candidates that do not come from a historically disadvantaged population, stand a slim chance of being accepted, even with exceptionally high marks. Achieving the minimum criteria for acceptance into a study course does not suffice at all. The secondary school learners that intend attending a university in South Africa are, generally speaking, under a lot of pressure.

Zoë suffers debilitating headaches and migraines. She has been having at least one migraine per week for a couple of years. When Zoë does not suffer a migraine attack, she generally has generalized headaches most of the time. Her mother also suffered migraines when she was an adolescent. Zoë's migraine attacks are particularly severe and render her incapacitated for the most part. She is unable to attend school or perform most of her responsibilities when she suffers a migraine. During the intake interview and in the process of gathering all relevant history and other information, it became clear that Zoë suffers anxiety that has gone unchecked for many years.

The training program that Louise compiled for her consisted of general biofeedback as well as neurofeedback training sessions.

Zoë did heart rate variability training in order to improve her ability to lower her arousal level while increasing RSA (respiratory sinus arrhythmia) while being taught coherent breathing by which the R-R interval on the ECG is shortened during inspiration and prolonged during expiration.

Electromyography (EMG) during which sensors were placed on frontalis and masseter muscles as well as temperature training sessions were included in Zoë's training program. She was taught visualization techniques that she could utilize and apply beyond the therapeutic setting.

Another biofeedback modality that has also been proven to reduce vagal tone is GSR/skin conduction which involves sweat gland activity, was also included in Zoë's training program.

The neurofeedback training protocols that were utilized included the following: alpha training on C4 and P4; alpha/theta training on Pz; frontal lobe training on F3 and asymmetry training on F3 and F4.

Alpha training generally has a calming effect and is often trained in the eyes open condition on the right side of the brain over the sensory motor cortex as well as on the right parietal lobe.

Alpha/theta training is generally done in the eyes closed condition during which lower frequencies conducive to relaxation and creativity are rewarded while higher frequencies associated with cortical involvement are being inhibited. Although alpha/theta training was originally applied in order to induce a hypnogogic state during which processing of complex emotional issues could be instigated, additional benefits were revealed through research. Alpha/theta training potentially holds benefits for alcohol induced anxiety and depression and is also often used for those who seek improved meditative concentration, reduced sympathetic autonomic activation, improved focus ability, sustained attention ability, improved working memory and improved neuroplasticity. Louise further justifies her decision of including alpha/theta training in Zoë's training program by emphasizing that alpha/theta training affects various neuroanatomical circuitries involving the arousal system, limbic circuits, affective, motivational and cognitive functions.

Zoë's training program was concluded with frontal lobe training to improve her attentional abilities and mood regulation. (The significance of alpha asymmetry in mood regulation has been researched extensively and elaborated on elsewhere in this book). The frontal lobe training sessions were ended off with rewarding 15–18 Hz on F3 which Zoë referred to often as her "sparky spot" due to the positive effects on her studying abilities.

As the training progressed, Zoë's headaches and migraine's became fewer and further apart until they subsided. She started realizing how the muscle contractions in her jaw and fascial muscles escalated to a headache and could regulate towards a more relaxed and calm state. She became aware of the physiological and emotional factors that contributed to her regular migraine's and could consequently avoid, regulate or correct those factors. Zoë's life without headaches and migraines is a life with so much more potential for joy and actualization. The best for last: Zoë managed to free herself from her dependency on analgesics.

12.3 Case Study: A 24-Year-Old Male with TBI

This case study is a contribution by Louise van der Westhuyzen.

Neal fell from the fifth floor of a building. Fortunately, a sky bridge interrupted his fall. Neal's injuries, including traumatic brain injury, two cracked ribs and a fractured scapula, changed life as he knew it.

Prior to the accident which occurred in 2016, Neal was a high functioning individual. He wrote his senior certificate examinations in 2012. Instead of the seven compulsory subjects, Neal had registered for ten subjects. He achieved A's (higher than 80%) in all of his subjects with the exception of Afrikaans First Additional Language. With these excellent results, Neal was accepted at the University of Cape Town (UCT), one of the most prestigious universities in South Africa, for a degree in actuarial science. During Neal's first two years of study at UCT, he passed all his subjects and passed all but two in his midyear exam in 2016. Neal had admitted to socializing too much and not paying enough attention to his studies.

Neal is described as having been quite a keen sportsman prior to his accident. He played both rugby and basketball. While playing rugby, he suffered two mild concussive brain injuries.

Six months after the accident, Neal was evaluated by Louise Van der Westhuyzen to ascertain the potential relevance of a general biofeedback and neurofeedback interventions.

Neal arrived at Louise's practice with a walking frame and added assistance. He had a full-time caretaker assisting him with bathing and getting dressed and other actions and activities he had difficulty in performing. He presented with right hemiparesis resulting in an uneven gait and limited use of his right arm and hand. Neal's speech at the time is described as having been indistinct with word finding difficulties. Neal also presented with memory related problems. Neal's reading fluency was limited and his reading speed was slow but it appeared that his reading comprehension was intact. Neal's attention span was five minutes and he even fell asleep during the interview. He also experienced difficulties with swallowing.

Following is a summary of relevant information from his initial QEEG report after a EEG recording done in December 2016:

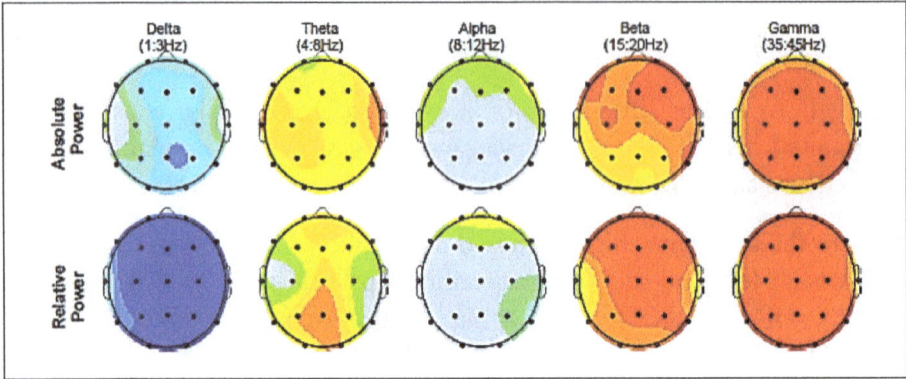

Figure 12.6: Absolute and relative power distribution across different bandwidths (Reprinted with permission from the registered software user). (Case Study 12.3).

A summary of the distribution of the power across the brain in single hertz bins is illustrated below.

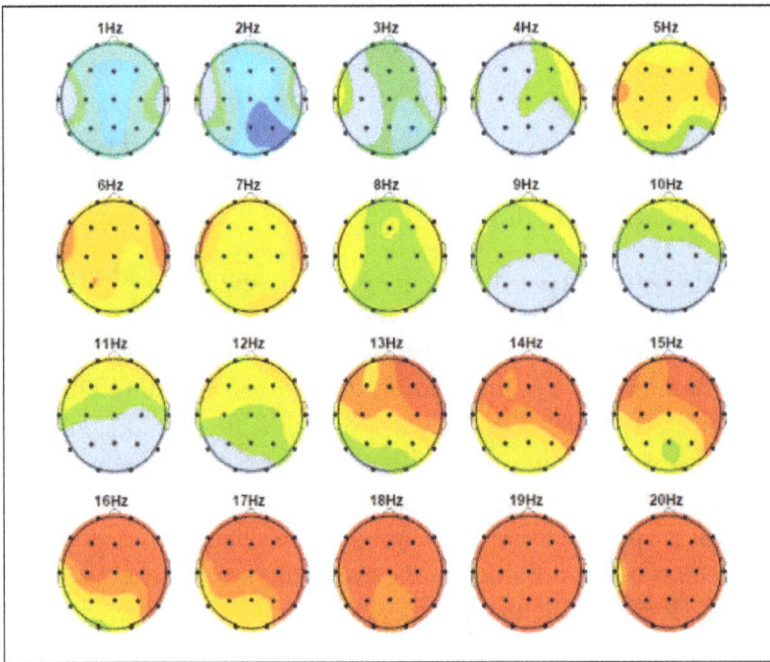

Figure 12.7: Distribution of power across the brain from 1 Hz to 20 Hz (Reprinted with the permission from the registered software user). (Case Study 12.3).

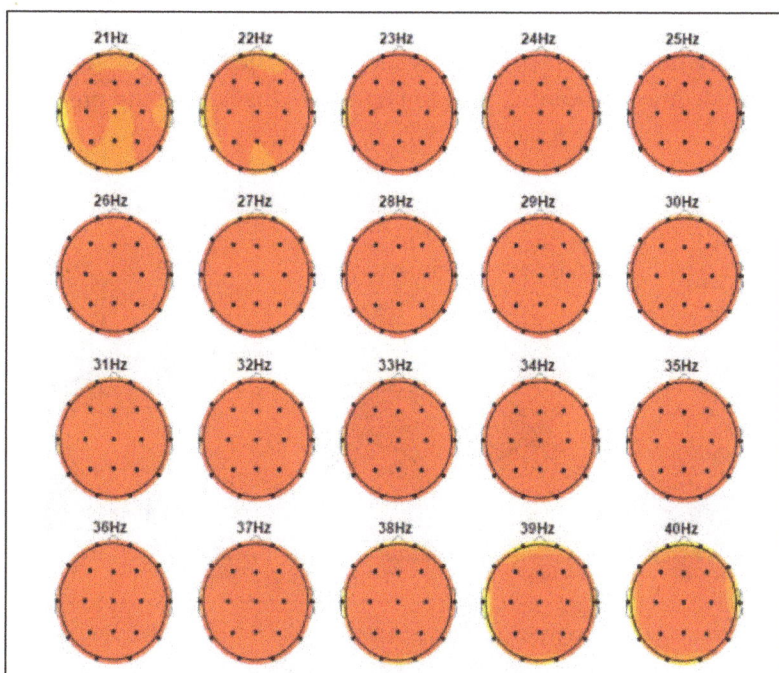

Figure 12.8: Distribution of power across the brain from 21 Hz to 40 Hz (Reprinted with the permission of the registered software user). (Case Study 12.3)

By the time Neal arrived at Louise's practice, he had received extensive rehabilitation therapy for approximately six months. The interventions included craniosacral physiotherapy, aqua-physiotherapy, and physiotherapy for his shoulder, occupational therapy, bio-kinetic therapy, psychotherapy, and career counselling. When Neal started with his general biofeedback and neurofeedback training with Louise, he continued with some of the above-mentioned therapies.

After neurofeedback training for two years, Neal's life is back on track with a few remaining challenges. Due to the right hemiplegia, Louise started with the neurofeedback training on C4. This right-sided training was followed by 10 sessions at C3 enhancing 13–17 Hz. Neal's walking started improving in terms of muscle output and minimizing walking aid. C3-C4 training sessions followed when Neal started walking with and without a cane. Louise then included two channel live Z-score training on C3, C4. As soon as it became evident that Neal was displaying improved regulation of his arousal levels and no longer fell asleep when inappropriate and yawning subsided, Louise moved on to 4 Channel live Z-score training for 20 sessions on C3, C4, P3, P4. The results of these training sessions are described as being remarkable. The subsequent training involved frontal, central, parietal, and temporal placements in different combinations.

Following are illustrations of relevant sections of the QEEG report following an EEG recording 22 months post the neurofeedback training onset in April 2018:

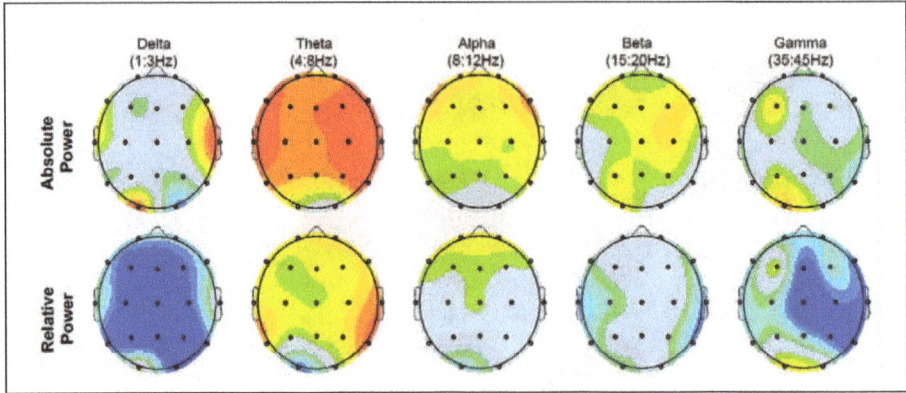

Figure 12.9: Absolute and relative power distribution across specified bandwidths (reprinted with permission of the registered user of the software). (Case study 12.3).

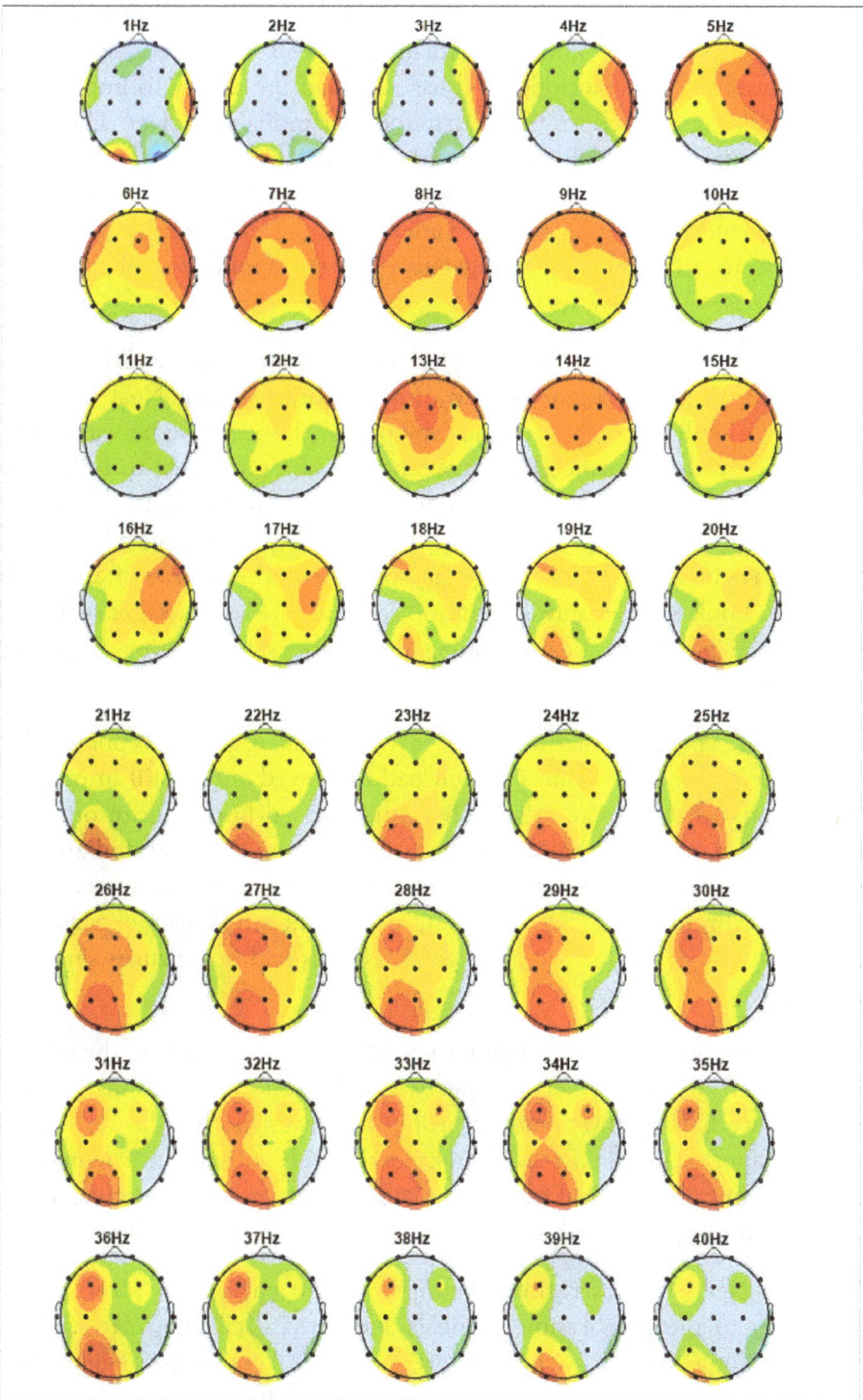

Figure 12.10: Distribution of power across the brain in single hertz bins (Reprinted with permission from the registered software user). (Case study 12.3).

The changes in the distribution of the power in the pre- and post-training recordings are drastic and self-explanatory. This brain was extremely dysregulated after the accident and has regained the ability to improve its own regulation as well as the distribution of available power. The most drastic changes are evident in the fast brainwave activity bandwidths. One feels privileged to have access to technology that enables us to witness such drastic changes in measurable outcomes and one feels equally privileged to be able to actualize such changes through the application of that same technology.

Neal is currently able to walk unassisted. He no longer uses a walking frame, a cane and no longer needs the aid of a foot brace either. Neal can once more write with his right hand and type on his phone which he was unable to do prior to his neurofeedback training. It is now possible to follow his conversations. He manages to remain focused on mathematical activities for two hours in a structured environment. Neal is able to manage all the basic activities required from an average person during the course of a day. He can read a book comfortably and compile an accurate and succinct summary on what he has read. Neal's reading comprehension has thus improved significantly.

In terms of symptoms that reflect Neal's experience, Louise reported that Neal indicated that his concentration had improved and is still improving. He reported that the excessive fatigue that caused him to doze off often at inappropriate times was something of the past. He indicated that his cognitive processing speed had not yet returned to where he experienced it to be prior to the accident. He stated that he no longer experienced any symptoms of anxiety or depression. He has had no seizures since the accident.

Louise also wanted to gain insight into Neal's behavior outside of the clinical environment from another perspective and requested that his mother would share her observations. According to Neal's mother, he sometimes makes inappropriate jokes and laughs excessively, often more than what the situation calls for. Neal has never been an organized or particularly tidy person, but he appears to be more disorganized than prior to the accident.

Although Neal still has residual hemiparesis, he engages in some chores pertaining to the preparation of meals and general cleaning. He has also registered for a distance learning course. When Neal completes assignments, he appears to be avoiding excessive reading and often attempts to deliver responses to questions without having studied the content. Most of Neal's free time is occupied by an array of ongoing therapies.

12.4 Case Study: An 18-Year-Old Female Learner with Developmental Delays due to Premature Fontanelle Closure

This case study was contributed by McGill Scott, the current President of the Biofeedback Association of South Africa (BFSA). McGill is also one of the three BCIA accredited neurofeedback trainers in South Africa and the international representative of BrainMasterTM. McGill is an educational psychologist registered with the Health Professions Council of South Africa. Her practice is in Cresta, a suburb of Randburg in Gauteng, South Africa. She is a neurofeedback practitioner with BCIA Board Certification. McGill has been incorporating neurofeedback into her practice for the past 16 years. McGill does wonderful work in schools over and above her work in her private practice. She is often a voice on behalf of BFSA members to the international fraternity pertaining to educational opportunities.

When McGill met Sue, Sue was a grade 9 (in South Africa grade 9 indicates the ninth year of formal schooling and it is the second year of the student's high school career) student at a private catholic school. The average age of grade 9 learners in South Africa is fifteen provided that you were never held back for a year. Sue however, had to repeat grade 1 due to developmental and learning difficulties that were already anticipated at the age of two.

When Sue was two years old, her parents noticed behavior that was not always age appropriate. It is admirable that the parents noticed delays because Sue is their first born and the delays were not gross delays. Because of their concerns, they had a consultation with a pediatrician who referred them to a neurologist. The neurologist suggested that scans of the brain be done which indicated that her fontanelles (the soft membranous gaps between the cranial bones in the skull of an infant) had closed prematurely. The fontanelles allow for rapid stretching and deformation of the neuro-cranium as the brain expands faster than the bone can grow. The implication of this news is quite drastic – Sue had inevitably already sustained some measure of brain injury. It could not be predicted with accuracy exactly how Sue's further development and her life would be influenced. The neurologist suggested that the parents be prepared to expect learning difficulties. Intensive remedial assistance was sought since the onset of Sue's schooling career. Sue had to repeat grade 1 due to the fact that all the learning outcomes had not been met by the end of her grade 1 year. Continued learning support was essential and the parents and the school did the best they could. Sue underwent a full psychometric evaluation when she was in grade 7. Her cognitive functioning fell into the low average range. The cognitive skills that measured lowest were her verbal skills, processing skills and working memory. A Cogmed course, aimed at improving Sue's working memory seemed moderately beneficial for a short period. By the time Sue had progressed to grade 8, she was really struggling academically. The role figures had a meeting during which the possibilities of having her repeat another year in her school career and placement in a remedial school, were considered. Sue's parents resisted both recommendations and requested her to be granted a grace period. And this is where Sue's journey with McGill and neurofeedback started.

McGill offers her services at schools in Johannesburg. Being an educational psychologist, she does not only offer neurofeedback but other learning support services as well. McGill's initial intervention program for Sue involved three neurofeedback sessions and two remedial intervention sessions per week due to the severity of Sue's learning needs. This program was followed for the first two school terms of Sue's grade 8 year and reduced to two neurofeedback sessions and two remediation sessions per week in term three. McGill thought it important to allow Sue more free time to engage in other activities that she wished to participate in.

Intervention Program – Year 1:

During the first year of Sue's neurofeedback intervention, McGill did exclusively power training, including training over the sensory motor strip and temporal lobes on C4, C3, Cz, T3 and T4. Amplitude training was also done on the parietal lobes on P3, P4 and Pz as well as on frontal sites (F3, Fz and F4). Training on some of the sites on the 10/10 placement system that indicates sites in between the 10/20 placement areas was also done. McGill also did bipolar training on inter- and intra- hemispheric sites, including C3-C4, T3-T4, F3-F4, P3-P4, C4-F4, T4-F4 and more. Training on homologous sites such as F3 and F4 separately was also done. Sue's symptoms and reactions to each training session were tracked carefully and played a significant role in McGill's protocol decisions.

Over and above the neurofeedback training, Sue's remediation plan was focused on improving reading speed, reading comprehension – with the emphasis on inferential comprehension – as well other receptive language skills. Sue was taught skills to assist her in the understanding of abstract language including the use of metaphors and other literary devices used in poetry and prose. Planning skills and study techniques were also included in Sue's learning support program.

The Inclusive Education Policy as well as the Independent Examination Board in South Africa makes provision for adaptations in evaluation methods for learners with specialized educational needs. The school allowed for additional time in which to complete test and examination papers, and also permitted an approved reader to read the question papers to the learner and offer planning aid.

Sue met the promotion requirements at the end of grade 9.

Intervention Program – Year 2:

During the second year of Sue's neurofeedback training, she also had two sessions per week. Live Z-score training, using four channels, was interspersed with amplitude training. Over and above the continued careful tracking of symptoms that influenced McGill's protocol decisions, tolerance levels were also considered with especially the four-channel live Z-score training. The following, are the main placements that were used for the live Z-score training:

- C3 C4 P3 P4
- C3 C4 F3 F4
- P3 P4 F3 F4
- F3 F4 F7 F8

In terms of remediation, the emphasis was on mathematics, geography and history based on the syllabus. The approved accommodations were implemented during the examinations and other assessments.

During her third year of neurofeedback training, Sue found the workload as well the pace of grade 11 very demanding. Consequently, she became more anxious and developed problems with sleep. She was introduced to heart rate variability and diaphragmatic breathing exercises and did relevant training daily with a biofeedback device at home.

ISF training was included in Sue's neurofeedback training program. (ISF training is discussed in chapter 5, under no 5.2.9). This training is usually very intense, and it can be difficult to find the optimal frequency. The placements that were used for ISF included T3/T4; T4/FP2; T4/FP1 as well as T3/FP2. Sue was receiving two training sessions per week at this point. Her training comprised of four Z-score training sessions for every one ISF training session.

The school once again allowed for the accommodations in assessments as previously approved. In South Africa, any adaptations in evaluations for the grade twelve year has to be approved by the Education Department or the Independent Examination Board in the case of private schools. This application involves a complete cognitive evaluation which was performed during the second half of Sue's grade eleven year.

The reader may be cognizant of the fact that intellectual potential as measured on a standardized intellectual scale generally remains rather fixed throughout one's lifetime until there is cognitive decline. The re-evaluation of Sue's intellectual capacity rendered the following results:

Tests	2010 (UK) WISC IV	2016 (UK) WAIS III
Language		
Vocabulary	8	11
Similarities	10	14
Comprehension	8	12
Information	11	15
Non Verbal		
Block Design	8	7
Picture Concepts	14	-
Matrix Reasoning	7	14
Picture Completion	6	8
Picture Arrangement	-	(10)
Other	-	-
Digital Span	6	8
Letter/No Sequencing	6	8
Arithmetic	6	12
Coding	6	12
Symbol Search	9	10
Scales and Indices		
VCI	93	118
POI	82	97
WMI	77	99
PSI	85	106
Verbal Scale	-	111
Performance Scale	-	98
Full Scale/GAI	-/87	105

The most significant improvement is in the language subtests. This improvement was reflected in her school report. All the role figures involved in Sue's life rejoiced at the improvement especially because it resulted in improved academic performance. Unfortunately the adaptations in evaluation methods were no longer permitted due to the fact that Sue's reading ability had improved significantly along with her improved scores on the cognitive battery. Sue had now finally reached grade 12 which is the final year of secondary school. Her neurofeedback and remediation program continued with sessions every second or third year. Learning support for her first additional language was added.

At the end of 2017, Sue obtained a University Entrance Matric and she is currently taking a gap year with her family in South America. She intends to return to South Africa and to enroll for a degree in psychology. McGill is very proud of her as are her family members. McGill commends her for her perseverance and diligence.

The author would like to commend McGill for the future of this young woman that now holds endless possibilities.

12.5 Case Study: The Story of Mark – The Young Man with No Past

This case study is a contribution by McGill Scott.

It is probably so that the practice of the average health care practitioner that adds neurofeedback to their services rendered changes. There are suddenly many 'firsts'. Mark was such a 'first'. McGill met mark soon after she had added neurofeedback to her practice. Back then, at the turn of the millennium, the options in neurofeedback were limited. Only amplitude training and alpha/theta training were available and there was no access to QEEGs and reliable normative databases in South Africa. Protocol decisions were based on the client's symptoms and the therapist's knowledge of brain function.

Mark was carried into McGill's office by his father. Due to a very serious motor vehicle accident in which he had suffered a brain injury, Mark had lost his ability to walk. Mark had also lost his identity. He had no recollection of any events prior to the accident. Without memories he could not have a sense of belonging, feel connections to his family members and friends or have a sense of self. McGill described him as a "free floating being with no attachments".

When they met, Mark was 17 years old and he would have been in grade

11, the penultimate year of high school. It was six months after the accident. McGill felt overwhelmed when she attempted to understand the full implications of Mark's situation. She had never dealt with a similar case in her entire career. Where would she start? Plans were in place for physiotherapy and bio-kinesiology and a caliper was to be constructed to assist with Mark's walking.

McGill was clear that a timeline of sorts had to be developed to ground Mark and make it possible for him to identify with his life. Mark's mother provided numerous photographs dating back to Mark's babyhood. With the help of photos and stories, identities of friends and family members were reconstructed and embedded into Mark's timeline to create a narrative. Once Mark had regained a sense of self, McGill and Mark started working on future goals. Mark wanted to enroll for his Senior Certificate Examination. McGill gained permission from the Independent Examination Board for Mark to be permitted to complete his matric year over two years and that special accommodations in terms of adaptations in evaluation methods would be granted.

In terms of neurofeedback, McGill did a variety of power training protocols over roughly a two-year period while carefully tracking symptoms throughout the process. McGill also assisted Mark with planning skills and other executive brain functions. Mark passed matric within the scheduled time.

After extensive Road Accident Fund court cases, it was suggested that Mark be institutionalized. After not having seen McGill for quite some time, he returned for neurofeedback in a severely depressed state. McGill offered both neurofeedback and Cognitive Behavior Therapy and Mark's life improved slowly but surely. Mark got engaged and he and his fiancée moved into a townhouse together. Mark had a creative flair and started painting and creating decorative objects. He learned to cook and took care of odds and ends in their home.

Mark completed his therapy six months prior to his wedding. By then his memory and executive skills had improved considerably. Mark had also become more aware of and sensitive to the feelings and needs of others and learned to keep his own counsel rather than becoming angry and speaking his mind.

12.6 Case Study: An 8-Year-Old High Functioning Girl Presenting with Poor Task Completion and Focus Skills.

This case study is a contribution by McGill Scott.

This is a very short report of the effect of ISF training after only four sessions. This case study is included mainly for the sake of neurofeedback practitioners that are considering including ISF training as another modality of neurofeedback for their clients where relevant.

A psychometric evaluation indicated that Jenny is a high functioning grade two learner. Her intellectual potential measures in the high average interval. Jenny struggles with task completion and also with remaining focused in class when required to do so despite her above average intelligence.

Jenny has a profile familiar to most therapists and many parents. This is typically a child that will be placed on stimulant medication – often without any other consideration.

Jenny was sent for a QEEG. Below are the Eyes Open and Eyes Closed maps with a linked ear montage from Neuroguide. The illustrations follow on the next page.

Eyes Open Information:

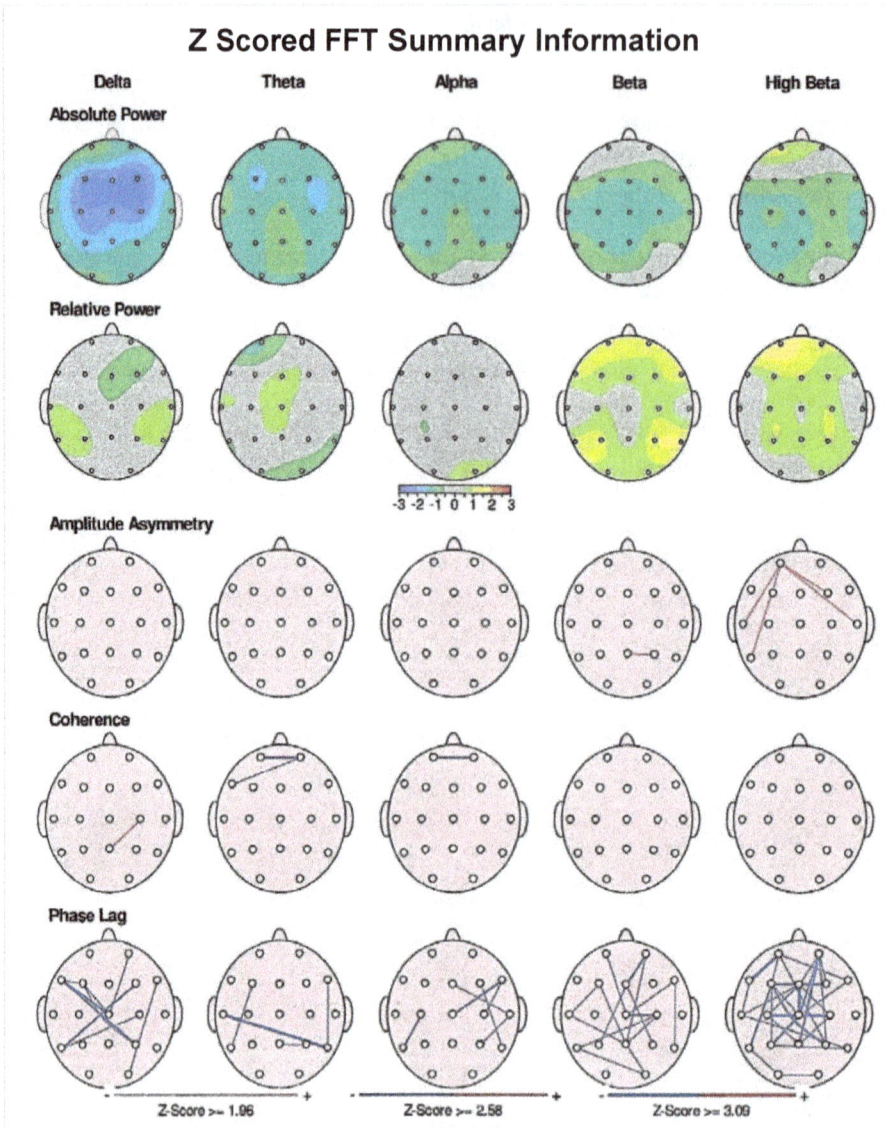

Figure 12.11: Summary information: Neuroguide, eyes open. (Case study 12.6).

Eyes Closed Information:

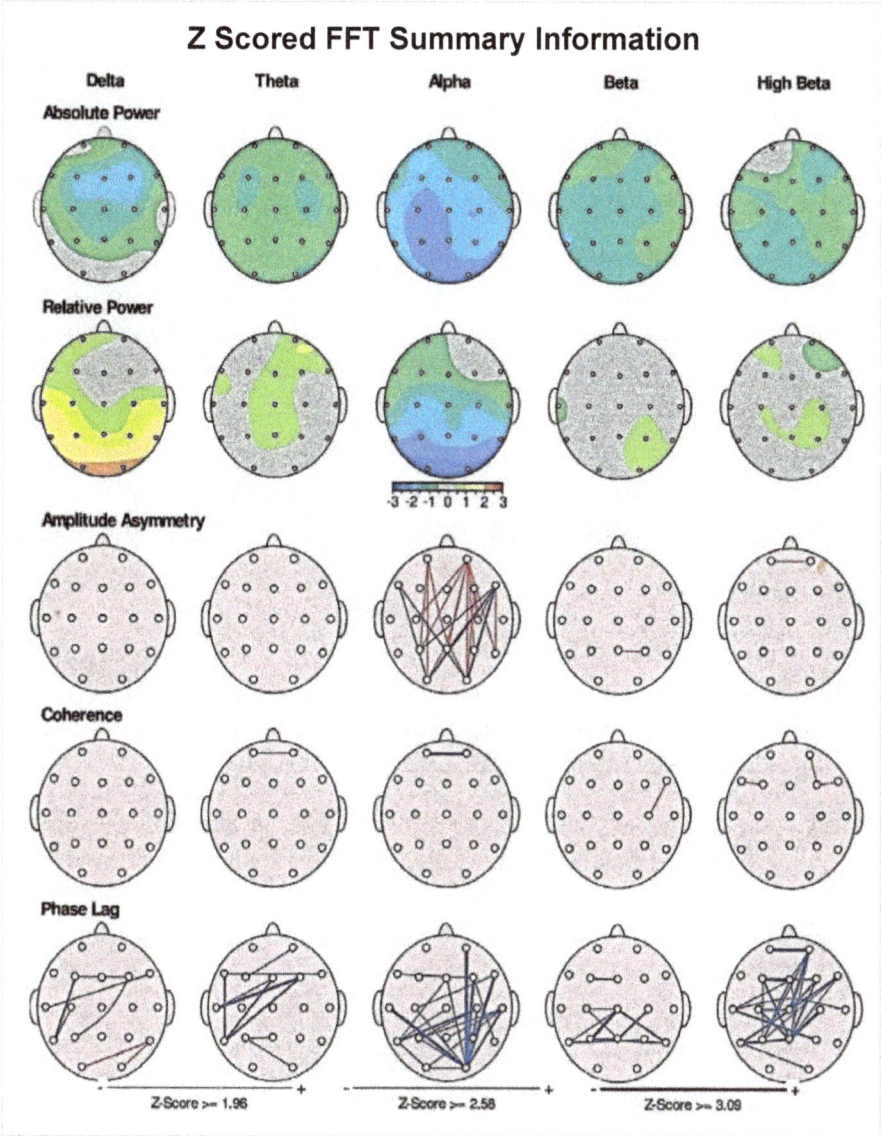

Figure 12.12: Summary information: Neuroguide, eyes open. (Case study 12.6)

McGill decided to utilize ISF training due to the magnitude of the power deficiency. (ISF training is explained in chapter 5). ISF works on the central nervous system at oscillations below the regular brainwave activity. There is generally a fairly rapid response to ISF training. McGill decided to start ISF training at placement areas T3/T4. ISF training often commences at 0,00030 Hz from which point an optimal frequency is determined based on the client's autonomic response to the training. By session four the frequency had been moved up to 0.00050.

Accurate observation and feedback is required for optimal success.

After the fourth session, the following feedback was received from Jenny's mother: "Jenny told me today that she was feeling top. No stomach or headache. Overall, she is much brighter. Her homework went much better. Normally a big struggle, but she managed to make sentences by herself. I was so proud of her."

12.7 Case Study: A 7-Year-Old Boy with Asperger Syndrome (Currently referred to as Autism Spectrum Disorder).

This case study is a contribution by McGill Scott.

Jake is currently studying Engineering. He was in grade 1 when McGill met him. Learners in South Africa are enrolled for their first year of formal schooling in a primary school in the year in which they turn seven years old. Prior to grade 1, they are enrolled in a Pre-Primary school.

Jake had been diagnosed with Asperger Syndrome by the time he was in grade 1. He had severe sensory modulation problems and could not cope with change (as is often the case with ASD – children). Jake would have major meltdowns if a cleaner had moved something on his school desk. Jake was highly intolerant of noise which posed a challenge in the learning environment. Jake presented with the typical social difficulties associated with ASD as well as with repetitive behavior.

The only neurofeedback training options at the time were amplitude training in either the eyes closed, or eyes open position. During eyes closed training, the alpha frequency is usually rewarded, and McGill did not consider that an option based on Jake's age.

McGill commenced with right sided training at CP4 which generally had a positive effect on Jake. In terms of frequency, McGill's approach was one in which she titrated down in small increments until Jake felt comfortable and calm. After regular training sessions at CP4 for one year, Jake could tolerate training on Cz and T3–T4. The frequencies at T3–T4 were kept constant because of the sensitivity of the temporal lobes.

Eventually, McGill managed to get Jake tolerant of training at Cz and Fz at 11–13 Hz when the beta3 activity was inhibited at between 20 and 25%. At the time there was literature supporting the relevance of shifting the reward frequencies up and down at Cz and Fcz with people who suffer OCD and rigidity in thinking patterns. McGill alternated between sessions during which the reward frequencies were shifted at the mentioned sites and training sessions at CP4 which she describes as the go-to calming site for Jake. After a further period of six months at a frequency of two sessions per week, significant changes were evident. Jake could now tolerate changes without having outbursts and his rigidity decreased.

McGill also worked with Jake on breathing and visualization techniques to help ease his discomfort. He was also taught to hold his right thumb which served as an anchor to remind him that he was okay.

McGill commenced with frontal placements. Jake could tolerate work being done on Fz as well as bipolar hook-ups on homologous sites F3–F4 and F7-F8. Jake could however not tolerate work being done on FP1–FP2.

The school Jake attended, upheld the principles of the Inclusive Education Policy which allows for certain accommodations for learners with special educational needs. Jake was permitted to be in McGill's office or in the library during break to be able to escape the hurly burly of break times. During sporting events Jake was permitted to sit in the tent with the teachers and assist with the scoring.

By the time Jake had reached grade 5, he was able to participate in the school's annual concerts without having a meltdown because of the loud music and noise. McGill also taught Jake basic life skills and helped him with being able to recognize his emotions. During Jake's last three years of primary school he went to McGill for neurofeedback and counseling sessions on a need to have basis.

McGill anticipated Jake might be affected by the changes associated with going to high school. He then attended sessions with McGill once every two weeks. In the senior secondary phase, Jake started talking openly about his condition and how lonely it often made him feel. McGill stated that that ameliorated somewhat when he could start holding onto his cognitive gifts.

McGill is convinced that the neurofeedback enabled a neurological flexibility that made it possible for Jake to cope in a regular mainstream setting and even assist learners that were less cognitively gifted than he was. Jake was even able to attend rugby matches and other sporting events as a first aid assistant after having completed a number of first aid courses.

12.8 Case Study: A 30-Year-Old Female with Trauma, Anxiety and Depression.

This case study was contributed by Justine Loewenthal, an Executive Board Member of the Biofeedback Association of South Africa (BFSA). Justine is a BCIA certified clinical neurofeedback practitioner. She is also a registered counselor under the board of psychology and a registered EEG technician with the board of clinical technology. Justine has been using neurofeedback in her practice since 2002. She has a keen interest in trauma, sleep problems, developmental delays, anxiety, and tic disorders.

Mary was 30 years old when she was referred to Justine for neurofeedback by a clinical psychologist in 2016. Mary was in dire straits. All previous efforts at alleviating her discomfort were in vain. She had severe adverse effects to different medications that were prescribed. Mary felt overwhelmed and hopeless. She was a prisoner of her feelings of being depressed, panicked and stressed. Mary had sleep problems as well pertaining to sleep onset and frequent wakening. It took her anywhere between one and a half to two hours to fall asleep and then she woke frequently through the night. Her concentration was poor and she had problems with her memory. All aspects of her life were impacted negatively by the constant discomfort she felt. At times Mary would have aggressive outbursts and failed to be able to describe what she was feeling. Mary's appetite was also affected by the state she was in– she struggled to eat at all. In addition, Mary was unemployed and in no condition to apply for a job and make a good impression during an interview. Mary experienced no joy and had nothing to look forward to. The best she could do was to attempt to survive.

Justine did a recording for a QEEG and it became evident that there were many frontal lobe irregularities. An analysis of the QEEG indicated increased alpha power in the frontal lobes, low delta, theta, and beta (12–15 Hz) power as well. A map of the eyes closed relative power distribution follows on the next page:

Z Scored FFT Relative Power

Warning: Absolute power must be consulted to interpret relative power

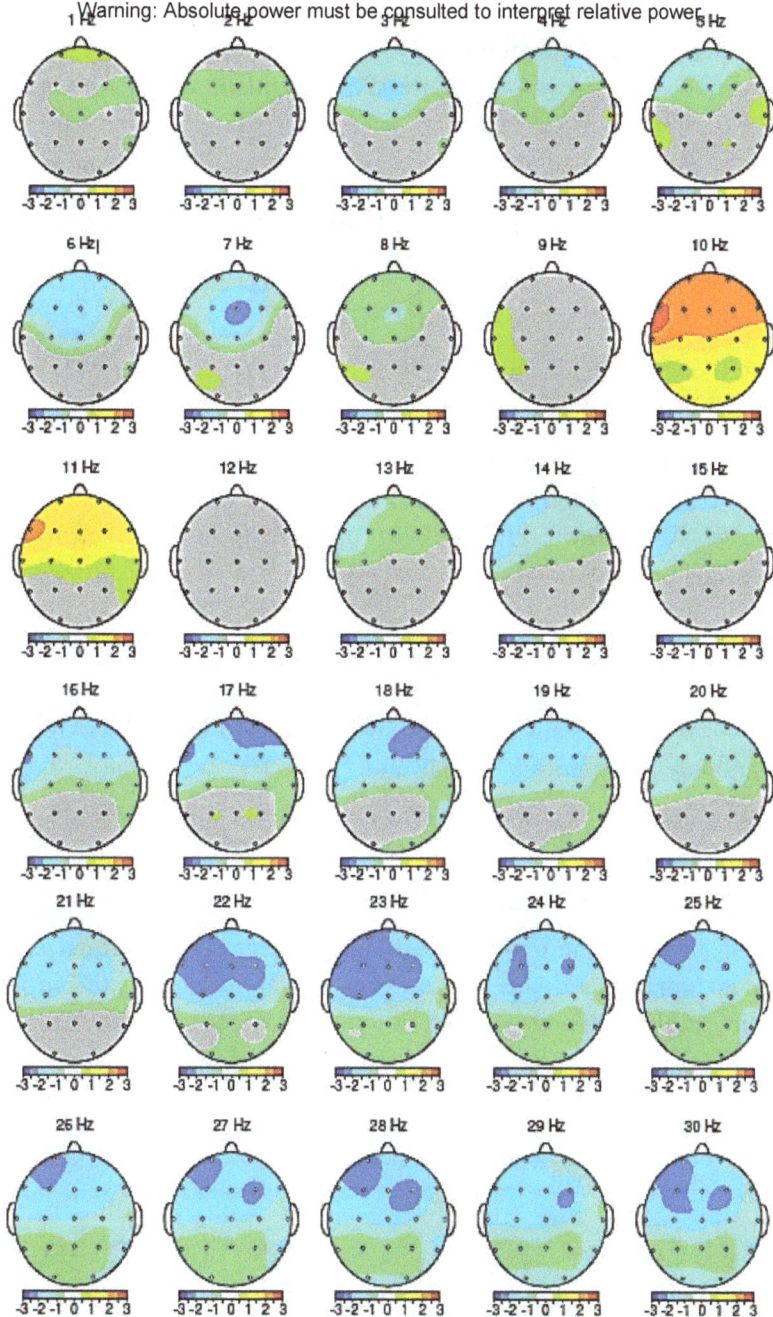

Figure 12.13: Eyes closed relative power. (Case Study 12.8).

Mary's routine EEG also revealed an excess of frontal and central alpha power.

After five sessions of neurofeedback training, Mary was clearly less tearful, and she reported improved concentration and quality of sleep. On average it now took her 45 minutes to fall asleep and she had significantly fewer awakenings during the night.

The first five sessions consisted of the following training protocols:

- 3 Sessions at Fz, rewarding both 3–7 Hz and 9–12 Hz and inhibiting both 9–12 Hz and 25–36 Hz
- 2 Sessions at Cz, rewarding both 12–15 Hz and 15–18 Hz and inhibiting both 9–12 Hz and 25–36 Hz

After 15 sessions Mary's anxiety had abated. She woke on average once per night, felt rested in the mornings and the score on the depression markers Justine used, had improved from 10 out of 10 symptoms present to 6 out of 10 symptoms present.

Sessions six through to 15 consisted of the following neurofeedback training protocols:

- 8 More sessions at Cz, rewarding both 12–15 Hz and 15–18 Hz and inhibiting both 9–12 Hz and 25–36 Hz
- 2 Sessions at Fz, rewarding both 12–15 Hz and 15–18 Hz and inhibiting both 9–12 Hz and 25–36 Hz

By the time Mary had completed 21 sessions of neurofeedback training, she was eating normally and sleeping peacefully. Her sleep pattern had been restored to normal and she was no longer waking during the night. She was feeling motivated and engaged in a quest for finding a job. She was not plagued by anxiety any longer, but she did feel down for short stretches every few days.

Sessions 16 trough to 21 consisted of the following neurofeedback training protocols:

- 6 More sessions at Fz, rewarding both 12–15 Hz and 15–18 Hz and inhibiting both 9–12 Hz and 25–36 Hz

After 32 sessions, Mary was no longer depressed. She did not experience anxiety neither did she have any problems pertaining to sleep patterns. She did not feel panicky at all any longer. She was calm, could think clearly with improved concentration and memory.

Sessions 22 to 32 consisted of the following neurofeedback training protocols:

- 11 More sessions at Fz, rewarding both 12–15 Hz and 15–18 Hz and inhibiting both 9–12 Hz and 25–36 Hz

After session number 32, Justine saw Mary for one session per month for four months. During this period, no regression was noticeable in both her symptoms and her EEG.

Sessions 33 to 36 consisted of the following neurofeedback training protocol:

- 4 More sessions at Fz, rewarding both 12–15 Hz and 15–18 Hz and inhibiting both 9–12 Hz and 25–36 Hz

Eight more sessions followed at irregular intervals using the following protocols:

- 1 More session at Fz, rewarding both 12–15 Hz and 15–18 Hz and inhibiting both 9–12 Hz and 25–36 Hz

- 7 sessions at F7, rewarding both 12–18 Hz and 15–18 Hz and inhibiting both 9–12 Hz and 25–36 Hz

From session four onwards Justine started her sessions with Mary with 15 minutes of heart rate variability training which helped to center and ground her. She then purchased a biofeedback device with which she could continue with HRV training at home on a daily basis for 10 minutes per day.

12.9 Case study: A 66-year-Old Female with Deteriorating Vision, Insomnia, Memory Problems and Tinnitus-like Symptoms.

This case study was contributed by Justine Loewenthal.

Jane was referred to Justine for neurofeedback by her optometrist. Jane's vision was deteriorating very rapidly. She also suffered insomnia for the past 11 years and managed to sleep no more than one and a half hours per night.

In January 2016, Justine did a routine EEG recording on Jane which indicated low amplitude fast EEG in the open eyes condition. Justine mentioned that this could be a normal variant with 7–10% of the normal adult population presenting with overall low amplitude or "flat" EEG. It appears to often correlate with a "busy brain" with competing thoughts and anxiety. A QEEG was also done. Jane presented with increased delta and alpha power as well as with decreased beta 1 power. See the maps on the following page.

Eyes Closed Information:

Z Scored FFT Relative Power

Warning: Absolute power must be consulted to interpret relative power.

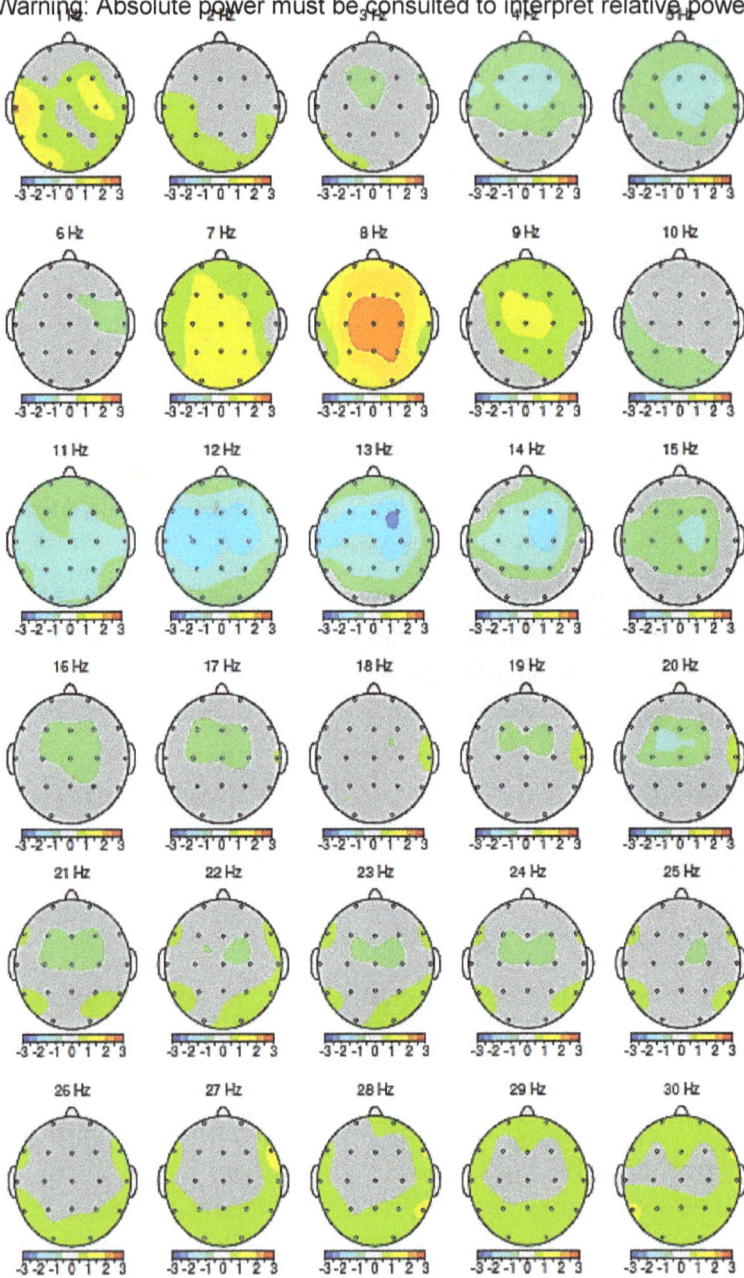

Figure 12.14: Z-scored relative power distribution – eyes closed. (Case study 12.9).

Eyes Open Information:

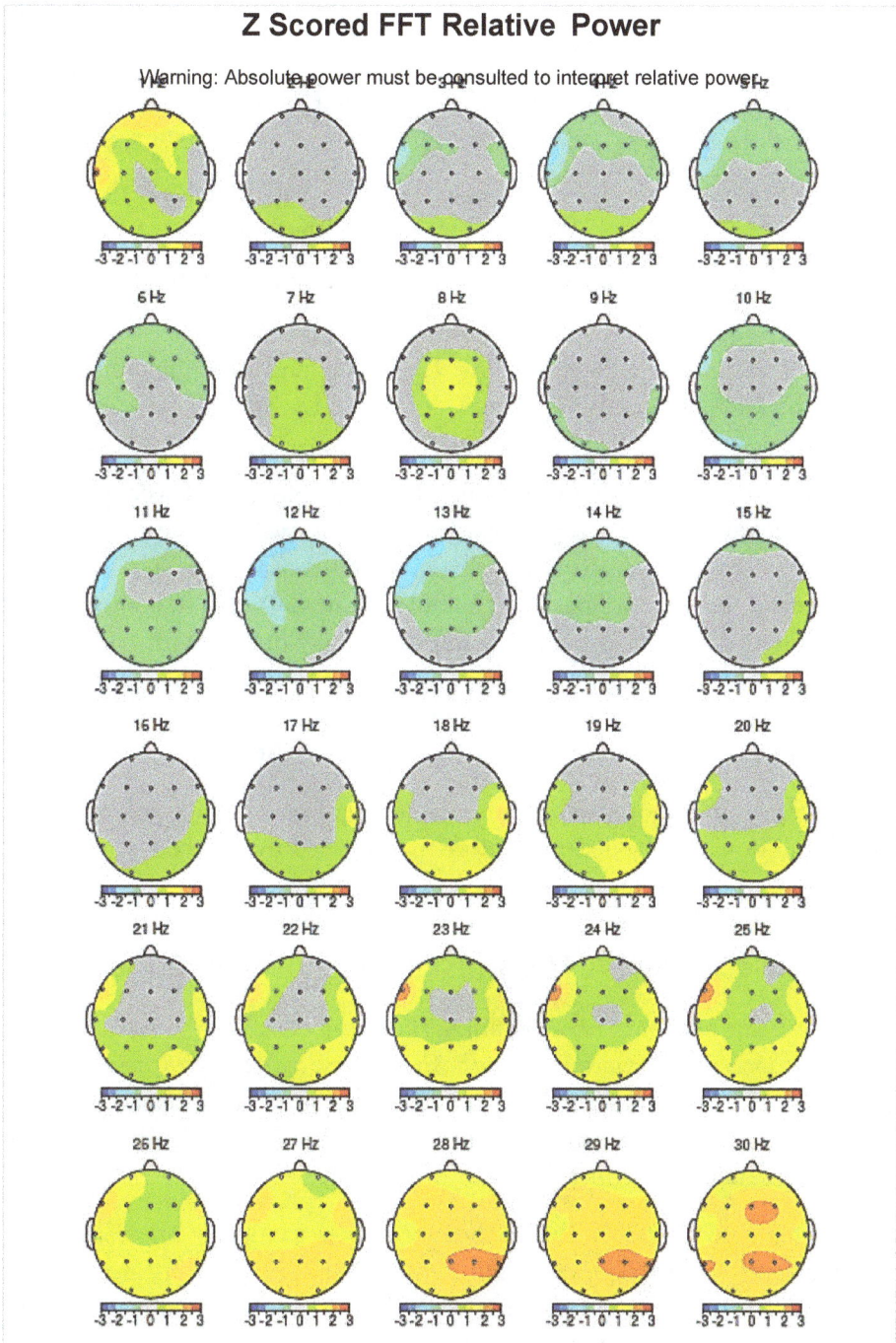

Figure 12.15: Z-scored relative power distribution – eyes open. (Case Study 12.9).

311

Justine did 34 neurofeedback training sessions with Jane using three different protocols. From session five onward up and until the last session, the sessions commenced with 15 minutes of regular biofeedback training followed by neurofeedback.

- The following neurofeedback training protocols were used with Jane:
- 8 Sessions on Cz, rewarding 10–15 Hz and inhibiting three bandwidths namely 0–3 Hz, 7–9 Hz and 18–30 Hz
- 8 Sessions on Cz, rewarding 13–16 Hz and inhibiting three bandwidths namely 0–3 Hz, 7–9 Hz and 18–36 Hz
- 18 Sessions on Pz rewarding 12–15 Hz and inhibiting three bandwidths namely 0–3 Hz, 7–9 Hz and 18–36 Hz

Jane started experiencing relief almost immediately. Her sleep started improving from the second session. She was able to fall asleep almost immediately and slept for a good six hours before waking. Towards the end of the process, Jane's quality of life had improved drastically. The incessant loud buzzing sound in her head had all but vanished. Owing to her improved self-confidence and concentration, she could play bridge with her friends once again. Her memory had improved markedly as well as her mood. Jane had no difficulty with word finding and her energy levels had normalized. Feeling tired and constantly drained was something of the past.

Three follow up appointments at a frequency of one session per month as well as a follow up three months after that, proved that there had not been regression.

12.10 Case Study: A Therapist's Story of Rehabilitation

This case study was contributed by Mitzi Hollander. Mitzi is a registered health care practitioner in Johannesburg, South Africa. She is a registered neurofeedback practitioner and EEG technician. Mitzi was one of the first neurofeedback trainers in South Africa and is therefore an important role player in the development and growth of neurofeedback in South Africa.

My journey into the field of neurotherapy was by accident – I literally mean "by accident". In 1995, a close family member was involved in a serious motor vehicle accident. As a family we had no idea of the dramatic impact this would have on our lives.

The victim was trapped in the wreckage of the car for two and a half hours. When the jaws of life arrived, they had to resuscitate the victim. On arrival at the hospital he had lost all his vital signs again and had to be resuscitated once again. The patient's Glasgow Coma Score (GCS) was four and remained there for approximately three weeks. For the following month the patient was kept in an induced coma. While trapped in the car, the victim had had a stroke which left him paralyzed on the right side of his body. He had also lost his speech as a result of the coma.

After approximately four weeks in the Intensive Care Unit, it was attempted to extubate him, but his lungs were too severely damaged, and he could consequently not breathe of his own accord. Many ribs had been broken during the accident and some had punctured his lungs. The smells and the sounds associated with ICU became very familiar to me. To complicate matters, there were many smaller emergencies interwoven into our reality that we had to deal with: There was a scarcity of blood due to the holiday season in December which is always associated with a high accident rate and a blood clot got lodged in the patient's arm that resulted in his arm swelling like a balloon – to mention two. The doctors informed me that treating the patient with blood thinners to dissolve the blood clot could dislodge more blood clots in the brain that could result in further damage to his brain. Further brain scans and EEGs were required to ascertain whether it would be feasible to administer blood thinners. Fortunately, it was possible and the patient's arm returned to normal.

The patient had been attended to by mainly Sotho speaking nursing staff in what used to be an academic hospital in Pretoria which is currently known as Tshwane. Very few white South Africans speak any of the African languages and the patient was definitely not one of those few. When the patient was extubated however, he spoke some words, phrases, or even sentences possibly, in Sotho. He was complaining to the staff that they were moving around too much in Sotho! I did some research and came across documented cases of pilots that that been gunned down and were comatose and could speak a foreign language of the caretakers when they became conscious.

Close to Christmas Day, the patient was transferred to high care and it became increasingly evident how extensive the brain damage was. We decorated the ward for Christmas Day and his two young girls were allowed to visit him for the first time since the accident. He recognized all of us, but he could not recall any of our names. We were then allocated a collective name: "appl"! After we had taken down the Christmas decorations, I asked him which day we had just celebrated and he did not have any comprehension of the event.

In an attempt to minimize the impact of the trauma on the children that would have been amplified by the fact that I would have to spend much time travelling to Pretoria every day, a dear friend, Linda, invited us to stay in her home. She cared for my girls as if they were her own and I will remain forever grateful to her. At some point the patient's language changed to a very flowery, poetic use of words. Our home language was Afrikaans but because the patient's main language pathway in his brain was damaged, his second language, which is English, was brought online. An example of this use of metaphors and poetic language is for instance in what he said one day: "Take me by my wings and lead me to my nest". What he was trying to say was that he wanted to be taken back to his bed.

Seven weeks in a coma, a poor prognosis, and limited resources fueled a frantic search for rehabilitation possibilities that supported the notion of neuroplasticity. We arrived home with a person trapped in a wheelchair, wearing nappies that did not have access to the words in which he wanted to express his needs. This was the same body of a person that could express himself so eloquently before the accident.

On this journey I was blessed by the kindness of many people. One such a person is Helen. Helen used to be our neighbor. She was a physiotherapist and gave of her time and expertise abundantly. She came by twice a day to initially work on improving the patient's lung capacity and then to enable the patient to get up out of the wheelchair. We could also start working on getting the patient more grounded now that he was back in a familiar environment. The main challenges appeared to be his memory, fatigue, and executive skills for many months ahead of us.

I approached his rehabilitation from a point of view of accessing all my resources and background in remediation and neurodevelopment. I also focused a lot on nutrition. I regarded oxygen, movement, balance, and rhythm to also be important points of reference in the rehabilitation process. Against the advice of the mainstream medical practitioners, I decided to access hyperbaric oxygen therapy and other alternative therapies such as acupuncture, sacral cranial and chiropractic therapy.

At some point during my research, I stumbled upon an article on neurotherapy in a local newspaper. The phrase that caught my attention was "internal locus of control". I was amazed to learn that I could change his brainwaves through a process of operant conditioning. I borrowed some money from the bank and off I went to Los Angeles to be trained in neurotherapy by EEG Spectrum who has since changed to EEGER. It felt very overwhelming at first but thorough training, mentoring and caring by many great people like Mike Cohen, Sebern Fisher, Dr Gary Schummer and Joy Lunt who supported me in my personal quest to be able to acquire all possible means of assisting in the rehabilitation, it became a life changing occurrence.

Soon after my return to South Africa, I started doing neurofeedback training on the children I was seeing for remedial assistance, as well. It then ensued that I invited Mike Cohen and Dr Roger De Beus to South Africa to assist with the training of other therapists in neurofeedback and in Quantitative Electro-Encephalograms (QEEGs) as well. In the meantime, I had qualified and registered with the BCIA as international trainer and neurofeedback provider.

Rehabilitation with the patient S continued for approximately five years. The process involved training on C3, rewarding 15–18 Hz for one year. This decision was based on the fact that the brain injury had left him with a very low arousal level.

I also introduced training on P3 for language processing and P3-F7 for language expression. Many other therapies focusing on balance, rhythm and timing were included in the rehabilitation program. S was frustrated and presented with many emotional outbursts and fluctuation in mood. Training on T3-T4 at 12–15 Hz reward, improved his emotional regulation.

Progress was steady and significant throughout. S had to reapply for his driver's license. A big challenge in this regard was that his three-dimensional spatial perception and orientation were significantly impaired. He could no longer judge distances accurately. He failed to be able to estimate the distance between his car and the car ahead of him or next to him. Training on P4 while rewarding 12–15 Hz improved his spatial orientation. He finally got to where he could be examined. He underwent a very extensive six-hour grueling evaluation and passed with flying colors. S was now independent once again.

My words can never do justice to the efforts of all who journeyed through this rehabilitation process with us – neither can they express the depth and the extent of my gratitude. Neurofeedback was the main tool in S's rehabilitation process and even more importantly it provided me with significant information when he could not express his needs in words. Neurofeedback offered a window into his brain. Once I had established baseline scores, I could ascertain how effective other support therapies were. With the hyperbaric oxygen therapy and the supplements, he used throughout therapy it was evident that the effects were positive judging by his brainwave activity.

Today he is a fully functional independent individual with an internal locus of control!

Over the years neurofeedback has become an established and recognized therapeutic intervention in South Africa. It is still an integral part of my practice. The introduction of QEEGs into the field has refined my approach. Having access to the statistical data the QEEG is based on, has increased the success rate and the efficacy levels of neurofeedback as an intervention. These facts along with the accessibility to functional medicine and nutrition, has made and integrative approach to rehabilitation possible.

12.11 Case Study: A 54-Year-Old Female with Conversion Disorder

This case study was contributed by Rika Scribante. Rika is a clinical psychologist registered with the Health Professions Council of South Africa. Her private practice is in Langebaan on the West Coast of the Western Cape She added neurofeedback to her practice in 2009 after her initial training in 2006. Rika is a member of the BFSA and other professional institutions. Rika works with both children and adults across a very wide spectrum of disorders and problems.

On 26 January 2018 a 54-year-old female patient showed up at Rika's practice informing her that she suffers seizures and that the epilepsy specialist neurologist had informed her that she had non-epileptic seizures. Natalie had severe seizures with dire implications and consequences for her health.

The neurologist had informed Natalie that she had suppressed events or problems to her subconscious mind and she needed to consult with a psychologist. She had severe sleep problems and suffered anxiety to the extent that she found it very difficult or even impossible at times to be amongst people. It had become impossible for Natalie to go to a shopping mall. After 15 minutes in the mall she would become disorientated and lose track of where she was and why she was there. Natalie started withdrawing more and more and mostly stayed home where she felt safer. Natalie had also lost interest in life. She felt depressed and didn't look forward to anything.

Natalie would have seizures at random times and would register only after the fact that she had fallen when she came to. The one seizure occurred in the general practitioner's office during a consultation which is when she was referred to a neurologist.

Rika started helping Natalie to identify triggers to the seizures. Initially it appeared that anticipatory anxiety played a significant role. When she anticipated people visiting, she would get a seizure. When she has had a seizure she just lies on the floor once she has regained consciousness. Her blood sugar levels were usually very high post seizure.

During Natalie's second visit in the first week of February, after she had had another seizure in the interim, Rika did a 15 minute neurofeedback training session on C3 with a 15–18 Hz reward and two inhibits of frequency bands 4–7 Hz and 22–36 Hz. She then gave Rika insight into her traumatic past.

Natalie had a difficult and complicated childhood. She grew up in East London (in the Eastern Cape on the southeast coast of South Africa) on the famous garden route. Her parents were not married and nothing else in her life was stable. They kept on moving from one address to the next. Natalie had learning difficulties and was placed in a school for learners with special educational needs until she was in grade 10. When Natalie was 10 years old, her father abandoned the family that consisted of Natalie's mother, an older sister, and a younger brother. Natalie's mother was then a single provider with three children. She was angry and refused for Natalie and her siblings to visit their father which they did do without their mother's knowledge or consent. Natalie's siblings eventually left home to embark on their own journeys and Natalie's mother attempted to keep Natalie at home with her. When Natalie met her husband her mother did not approve of them getting married. Natalie describes her experience of her married life as always having to be in the middle of some quarrel or disagreement. Her perception was that everybody was forever fighting and she felt torn.

After another neurofeedback training session on C3 with a 15–18 Hz reward and the same inhibits as before, Natalie reported that she had slept much better and felt more energized and motivated.

Natalie had not had contact with her mother for many years until one day she contacted Natalie and wanted to visit them. Natalie felt fearful and stressed. On the fifth day of her mother's visit, Natalie's mother and Natalie's husband finally made their peace. Natalie's mother appeared to have been sleeping later than usual the following morning, but when Natalie had gone to check in on her, found that she had died in her sleep. She had suffered a heart attack. Natalie describes the time she had with her mother and her husband as the happiest time of her life. The positive rephrasing was that her mother had come to make peace before she died. After her mother's death, Natalie's sugar levels were exceptionally high. During the third week in February, Natalie did another neurofeedback training session on C3 at the same reward, and inhibit frequencies. Natalie reported that after the session she felt less anxious and that her sleep had improved. She also did not have nightmares as frequently as before. She had not had another seizure since the onset of the therapy although she did have muscle contractions once but did not lose consciousness. Natalie reported that she could even go to the shopping mall without feeling fearful or anxious. Her neighbor also reported that she witnessed a significant positive change in Natalie.

In the following session more information Natalie attempted to suppress was revealed. When Natalie was a young teenager, her sister's husband harassed her sexually. He would sneak up behind her naked and waited for her to turn around and see him. Nobody was willing to believe Natalie when she reported these incidences. She consequently felt that she had no voice and wondered why these things should always happen to her. She felt that she was on her own and that she was always being bullied.

After yet another neurofeedback training session on C3 during the last week of February, Natalie reported that she felt so much better. The nightmares had dissipated, her sleeping patterns were normal and she was motivated to involve herself in all different chores in and around her house. She no longer felt guilty to engage sexually with her husband.

After her first session of neurofeedback training during the first week of March on C3 for a longer period of time, Natalie reported that she no longer suffered anxiety and has not had any seizure activity or even an aura of an attack. She felt happier, motivated and energized. Her blood sugar levels no longer spiked either. She suggested that the frequency of the training sessions and the psychotherapy be spaced to fortnightly sessions due to money constraints.

Natalie had her following training and psychotherapy session at the end of March. There had been no regression. She could travel on her husband's motorbike with him and had no anxiety whatsoever.

When Rika consulted with her again during the second week of May, there had unfortunately been a relapse due to (most probably) the lapse in time since her previous session. Natalie's sleep had started to deteriorate again but she had fortunately not had any seizures. She had the intention of going to Port Elizabeth with her husband at the end of the month which had the implication of travelling on the back of the bike for a long distance which could potentially be stressful. Rika recommended that they should revert to weekly sessions once again.

Everything was back on track in terms of Natalie's sleep patterns, her energy levels, and her mood by the end of May. There were no indications of any pending seizure activity.

Rika reports that Natalie had been transformed from a scared and vulnerable woman to a person who can once more enjoy life with her loved ones. Her blood sugar levels never spiked again, she never has nightmares and she feels happy and content.

The author has included information on non-epileptic seizures (NES) obtained from a neurologist, courtesy of Dr James Butler, for the perusal of all neurofeedback practitioners and all readers alike.

Non-epileptic seizures (NES)

Non-epileptic seizures are indeed neurological events that resemble epileptic seizures but they are not epileptic seizures. Epileptic seizures originate in the grey matter of the brain which includes the outer few millimeters of the brain known as the cortex. Epileptic seizures are caused by abnormal electrical discharges in the brain. NES are not caused by abnormal discharges in the cortex and are related to mechanisms in deeper brain structures and more specifically structures in the subconscious brain. These events are thus beyond the voluntary control of an individual.

When NES is diagnosed, an epileptologist ought to do a thorough investigation into the symptoms of the seizures. Video-EEG recordings are required for an accurate diagnosis during which it is determined if the discharges that distinguish epileptic from non-epileptic seizures are present or absent. Such recordings require hospitalization and although costly, this course of action is safest on the long run to avoid the prescription of anti- epileptic drugs and encourage appropriate therapies.

NES is usually caused by subconscious conflicts or psychological problems. NES is one of the conversion disorders. The term "conversion" has its origin in Freud's teachings that anxiety is converted into physical symptoms. The conversion disorders used to be referred to as hysteria.

What is very important to understand is that the person that suffers a conversion disorder has no control over the conversion process. There is no pretense or faking of symptoms. A NES is a coping mechanism of the brain to deal with emotionally traumatic events. People with a history of sexual abuse or who have suffered other trauma are more at risk of developing a conversion disorder. NES ought not to be dealt with in a dismissive way. It affects a person's quality of life just as much as epilepsy does.

The sufferer ought to be guided to acceptance and understanding of the diagnosis at the onset of the therapeutic intervention.

12.12 Case Study: A 22-Year-Old Male with Depression

This case study was contributed by Rika Scribante.

Rika met Noah when he was a 22-year-old second year pharmacology student at a university in the Western Cape. His father accompanied Noah to their first meeting. Rika experienced him as having the appearance of a depressed person. He was unkempt and reserved.

Noah's father took the liberty of explaining his perception of Noah's problem. His father explained that Noah has had health issues for the past two years. His son is withdrawn and has been avoiding people whereas he had many friends before. In 2018 Noah was repeating his second year due to difficulties with chemistry and pharmacology. He used to obtain good results at school. Noah had been staying with his uncle who lives in close proximity of the university and he has noticed that Noah was failing to take care of himself. He went to see a psychologist at the university who diagnosed him with major depression disorder. Noah was in his father's words: "falling apart" and had had a nervous breakdown. Anti-depressants were prescribed. In Noah's father's opinion his son was addicted to computer games and he understood that it would be difficult to just end an addiction.

When Rika requested the patient's own take on where he was at he reported that his father had pretty much laid out all the cards on the table and that he was not good at communicating. He did mention however, that he had problems with sleep and that he suffered severe panic attacks. He stated that he was used to being the top student in the group and when reality contradicted that, it caused much discomfort because it affected the image he had of himself. Due to his lack of success in his studies he could not see a way forward and had no idea what to study instead if he had to change his course. He also stated that he had fantasies of ending his life and that those visualizations and thoughts waxed and waned.

Noah said that he queried his own existence.

Nothing stood out as red flag from Noah's background. He had had a sheltered childhood and his parents got divorced when he was 12 or 13 years old. He never had many friends but only mainly because he was introverted and preferred it that way.

When Rika attempted to establish the onset of the depressive like symptoms it became evident that he started feeling depressed in May 2017. He remembered that his energy was very low and that he wanted to stay in bed all day. He cried a lot and had no desire to leave his room. In November Noah became suicidal for the first time and related that he had become "messed up' . He started experiencing panic attacks and found it increasingly difficult to focus and study and he stopped caring about his future. He achieved an aggregate of between 50% and 60% which to him was not nearly good enough. He started feeling hopeless and overwhelmed. He worked hard at motivating himself to attempt to design a computer game or to compose music or to write a book but all amounted to nothing and he regarded all his efforts to be pointless. He voiced that he had been setting himself up for failure. He passed his time with anime (Japanese hand- drawn or computer animation) and other forms of sketching to escape from his negative thoughts. Rika made Noah aware of his negative belief about himself and suggested that neurofeedback training be part of his therapy which may be helpful with much of the discomfort that he was experiencing.

Rika commenced with a neurofeedback training program for Noah in January 2018. After the first training session with a 15–18 Hz reward frequency on placement area C3 with two inhibits at 4–7 Hz and 22–36 Hz, Noah reported that his sleep had improved although he still woke on average twice during the night. His mood had lifted and he felt more energized. He could also sense a significant improvement in his focus and concentration which lasted for approximately 24 hours. One week later Rika repeated the same training protocol at an extended training time which was now 18 minutes and the same positive outcomes were experienced but at a higher intensity. The training times were increased at increments of three minutes on a weekly basis with consistently positive outcomes. When the training time was extended to 24 minutes, Noah suffered a panic attack during that week. He had managed to spend time with his friend though and had enjoyed it very much. When he was exposed to heavy traffic and many people he felt irritable and experienced the noise to be overwhelming.

Noah gained the insight that he cannot tolerate high noise levels and that noise was a trigger for a panic attack.

Rika explained what the implications of a low arousal level are to Noah specifically. When his arousal level is too low, he isolates himself, he has negative inner chatter, he experiences low self-esteem and it causes confusion.

Despite the panic attack that Noah had had that may have been indicative of an arousal level that is too high and unusual for Noah to be able to navigate himself calmly and safely, Rika understood the importance of getting Noah to a space where he could function at a healthier arousal level. She thus continued with left sided training over the sensory motor strip at 15–18

Hz with the same inhibit frequencies as before for training periods of 27 minutes over 10 consecutive weeks at a frequency of one session per week.

After the fifth session Noah's suicide thoughts abated. After the ninth session, Noah did not get panic attacks any longer but he still isolated himself. Rika explained the importance of building pathways to destinations and goals that he wanted to achieve. Noah decided that he wanted to write a book, work at his drawings, and start a blog. He also assisted his father with renovations for which he earned some money. He enjoyed the physical work. Noah also enrolled for English at UNISA (a correspondence university in South Africa).

After the tenth neurofeedback session using the same protocol, Noah's focus ability was no longer problematic, he no longer woke up during the night and he started making conscious efforts to communicate with people more often – even with strangers he would come across in the mall.

Noah also started reporting on how his artwork seemed to be evolving and how inspired he felt. He became more aware of his environment and mentioned that he had noticed the beautiful reflection of the clouds in a pool of water. Noah by now had come to the realization that he had lived his life without engaging with the beauty that surrounds him. He reported that a friend had mentioned to him before that he was living his life with his eyes closed and he realized that he had had what he refers to as a "narrow vision" and that his experience of life had changed dramatically.

After Noah's eleventh session of neurofeedback with the same protocol, he reported to Rika that he had gone out with some friends and "spotted an anxiety attack coming but I was able to get it under control' . For the first time in his life, Noah was looking forward to his studies. He had also come to the realization that he used to base his decisions on his father's expectations and that that had changed. He could now determine what he wanted and honored himself in his decision making.

Then the unexpected happened: Noah had a severe panic attack which left him and his father very despondent. It felt to them that the positive changes were short lived. Rika then did a session of six minutes right sided training rewarding 12–15 Hz on C4 and 21 minutes on C3, rewarding 15–18 Hz. Although Noah felt much calmer after that training session, his sleep deteriorated drastically. The following week, Rika reduced the training on the right side of the brain by one minute and increased the training time on the left side on C3 by one minute. Noah woke only once during the night following the training date and reported that he felt very good. The following week the training time on C4 was reduced further by one minute to four minutes and the training time on C3 was 23 minutes.

Noah was now confident again that he was on the right track. He continued with spending much time on his art work and was eager to discuss his dream with Rika because his dreams provided the inspiration for his art.

The following three neurofeedback sessions consisted of three-minute training at C4 at 12–15 Hz reward and 24 minute training on C3 at 15–18 Hz.

Rika sums Noah's progress up as follows: Noah was transformed from a neglected, deeply depressed young man into a person that believes in himself and knows what he wants from life. He grasped his dream with both hands: he is now studying to become an author and illustrator of his own work. He is now following his own happiness and no longer attempts to follow his father's dreams. Although Noah is introverted, he is reaching out to people more and more and he is living his life with passion and joy.

12.13 Case Study: A 60-Year-Old Female with PTSD

This case study was contributed by the Author.

No human being should ever have to suffer the atrocities Marna did on that fateful day in 2014.

I met Marna in November 2017, more than three years after her hijacking and kidnapping. Her discomfort and unease were almost tangible. She was on high alert, nervous and trembling. She had been referred to me by her chiropractor that said that he was not managing to bring relief to her tense muscles that were causing chronic headaches and generalized pains.

Marna's first words to me were that she constantly felt as if something terrible was about to happen. It was virtually impossible for Marna to relax. She also made it very clear that she did not want to talk about what had happened to her – she just wanted the discomfort and the pain to dissipate. Marna did talk – in fact, Marna wrote her story for the purpose of this book so that others like her in South Africa that suffer trauma, can know that there can be a normal life after trauma. Marna is a very conscientious and diligent worker and has been thus for her entire professional life. She works in the finance department for a company that transfers perishable foods. Due to odd delivery times and to the fact that Marna was never one to sleep late, she arrived at work at 3:30 am every morning. She was always first to arrive. Marna never used to be a fearful person either and was not concerned about security and safety issues.

On this direful day in 2014, Marna parked her pink Smart Car and as she got out of the car and walked around to the passenger side to fetch her handbag, she noticed two men heading her way. She started making her way back to the driver's seat but one of the assailants ran towards her and grabbed her by her neck from behind. The second assailant had caught up with them and they were nervously shouting instructions at one another. The one was shouting to the other to shoot her and the other shouted to shove her into the boot of the car. Marna recalls that she was only aware of a desire to survive. She felt a gun to her head and became aware that she was struggling to breathe because of the strangling grip she was in. She was shoved into the boot and much chaos and shouting ensued. According to the camera footage, that which had felt like two hours was in fact only minutes. Two minutes after the chaos commenced, she was now in the boot of her car at the mercy of whoever was racing her little car as fast as it would go over pavements, on the wrong side of the road without obeying any traffic rules. At that point Marna was convinced that both the assailants were in the car with her. It turned out that the one with the gun was not with them. The driver shouted to Marna to get into the passenger seat which was virtually impossible to do from the boot of the car without stopping. He kept demanding that she would make her way to the passenger seat and out of fear she actually managed to squeeze through the very small space between the seats and the roof of the car which resulted in significant injuries.

What followed was a harrowing seven and a half hours of threats, racing, stops at drug merchants where she was forced in and out of the car, trips through informal settlements with burning tires in the streets and unimaginable fear. Marna reported that the uncertainty of it all was agonizing. The threats and shouting would range from that she was going to be killed soon and that she would be returned to her place of work later. At one of the drug merchants' houses where her assailant had ordered Marna out of the car, she was taken into a room where she had to sit on a bed. She was petrified and just stared at the floor while people were coming and going and getting dressed and undressed. Marna was ordered back into the car and other men also got into the car to get a lift to another drug merchant's house. It appeared to Marna that her assailant did not have a clear plan and was possibly attempting to muster up the courage to kill her. He smoked Cannabis over which he had crushed a pill which was probably a drug to enhance the effect of what he was smoking. It was established later that he had recently joined one of the most notorious gangs from the Cape Flats and that she had been targeted for his initiation "project".

He drove Marna to a deserted place called "wolfgat" and ordered her out of the car. He asked her if there was a sharp object in the car with which

324

to kill her. This was the first time that Marna realized that he did not have a firearm. The assailant that had held the gun to her head did not get into the car with them when she was abducted. He then instructed her to walk and kneel so that he could crush her skull with a rock. Marna walked with her head down and prayed. She recalls thinking that it was probably ten paces towards her death that she was   walking.

A patrol car arrived as if by miracle and Marna was rescued. At the police station a trauma debriefing officer instructed that she be taken to a doctor immediately. Marna's two children had been contacted and met her at the police station. They took her to her general practitioner of 36 years. What transpired there was a total violation and negation of Marna's ordeal that had prolonged negative consequences. The medical practitioner said to her that fortunately nothing serious had transpired and she was very fortunate to have escaped with her life. He suggested that she should take a mild sedative for a while. It is hardly surprising that it took Marna three years and a nudge from her chiropractor to seek help at an emotional level.

We commenced with Marna's neurofeedback training sessions in November 2017.

Marna completed a PTSD checklist, the Amen Depression and Anxiety questionnaire and a Symptom Tracking Form based on the arousal model. At the time of her intake there was no access to QEEGs in Cape Town. Symptoms were very carefully tracked throughout as well as amplitudes in all frequency bands. We did 30 weekly sessions after which we tapered down to one session per month. All sessions were amplitude training sessions. The following protocols were used:

Session 1: C4	Reward: 12–15 Hz	Inhibits: 4–7 Hz and 22–36 Hz
Session 2: T4-P4	Reward: 10–13 Hz	Inhibits: 0–7 Hz and 22–36 Hz
Sessions 3–10: P4	Reward: 8–11 Hz	Inhibits: 4–7 Hz and 22–36 Hz
Session 11: C4	Reward: 12–15 Hz	Inhibits: 4–7 Hz and 22–36 Hz
Session 12: Pz	Reward: 8–11 Hz	Inhibits; 4–7 Hz and 22–36 Hz

Session 13: C3 1 Min C4 26 Min	Rewards: 15–18 Hz 12–15 Hz	Inhibits: 4–7 Hz and 22–36 Hz
Session 14: P4	Reward: 8–11 Hz	Inhibits: 4–7 Hz and 22–36 Hz
Sessions 15–31:T4- P4	Reward: 10–13 Hz	Inhibits: 4–7 Hz and 22–36 Hz

There was no significant relief after the first two sessions. After session number three Marna overslept which is very unusual. We agreed that it was a good sign. Her sleep had been more peaceful and it was possible for her to abandon herself in sleep for the first time in a very long time. Marna also started becoming more aware of how her body responded to anxiety and stress.

After session number four, Marna's sleep had improved significantly. Whereas before she regularly vomited in the mornings (which she had grown so accustomed to, that she did not link it to the anxiety associated with having to go to work while it was still dark and expose herself to the same circumstances of the abduction) that was no longer the case. Despite the fact that there was a trigger that would ordinarily activate a stress reaction, Marna did not feel anxious or stressed.

Marna started sharing a lot of information pertaining to her childhood as well as her current circumstances. There were many traumatic events that occurred during her childhood as well. Marna was still suffering debilitating headaches and continued seeing her chiropractor in this regard. He reported that it had become possible to make progress in his work with Marna since the onset of the neurofeedback training.

Marna became more and more open to suggestions of meditation techniques and the use of positive affirmations. We focused a lot on self- worth and the importance of honoring oneself. It was emphasized how unacceptable the behavior and approach of the medical practitioner was that had diminished Marna's experience to a fortunate escape from death. Options of how to deal with the occurrence in an empowering manner were discussed. Communication with the prescribing psychiatrist regarding anxiolytics also ensued.

In January 2018, Marna started becoming more consciously concerned about the stretch of the harrowing abduction trip that appeared to have been wiped from her memory. We started looking at road maps and reconstructing the route her kidnapper had taken her on which before was avoided at all cost. Soon after the surfacing of those memories, Marna started feeling depressed and did not want to go to work in the mornings. We figured out that it was not only the surfacing memories but also the fact that there were construction workers working close to her house which made her feel unsafe. I suggested that she should go and spend a few nights at her son's house.

When we started with a trauma protocol used with great success by Sebern Fisher in March, Marna starting sharing details of the ordeal she had suffered. She also joined a dance group which she enjoyed tremendously.

In April Marna reported a significant event. A street beggar approached her in her car and her legs did not start shaking uncontrollably and no headache developed. She was no longer on the lookout – constantly anticipating any potential danger and planning an escape route. The street beggar was a street beggar – Marna did not perceive him as a potential assailant or murderer.

We started discussing dreams Marna had about other significant events and traumatic experiences from her past. Marna did not want to add any other therapy to her neurofeedback training or see any other health care practitioner for added support.

Towards the end of April of 2018, Marna reported that she had gone on a three kilometer hike in a forest on her own and she was not scared at all. Before I met Marna, she related an incident during which her son and his girlfriend invited her on a hike in a safe area because they knew how much she had enjoyed hiking before. When another hiker approached them from the opposite direction, she got a panic attack. Marna was pretty much house bound after the incident. She had added some security measures to her home and felt safe only in her house or when she was driving in her car.

By August 2018, Marna reported that she no longer had headaches. Marna started developing a need to assist her children with the processing of what had happened to her. Both her children are adults and the abduction was never discussed. Marna became aware of how protective her son had become of her and also that he had suppressed anger. Marna was no longer in survival mode. She started engaging with life and her loved ones in a more balanced way. On 13 September 2018 Marna reported that she had said the following words out loud to herself: "I am healthy. After four years I can say that I am fine. I can talk about anything without getting any anxiety or panic attacks".

In her write up, Marna thanked me for having her life back and I wish to pay the gratitude forward to Marna for her perseverance and beautiful spirit. And then I wish to thank each and every neurofeedback practitioner and neurofeedback researcher that enables these miraculous recoveries through their diligence and character.

12.14 Case Study: A 13-Year-Old Boy with an Array of Diagnoses and Ritalin.

The author requested Angelo's (pseudonym) mother to describe the meandering journey from specialist to specialist to neurofeedback.

Angelo is the younger of two children. He was always a happy baby that smiled often. He reached all his developmental milestones early. He was full of energy and wished for the days to be longer. He resisted bedtime and attempted to postpone his sleep time with clever plans.

At the age of five, Angelo was enrolled at a play school for three mornings per week. He did enjoy being with friends but still preferred being at home with his toys. Eventually Angelo had to go to Gr R which is what the preschool year is called in South Africa. The parents chose a preschool on a farm where the children had the opportunity to have access to the farm animals and enjoy a lot of time outside in nature. Concerns started developing with educators about Angelo's handedness and his lisp. Speech therapy was recommended and home programs were provided. After a while Angelo did not feel comfortable and happy at school. He found it difficult to mingle with his peers at school. Often he would feel that the school day is too long and then he would sit outside the classroom and wait for his mother to fetch him from school.

Angelo was enrolled in a different school for his grade 1 year. His mother reports that the grade 1 teacher was very understanding and supportive. She often walked him to his mother's car in the afternoons to have a quick chat with her. She mentioned that Angelo would often daydream in class and not be focused on the activity at hand at all. She observed that Angelo loved drawing and that he was very talented and creative. He loved drawing characters from the transformer movies and would then engage in imaginary play. According to the teacher Angelo's reading and spelling skills were not on a par with his peers and it was decided that remedial intervention was necessary. Occupational therapy was also suggested based on some midline crossing issues and the fact that Angelo's handedness had not been established. He benefited from the occupational therapy.

For what followed then, Angelo's parents were not prepared: Angelo was said to have an interest in Satanism! His parents were shocked and even considered that they may have missed something. The allegations were based on Angelo's drawings of the transformer characters! Angelo was taken to a psychologist for a professional opinion. The parents were confused by how such an inaccurate perception of Angelo could have transpired. He was perceived by friends and family as an exceptionally gentle, kind, and loving person. Then followed the following shocking news: The psychologist diagnosed Angelo with ADHD (mainly inattentive presentation) and autistic tendencies. After a few sessions with the psychologist, Angelo's parents decided to terminate the therapy because the findings and the approach just did not add up to what they knew about their child. They felt confused and bewildered and filled with self-doubt but intuitively they knew that their child was not on the autism spectrum.

In grade two, the school recommended that Angelo be placed on stimulant medication. By then Angelo's mother had tried out all the supplements and natural substances that were suggested in the literature and by an array of people. They went to see a child psychiatrist (referral done by the psychologist that had seen Angelo before) for a prescription. The psychiatrist confirmed the diagnosis of ADHD and also suggested that Angelo possibly had an autism spectrum disorder. Angelo's mother recalled details about the visit to the psychiatrist that I choose to include for the purpose of enabling the reader to get a sense of this interesting child. The psychiatrist suggested that they should go and look for dinosaurs on the hill visible through the window of his office. Angelo replied that that would serve no purpose because they were extinct. The psychiatrist then suggested that they could possibly go and search for dinosaur eggs then to which Angelo responded with that that was rather a lame trick because dinosaurs never existed in that particular area. The author wishes to add that she got to know Angelo as a child with a beautiful sense of humor and a wonderful imagination and that his responses that day were not an indication of a tendency to literal interpretation associated with the diagnoses in question.

Ritalin 10mg LA was prescribed and there was no noticeable improvement in Angelo's academic performance. What was noticeable however was that Angelo became systematically more and more withdrawn. The class teacher informed Angelo's parents that he was no longer participating in discussions and that he had become very withdrawn. Angelo's mother called for a meeting with the class teacher, the psychologist, the remedial teacher, and the psychiatrist. She was very concerned about the effect the medication was having on her child. He was no longer the happy child he used to be. His whole demeanor when he approached his mother waiting for him in the car after school was that of a depressed child. Angelo had since developed problems with sleeping. Sleep deprivation was starting to take its toll. The outcome of the meeting: Everybody, with the exception of Angelo's parents, recommended that Angelo would continue using the stimulant medication.

Grade 3 was approached once again with a positive attitude. Angelo's grade 3 teacher was a dedicated and kind teacher. She gave positive feedback about Angelo's performance and his behavior. Angelo's concentration was still a reason for concern according to the class teacher, however. The stimulant medication dosage was increased to 20mg LA.

Angelo's grade 4 year was once again problematic. There was consistent negative feedback and suggestions of further evaluations and confirmation of existing and possibly other diagnoses. Angelo's parents were confused and exhausted. They could not understand how it was possible that they did not see the same reasons for concern in Angelo's behavior at home.

The parents had to return to either the psychiatrist or a general practitioner every couple of months for a renewal of the script. During a visit to the general practitioner in Angelo's grade 4 year, the general practitioner informed Angelo's mother that Angelo definitely had an autism spectrum disorder based on the fact that he had another patient that also giggled when he examined him and that that child was autistic. The parents were once again devastated.

In Angelo's grade 6 year, he was brought to the author's practice for an evaluation. He was evaluated on the South African Individual Scale-Revised (SSAIS-R). Reading, spelling, writing, and arithmetic skills were also assessed. Angelo was busy with the evaluation process for an entire morning which enabled the author to do a thorough clinical observation as well.

The candidate's subtest scores on a twenty-point scale on the SSAIS-R were as follows:

Verbal Scale	
Vocabulary	10
Comprehension	14
Similarities	12
Number Problems	19
Story Memory	5

Non Verbal Scale	
Pattern Completion	17
Block Patterns	15
Missing Parts	12
Form Board	11
Additional Tests	
Memory for Digits	11
Coding	6
Summary	
Global Scale	Superior
Verbal Scale	High Average
Non Verbal Scale	Superior

Feedback regarding symptoms pertaining to Attention Deficit Hyperactivity Disorder was requested from the school and the parents. Feedback from the school indicated that Angelo was very passive in class and that he presented with five symptoms pertaining to inattentiveness. He presented with no symptoms pertaining to hyperactivity and impulsivity. In the home environment he presented with six symptoms pertaining to inattentiveness in a low degree and two symptoms pertaining to hyperactivity in a low degree. Angelo's performance on the Story Memory subtest was very significant. The Story Memory subtest is a clear marker of auditory attention. His relatively low score on the Coding subtest is also an indication of a concentration problem. Angelo's performance on the Schonell Spelling Test indicated the existence of a spelling problem. Concession recommendations were made to the school and we commenced with a neurofeedback training program.

Although no conclusive evidence regarding the existence of an autism spectrum disorder can be inferred from a cognitive profile, an analysis of the single item responses does give an indication. Neither in his responses to the test items nor in clinical observation of his test behavior, did the author notice any tell-tale signs of anything that resembles autism. The author was of the opinion that many of the complaints and concerns that have been raised over the years were possibly a result of the discrepancy between the learner's verbal and non- verbal skills. Learners with these cognitive profiles often underachieve and typically achieve better results once they get to choose subjects (in grade 10) that are more practical. In terms of Angelo's behavior– that different people have found unusual or strange – it is true that Angelo is not a mainstream learner, but in a very interesting and endearing way.

It was evident that there was indeed a concentration issue and that Angelo appeared to be one of those learners that did not respond favorably to stimulant medication.

The goals of the neurofeedback training program were thus to improve Angelo's concentration ability so that he would not need to use stimulant medication and to improve the balance between his verbal and non-verbal skills by attempting to improve his overall verbal and left brain functioning.

The following neurofeedback training protocols were followed:

Sessions 1–4: C3	Reward: 15–18 Hz	Inhibits: 4–7 Hz; 22–36 Hz
Session 5: C3+C4	Reward: 15–18 Hz 12–15 Hz	Inhibits: 4–7 Hz; 22–36 Hz Inhibits: 4–7 Hz; 22–36 Hz
Sessions 10–19: C3	Reward: 15–18 Hz	Inhibits: 4–7 Hz; 22–36 Hz
Session 20: Cz	Reward: 16–19 Hz	Inhibits: 4–7 Hz; 22–36 Hz
Session 21: F3+C3	Reward: 15–18 Hz	Inhibits: 4–7 Hz; 22–36 Hz
	16–19 Hz	Inhibits: 4–7 Hz; 22–36 Hz
Sessions 22–25: Cz	Reward: 16–19 Hz	Inhibits: 4–7 Hz; 22–36 Hz
Sessions 26–27: C3	Reward: 16–19 Hz	Inhibits: 4–7 Hz; 22–36 Hz
Session 28: Cz	Reward: 16–19 Hz	Inhibits: 4–7 Hz; 22–36 Hz
Session 29:	4 Channel Live Z-score at F3, F4, P3, P4	
Sessions 30–37:	2 Channel Power Training at C3 + C4	Rewards: 15–20 Hz and 12–15HZ Inhibits on both channels: 4–7 Hz and 22–36 Hz

Angelo appeared to be more responsive and started participating more in class from the onset of the training sessions. When the reward frequency was lifted to 16–19 Hz at session 20, the overall response in terms of the same markers the author uses for every training session, was even more positive. The parents and often the teacher as well are requested to rate the trainee's behavior in terms of sleep, task completion, concentration, energy, headache, activity level, mood, physical symptoms and tics on a standardized feedback form twenty-four hours after every training session. It was evident that the learner's arousal level had been too low at the onset of the training which made it difficult for him to focus and caused his energy levels to be low. After session five during which only one minute right sided training was done at the SMR reward frequency, it was evident that he could not tolerate right sided training at all. His energy levels and overall mood were lower after just one minute of right sided training.

By the time the two channel power training was introduced, the amplitude of the trainee's 16–19 Hz activity at Cz measured higher than 8 microvolt in comparison to 5, 7 microvolt at the onset of the training. Angelo's mother decided to stop administering the stimulant medication at session No 26. The feedback had been consistently and increasingly more positive for a long time. The teachers found Angelo much more spontaneous and responsive. He often had the whole class group in stitches with his fine and clever sense of humor.

Angelo's mother reported that Angelo transformed into the child that they had always known they had. She described Angelo as always being receptive and ready for a joke. His relationship with his brother has improved significantly. Angelo can now shine forth as the happy, content, funny, gentle, and kind person that he is that makes the world a better place.

Angelo no longer appears to have a concentration problem. His marks are slowly but surely improving. A re-evaluation at some point would be interesting in order to ascertain if the discrepancy between his non-verbal scaled scores and his verbal scaled scores has declined. Such a re-evaluation would be deemed unnecessary though should Angelo's performance continue improving unless it were to satisfy curiosity or serve as a testimony to neurofeedback from a different perspective as well.

12.15 Case Study: A 62-Year-Old Male with Cerebrovascular Accident

This case study was contributed by the author.

I met Bernard two years after he had suffered a massive stroke towards the end of 2015. A MRI of his brain showed a large left middle cerebral artery ischemic infarction.

Bernard lives in a remote rural village called Bray in the North West province of South Africa situated on the border with Botswana, 1 400 km from Cape Town. Bernard used to be a competent high ranking military officer until he took to the business world where he left his mark as a successful and honorable businessman. He was known to be a well organized man and rather set in his ways. In September 2015 the lives of Bernard and his wife Caroline changed dramatically. But there had been early danger signs.

One evening in June 2015, Bernard and Caroline were on their way to join their son for a birthday dinner at the nearest town when Caroline noticed that Bernard behaved strangely when he exited the apartment they were staying at. He opened and closed the front door repeatedly almost as if he were stuck in the repetitive motion for a few seconds. At the restaurant he started perspiring profusely and his muscles contracted causing him to lean towards the right and then he lost consciousness. He was admitted to hospital and kept overnight for observation and discharged the following morning with a vague explanation that he had suffered some chemical reaction and that there was no reason for concern. In September 2015 Bernard and Caroline had to go to the same town where they had met their son a few months before to purchase stock for their shop in Bray. Bernard seemed very tired and slow and rested at the apartment they had rented while his wife did the shopping. On her return she found him lying on the ground and called an ambulance. Bernard was admitted to the same hospital in Vryburg he was admitted to in June. One hour after his admission he had a seizure. Caroline made arrangements for Bernard to be flown to a well-equipped hospital in Bloemfontein which is 320 km away. The attending physician at the hospital in Vryburg informed Caroline that her husband had suffered a major stroke and that it was very unlikely he would ever be able to walk or speak again and would probably be incontinent for the rest of his life – if he survived.

Caroline stayed at Bernard's side day in and day out when he was moved from the Intensive Care Unit at Bloemfontein to a general ward. After three weeks in hospital, Bernard was transferred to a rehabilitation center. At that point it was evident that Bernard had expressive and receptive dysphasia. It appeared that the speech therapy, physiotherapy and occupational therapy had little or no effect. Bernard was unresponsive and showed no sign of interest or comprehension.

Caroline took her husband home to their farm in Bray and started the long and lonely journey of attempting to get access to her husband's needs and desires and getting him to start engaging with life once again. Caroline often mentioned the frustration she experienced in constantly having to explain that Bernard was not hard of hearing.

With the assistance of the physiotherapist Bernard started walking. It was more of a shuffle than really walking. Caroline had to get power of attorney to manage business affairs that she had not been involved in prior to Bernard's stroke. She met with a lot of resistance and enjoyed very little support from banking officials and clients. Bernard slowly started showing signs of improved memory and could eventually calculate the salaries of their employees.

In February 2016, Bernard had to be hospitalized for a month for major depressive disorder.

At the time Bernard commenced with neurofeedback training sessions at the author's practice in November 2017, he had expressive dysphasia, but it appeared that he had relatively intact receptive language skills. He could not express himself in speaking or writing. His balance and coordination were poor with marked right sided hemiparesis. His eating utensils had to be strapped to his hand or else he would drop the knife or the spoon he was holding in his right hand. Bernard choked regularly when he ate or drank and lost consciousness sporadically.

Bernard has thus far responded well to the neurofeedback training sessions on the following protocols:

Session 1: Cz	Reward: 15–18 Hz	Inhibits: 0–7 Hz; 22–36 Hz
Session 2: C3	Reward: 15–18 Hz	Inhibits: 0–7 Hz; 22–36 Hz
Session 3: T3	Reward: 15–18 Hz	Inhibits: 4–7 Hz; 22–36 Hz
T4	Reward: 12–15 Hz	Inhibits: 4–7 Hz; 22–36 Hz
Session 4: F7-C3	Reward: 15–18 Hz	Inhibits: 4–7 Hz; 22–36 Hz
	Reward: 15–18 Hz	Inhibits: 0–7 Hz; 22–36 Hz
Session 5: F3-C3	Reward: 15–18 Hz	Inhibits: 4–7 Hz; 22–36 Hz
	Reward: 15–18 Hz	Inhibits: 0–7 Hz; 22–36 Hz

Session 6:	4Channel Live Z-score on T5, T6, Fz, Cz	
Session 7:	4Channel Live Z-score on T5, T6, Fz, Cz	
		Inhibits: 4–7 Hz; 22–36 Hz
Session 8: F7-F8	Reward: 12–15 Hz; 14–17 Hz; 15–18 Hz	Inhibits: 4–7 Hz; 22–36 Hz
Session 9–11: F7-F8	Reward: 12–15 Hz	Inhibits: 4–7 Hz; 22–36 Hz
Session 12:	4Channel Live Z-score on T5, T6, Fz, Cz	
Session 13: F7-F8	Rewards: 15–18 Hz; 12–15 Hz; 10–13 Hz; 15–18 Hz	
Session 14:	4Channel Live Z-score on F7, F3, F4, F8	
Session 15: Cz	Reward: 15–18 Hz	Inhibits: 4–7 Hz; 22–36 Hz
Session 16: F7-F8	Reward: 12–15 Hz; 15–18 Hz	Inhibits: 4–7 Hz; 22–36 Hz
Session 17: Cz	Reward: 15–18 Hz	Inhibits: 4–7 Hz; 22–36 Hz
Sessions 18–19	4Channel Live Z-Score on T5, T6, Fz, Cz	
Session 20: Cz	Reward: 15–18 Hz	Inhibits: 4–7 Hz; 22–36 Hz
Session 21:	4Channel Live Z-score on T3, T4, Cz, Fz	
Session 22: Cz	Reward: 15–18 Hz	Inhibits: 0–7 Hz; 22–36 Hz
Sessions 23–24:	4Channel Live Z-score on T5, T6, Fz, Cz	
Session 25: Cz	Reward: 15–18 Hz	Inhibits: 0–7 Hz; 22–36 Hz
Sessions 26–28: C3	Reward: 15–18 Hz	Inhibits: 0–7 Hz; 22–36 Hz
Session 29:	4Channel Live Z-score on C3, C4, T3, T4	
Session 30: Cz	Reward: 15–18 Hz	Inhibits: 0–7 Hz; 22–36 Hz
Session 31:	sLORETA Z-score Brodmann 45 and 46	
Session 32: C3+C4	Reward: 15–18 Hz; 12–15 Hz	Inhibits: 0–7 Hz; 22–36 Hz; Inhibits: 0–7 Hz; 22–36 Hz
Session 33:	sLORETA Z-score Brodmann 45 and 46	

Due to the distance Caroline and Bernard had to travel, they would stay in a guesthouse very close to the author's practice for one week at a time and have either one or two sessions per day depending on Bernard's tolerance and also on the particular protocols used. The protocol decisions were based on the available reports and scans of the CVA, extensive research, the responses to many questionnaires, the most prominent discomfort at the time, very careful tracking of symptoms using standardized markers, feedback from Bernard's wife of his response after every session and clinical observation. Meticulous records are kept on all noticeable and potentially significant changes on the EEG which are analyzed and compared with the collateral information.

The first observable changes occurred right at the beginning of the training program. Bernard's energy levels improved, and his mood became more positive. After session no four it became evident that Bernard's balance was improving. He was also more willing to attempt to speak albeit with a slur. His expressive language then started to improve systematically. He was more willing to participate in the language exercises that his wife had been presenting to him diligently for the past two years. Bernard once again started being concerned about his appearance. Once a very well kempt and tidy man always looking neat and clean, all of that changed after his stroke and now for the first time, Bernard was once again choosing his clothes with care and dressing with a sense of pride.

By the time we had completed session number six, Caroline reported that Bernard's reading was beginning to improve. The one constant factor in Bernard's neurofeedback process is that his balance kept on improving.

Once we started working with the connectivity measures in the 4 Channel Z- score training protocol, it became apparent that the Fz, Cz coherence scores showed deviances above six standard deviations above the norm across all frequency bands. These scores all moved much closer to the normative mean within one session. Bernard was extremely tired after that session and wanted to sleep much longer than usual. It was noticeable after that session that his balance had improved significantly.

After the training sessions on F7-F8 (bipolar hook-up on single channel) Bernard's speech intonation improved to the extent that I could begin to hear his words without requesting his wife to interpret what Bernard was attempting to communicate. His balance however started deteriorating and the dexterity of his right hand deteriorated. He started dropping the pencil with which he would practice writing for instance. After more training on Cz this improved significantly. The only training session to which Bernard had a marked negative response in terms of most markers that were being monitored was the 4 Channel Z-score training on F7, F3, F4 and F8.

By session number seventeen, Bernard was no longer eating with special adapted eating utensils but with a normal knife and fork.

Bernard's first wife had passed away in a motor vehicle accident in 2002 and his daughter from that marriage passed away in a motor vehicle accident in 2005 in the same area. Although Bernard could remember his daughter, he appeared to have no recollection of his late wife. After the 4Channel Z-score training on T5, T6, Fz, Cz, Bernard started recalling fragments of information of what had appeared to have been blocked out.

By session 26 Bernard's expressive language skills appeared to have improved in terms of vocabulary and pronunciation although he was still using a lot of gestures and short phrases, single words and writing of words in the air.

Before neurofeedback training, Bernard fell often and lost consciousness often. It was not always clear which came first and not easy to get information from Bernard to ascertain whether he fell because he lost consciousness or whether the knock on his head when he fell caused him to lose consciousness. Unfortunately, after session 26 Bernard fell again, knocked his head (left frontal) and lost consciousness. This was the first time he had fallen since the onset of neurofeedback.

I discussed the possibility of sLORETA Z-Score training with Bernard and his wife on their return to Cape Town four months later.

In the meantime, Bernard's wife reported that he had resumed previous habits of always straightening objects and moving everything into orderly and neat patterns. He insisted that dirty dishes be taken to the scullery immediately after use and that everything in their house be spic and span.

Bernard was doing well and seemed more energized and driven.

In the sLORETA Z-score training sessions, Brodmann areas 45 and 46 in the lateral posterior frontal lobe (Broca's Area) and the dorsolateral prefrontal cortex in the dorsolateral frontal lobe, were specified due to their relevance to language function.

After the first session I informed Caroline that I would give her a call later that day to ascertain how Bernard was feeling after this new protocol that we had not utilized before. When I called later that day, there was no reply. After repeated attempts, I felt worried. Fortunately, Caroline had informed me which guest house they were staying at so I paid them a visit there that evening to check in on them. I was very pleasantly surprised to find a chirpy, happy Bernard of whom Caroline reported that he had not stopped talking since the afternoon session. As soon as he saw me, he came towards me with a smile and started saying names of people. Caroline explained that those were the names of their employees that he could prior to that day neither recall nor say. He continued into the night with requesting information about different relevant groups of people and repeating different groups of names. It was evident that certain brain functions that had remained in "limp mode" since the stroke were now activated.

The second session using the same protocol did not have the same profound

effect, as we so often experience in neurofeedback. A particular protocol does not always render the same response from the same individual. It is logical to assume that the reason is simply because of the neuroplasticity of the brain that allows for changes with the implication that the brain is different by the time of the next session. Many of these changes we can measure, and some involve such intricate dynamics that we may never be able to measure and will leave us in awe possibly to the end of time.

Bernard's journey with neurofeedback continues and he will probably bear testimony to the field of neurofeedback with rippling effects.

At the time of this book going to the press, Bernard had unfortunately suffered a few more severe strokes. Sadly, he was bed ridden since November 2018 and passed away in February 2019. His wife offered her unwavering support throughout.

Chapter **13**

Attestation Statements

13.1 The Unedited Testimonial of "Rose"

This case study is a testimonial contributed by 'Rose'. The client chose her pseudonym. All names other than the name of the author have been changed.

Rose was thirty-eight years old when she started a neurofeedback training program with the author in 2017.

People often ask me what happened. They look in disbelief and just can't seem to process or create a story in their minds of why I move the way I do, why I talk the way I do. Perhaps being different also looks different or people are genuinely concerned or perhaps just curious.

My story started in 2008 after I gave birth to a beautiful boy. I was on maternity leave when I dropped a mug on the floor. This seemed odd to me and since I've always been in tune with my body, I stored that incident in my mind, not realizing I would have to regurgitate it soon after. My right hand and arm seemed to have become weaker and slower. It almost felt silly – as though a mom would tell her child not to act silly, I was telling my arm the same. Eventually I decided to see a doctor who then sent me to the hand doctor who injected my wrists with steroids. All the steroids did was to cause me to drive home in a very weird manner – I was driving with my wrists. The doctor was of the opinion that it possibly was carpal tunnel brought on by pregnancy. Nope, that wasn't it! Months went by and my arm was still the same. I just decided to live with it and thought that the pregnancy probably threw my body out of balance and soon I'd be back to my normal self. That didn't happen. This disease just progressed.

One year I decided to buy myself running shoes with which to train because I was going to attempt the Two Oceans Marathon. The Two Oceans Marathon is a very popular annual ultramarathon (56 km) and a 21 km half- marathon in Cape Town, South Africa over the Easter weekend. This marathon is referred to as the world's most beautiful marathon. I've always enjoyed running, I would start it for a while and then stop: life kept happening. This was the year! I convinced my colleague to join my quest telling him it would be a great bucket list item. Not much convincing was needed and off we were jogging. I noticed that my right foot would often trip me, but I would recover and just continue. Then it started happening that my right foot would trip me over and over again and again I would recover and continue running until one day I didn't recover and landed in the dust. That was the end of the running.

I decided to raise this with my GP who referred me to my first neurologist. Yes, I've seen many doctors: a lady once beaming with health now needed a specialist's help. Dr O believed that I had a tumor that was causing the funny handwriting and the slow arm and the right leg that was tripping me. After an MRI of my brain and of the spine there was no explanation for what was happening. You could see that something was wrong, but it had no name. I had a disease called The Unknown. Dr O then referred me to the head of Neurology at Tygerberg Hospital, Dr C. What a lovely man. I was always fascinated by his little bowtie he would wear and how he would talk and barely make eye contact, but he was caring, that much I could see, I could feel. He was as perplexed as Dr O and eventually this disease had its first name: Stress. Dr C believed it was stress and I considered to a degree that stress could affect me, but I still felt that this was just something else. Dr C saw me often and as the disease progressed, he realized it was not stress. One day he apologized to me and said it was definitely not stress but that I needed to bring my husband to my next appointment. I knew this was dreaded news—his demeanor had written it so clearly. He looked sad — I could see it and I could feel it. For the next appointment my husband accompanied me. That day this disease received its second name: Cerebellar disease. We were told that I would be in a wheelchair in five years and that it would just get progressively worse. There was no cure, no hope. I couldn't hold back the tears. Brandon and I walked back to the car in complete silence and for a moment we just wanted to forget what we had just been told. I wanted to return to the time when life was amazing, when I had just given birth to my second healthy son, when my marriage was beautiful, my career was booming and my husband loving and happy. Life was amazing just now. I wanted to be there.

After my encounter with Dr C, I decided that no doctor would have the final say because I serve a God of miracles and so off I went to Mini and bought my dream car, brand new: Mini Cooper in pepper white. Dr C wanted to give me relief, I was then sent to Dr H. Dr C didn't feel I belonged in Tygerberg hospital so he wanted me to have private care. I suppose it was a consolation to him for not being able to fix me. The day I met Dr H, I confidently walked into his office wearing my favorite color, yellow, and high heels. Oh, how I love high heels! He too examined me, and he too was perplexed. He couldn't understand what was wrong with me but over and above that he also couldn't understand how someone with such an issue would walk around in high heels and a bright colored t-shirt. He believed it was psychological. He believed that I was causing this myself, that I would choose to have a less than amazing life, choose not to run with my boys, choose not to go bike riding, choose not to play hide and seek. I had a dream when I was young, and my dream was to have an amazing life. I had that – an amazing life! And here was a doctor telling me that I somehow chose to contaminate that dream!

One day I took my boys for their six-monthly dentist check-up. My dentist and I were Facebook friends and we could speak about things other than floss and root canals. When we were done he came towards me and asked me what was wrong. I could see the pain in his eyes. I told him I didn't know, and he then asked me to just go and see his GP, Dr M O. I went to see her and her opinion was that I had MELAS. That blew my mind because that was fatal. She referred me to her neurologist, Dr. R. Before she was done, I asked her to draw bloods for my thyroid. I was due to have my levels checked. She then also had my thyroid anti bodies checked. She called to say that my thyroid anti bodies were so high that the reading wasn't available, and my disease received its third name: Hashimoto Encephalopathy. I felt relieved, this was treatable, I would be able to live my dream-I would have that amazing life after all. That was short lived too. There were no improvements. I was taking 18 tablets a day, some steroids, and others auto immune suppressants. I wasn't feeling good. I then had another go at intravenous steroids but there was no real impact. I think at this point I was so desperate that I made myself believe that I was getting better, but that was sadly not the case.

Somewhere in between all of this I decided to give ViiV Healthcare a go. It is a pharmaceutical company specializing in the development of therapies for HIV infection. A friend had mentioned that this was great, that they did a test on your blood and could tell you exactly what was wrong with you. Well that process was expensive, and it just added more tablets to my day. Though it didn't make me feel better, it wasn't making me feel worse. If anything, taking more tablets was messing up my psyche. I felt that taking tablets just showed how sick I was and I did not want to be sick. I didn't want to speak that of myself, that was negative talk and I was not about that life. Somewhere in-between all that I decided to try acupuncture and my Chinese acupuncturist felt that stress too played a very important role in my condition, that if I left my stressful job, I'd get better.

At some point I asked Dr R for a second opinion. This wasn't really a second opinion since Dr R was by far not the first doctor I had seen. He referred me to Dr. H at UCT Hospital. She assessed me and my disease had its fourth name: Primary Lateral Sclerosis (PLS). She believed that all my symptoms pointed to this and it definitely was not Hashimoto Encephalopathy. Somewhere in-between all of this, my best friend, Hannah, who has walked this journey with me from the start, who with me has cried many tears, laughed many laughs and shared jokes to lighten the thought of my body failing me, spoke to one of her friends who said that I had to go and see Dr B at Panorama. I had nothing to lose, at this point, I had everything to gain and there was always hope. Each time I would stay in hospital or see another doctor, there was always hope that one of them would discover what was wrong and that it would be so simple that we would all laugh it off. I even envisioned myself throwing a: "It's been discovered"-party. Any doctor or stay in hospital was a possible precursor for that big party, so there was always hope. Dr B too thought that it was PLS. He sided with Dr H so what now?

Back to the drawing board and back to Dr R and C with the news. Dr C did not believe in the PLS diagnosis at all and asked me if he could see me again. Hannah decided to join for this consultation. When I arrived I was amused at Dr C's greeting to Hannah and I. "The ladies of Kensington, we have been waiting" while holding out his hand to show us which room to enter. "We?" what was "we" who was "we"? Dr C had a great sense of humor. As we entered, we were in a small auditorium packed full of doctors. There must have been about 25 doctors all in varying degrees of experience, status, and importance. Some were students, some were young neurologists, some were veterans at this game and one of them was the leader in research in PLS. Dr C had asked Dr XXXX who was the, as Dr C described him, "the best with PLS". I was put on show. Doctors were shouting terms and Dr C or any other doctor would then almost debate it and they would discuss, decide and move on. This went on for about one and a half hours. I had to do various hand and leg movements; all the while Dr C would ask if I was ok. They all unanimously agreed: Not PLS.

Some time went on and Hannah was still trying to speak to whomever she could. I would paint myself a picture of ladies sitting and discussing the latest fashion with a cup of tea in the hand, a little scone on a side plate on the lap with a beautiful view of the ocean and Hannah would say "You know my friend, her name is Rose and something terrible is happening to her body, she can't walk properly, can't talk properly, falls over what do you think it can be". I'd quietly smile in appreciation, and knew she really cared. Finally, over a cup of green tea someone mentioned that their dad had a lot of confidence in a neurologist, Dr. K. He was in the southern suburbs of Cape Town; I hadn't really given any of the southern suburb doctors a chance to solve the mystery of Rose. Once again Hannah and I went, full of hope. Maybe Dr K would be the one and we would be planning that victory party on route back from his rooms. That didn't happen, quite the contrary happened. We spoke about my condition; I related the story.

He examined me, did some research on the internet and then said "I definitely agree with the Spastic Paraplegia, it will never go away, it will progress. You need to stop doctor hopping. You need to mourn your health as someone who mourns the passing of their mother and move on". I was stunned, shocked, and felt almost empty. Those words made no sense to me – they were empty and hurtful. Of course, I understand that doctors have to detach emotionally, but to such an extent? Hannah started crying profusely. Dr K had shattered the hope we had. I started crying as well and didn't say much after the devastating news, walked out of the rooms to stand outside and just tried to make sense of what had just happened. Hannah paid for the consult while I was standing outside. The receptionist came outside to hug me. She had the empathy that the doctor was lacking. She just said "sorry" and that was all I needed her to say to understand exactly what she meant. That was a very low day for me. I've had many low days, but only two really stand out and this was one of them. I cried and cried. I would play those words over and over in my head and cry. My heart was aching. Physical pain resounded in my chest and I didn't think I would get over it. Every ounce of hope started dissipating. How would I pick myself up? I spoke to Brandon and cried. I spoke to my mother-in-law and cried. I spoke to my dad, my heart ached more. No parent wants to hear of something they can't fix and this my dad could not fix, he couldn't even offer relief. This was sad.

A few days passed and I had to be "happy" for my boys. They didn't understand all of this. Sometimes I wonder if we ever did. How would we explain something so weird, something that had so many names? How do we describe this without sounding like this was part of a sci-fi script? We couldn't. I had two choices: Live or Die. I chose to live; I didn't work so hard at everything to allow something like a disease to define me. I would define me, and I would live the best life I could. I decided that no doctor had the final say but that I believed in something greater that could in one spoken word or one touch heal and take away this disease. He would rescue me, and so my hope returned but this time it was not rooted in man but in God. I realized that I had been seeking answers and healing from people instead of asking God to send the right people my way or just come Himself. I started to more earnestly seek His word and in doing so found solace in that I was otherwise healthy, had two healthy beautiful boys and had a loving husband whom I have loved most of my life and who loves me back, mysterious disease and all. Talk about "in sickness and in health": we were living this daily. We were being true to the vows we said on the windy day of 20 December 2003. God had a greater plan for us and this was part of it. I started surrounding myself with positivity, after all, that was who I was, the ultimate optimist. I started reading books that would make me think of ways to keep positive but also realistic, podcasts that would make my day start off on an amazing note and have conversations that would just boost my day. In all of this, I would have some off days but all of a sudden, I would easily pick myself up. My pity parties no longer lasted longer than they needed too. I would feel sadness because we are all allowed to feel all emotions. The trick was to identify the emotion and then to deal with the emotion accordingly. I started doing that daily and it was a struggle at first. I wished it was over and I was at the end of the tunnel. That wasn't how it worked, I couldn't go over or under this struggle – I had to go through it. The beauty of going through something is the unknown arts that you discover. There are many things I discovered about myself, I'm still discovering, and the journey is beautiful. One very important lesson I learnt was that nothing was more important than living in the moment you have been given. Just to sit quietly and be, was something that was foreign to me, it felt as though I was wasting time but now I started reading again but not with the goal of finishing so many books by that date, but to enjoy and savor every word and profound phrase that presented itself to me. In all this there were boundless blessings and living in the moment was one of them.

My life was always rushed. A people pleaser never gets tired and spends far too much energy on others: that was me. Perhaps this disease was meant to have me pause and enjoy life, enjoy my boys, enjoy my husband. I started taking in the scents of my boys and husband with the intention of storing the scent in my subconscious mind so they would be with me forever. Work was a means to an end and not an all- consuming need to prove myself to anyone. I was being true to myself only. This felt fantastic.

I remember how someone told me to get a disabled disc for my car and I refused to treat this as though it was a disability. I was not disabled. I didn't want to label this or give it power. As soon as the pride subsided I realized how much easier and safer it would be for me if I had a disabled disc. I'd not have to worry about crossing the road or worry that if it was raining,

I'd have to park too far so I decided to apply for the disc. It's quite a process but I suppose if it wasn't then anyone would be applying for discs. It's really something innate in human beings to want things to be easy. Don't get me wrong, I too was like that – I'd circle to get a closer parking rather than just park and walk a few extra steps. Now I appreciate walking a whole lot more. So I eventually received my parking disc. The disc was a blessing and a curse. People would stare at me, talk under their breath, I even had a guy knock on my car and then approach me at my window to reprimand me for using a disabled parking space. I then realized that it seemed disability had its own face and I clearly did not portray that face. What does disabled look like? Can disabled not drive a mini? Can disabled not be young? Can disabled not wear make-up? What did this person's disabled look like? That day when the man with the prosthetic leg knocked on my window, I showed him the disc and said to him to trust that I wouldn't park in the bay if I didn't need too. I didn't want any attention on myself. One day I had just pulled into the parking bay at Woolworths' parking lot when a gentleman (not quite so gentle) said something about parking in the disabled bay. He said   it loud enough for me to hear but soft enough to make it seem as though he was speaking to himself. I had had enough. I marched myself into Woolworths to find him and as I approached him, he started apologizing whilst looking down at the floor. I trust he would never do that again. Though I really don't mind people questioning me about parking in the bay since it is reserved for those who are disabled, there is just a way to speak to people. One does not have to be rude. So now I'm the one asking people who park in disabled bays if they have discs because I've found that people would park in the bay to quickly run to the shop or go to the bank.

One day I was at work and chatting about my son Tristan and how focus is an issue for him and how he struggles to focus for longer than 20 minutes. The greatest frustration wasn't his focus as much as his results that just didn't fit his excellent mind and memory. He could regurgitate facts on demand but when put in an environment where he had to answer questions, the response was vastly different. My friend, Jeanne, another of my sister's in Christ, then mentioned that her sister had the same problem and that she had started seeing Helena, a neurotherapist. Jeanne went on to explain that before neurotherapy her sister wouldn't focus, disliked reading and was average at school but that she now loved reading and had even started her own business at the tender age of 22. This was good news because much of what I was experiencing with Tristan, Jeanne's mum was experiencing with Kirsten. I listened but didn't jump into action. We had been through so many various ways of helping Tristan to focus that I wasn't eager to rush into another form of help. Weeks passed and Jeanne came walking into my office, rather excited, she had something to share. I enjoyed sharing, it just reminded me that we are all doing life and all our lives have similar key events. Jeanne came to tell me that she had shared my story with Helena and that Helena would like to meet me and see if she could possibly help me. I was at first skeptical, this is understandable given my history of discovery. I decided to give neurotherapy a try and what I discovered was profound.

When you walk into Helena's rooms, there is an immediate calm, every wall you thought you had around you just waits outside as you step over the door frame into the reception area. A friendly face greets you, and you begin to wonder if it's something in the air. You see a water fountain ahead of you trickling away putting you into a dreamy state. I wait to meet Helena, who I've by now googled just to paint my own picture of. Why do we even do that? It's like finding your gift before Christmas. Helena comes to meet me, there is a way about her I just can't explain but all I know is that I was about to have verbal diarrhea and spill it all. As soon as I started speaking, I started crying. I couldn't understand why. I've told many people my story and those who haven't known me before this happened were the easiest to tell because there was no hurt or pain in their eyes once they compared me now to me then. Nonetheless I was crying – that heartache was back and I think for once I felt ok to let it out after those dreaded words from Dr. K. I started my sessions and though I had no anxiety or ADD/ADHD, I felt more confident, my thoughts were clearer. I felt as though I could easily and effectively compartmentalize life. This was amazing. After a few months, I decided to give Tristan a go at neurotherapy. The change in Tristan was immediate. I was blown away. All of a sudden, he could focus, he was no longer over emotional and he was just so much easier to get along with. You see, Tristan isn't as mature as his peers and since he is emotional, these two attributes weren't beneficial to a 10-year-old at the time. Tristan also enjoyed going to Helena because she would coach him over and above his neurotherapy. He just needed to offload. Tristan is almost done with all his sessions and will be doing maintenance sessions soon but the change in Tristan is phenomenal. He has grown so much since starting neurotherapy, it has changed our lives and we will be eternally grateful.

I had a baclofen pump surgically inserted into my abdomen area which then, via a tube that runs from the pump up my spine, releases medicine at a calculated time. When I woke up after surgery, I was started on 200 micrograms per day. This pump was supposed to offer relief to the spasticity. The trial was amazing and it showed promise but what I hadn't realized was that the dosage I needed was far more than the trial had given me. The trial was quick relief but the pump had to be constant relief. I was disappointed because though this couldn't heal me, the relief might mean that I could run with my boys, something I've dreamed of ever since I was a teenager. I wasn't complaining because the meds eased the walking on my toes. I was walking flat footed, albeit it was still slow and stiff, it was a whole lot better than before. Gradually we increased the dosage of the pump and eventually I was up to 420 micrograms per day. This didn't come without side effects. I had a constantly hairy tongue that would be there no matter how much I would brush or how much gum I'd try to eat or how much liquids I'd try to drink. My urine had a foul smell. I was too embarrassed to use the bathroom at public places. My toes would feel numb and sometimes I'd wake up with my feet having pins and needles. Try getting out of bed with your feet still sleeping, not a pretty sight at all. My fingers would be numb too, but I tried to alleviate the agony by sleeping differently or making sure I wasn't reading for too long or that I wasn't lying in bed on my back which for some or other reason would cause my feet to go numb. It was frustrating but after all I'd had to bear, this was ok.

June 2017 I noticed something strange, I was having consecutive good days.

Those were rare. I was used to having a good day then a string of bad days. That was the routine but this time I had one good day and then another good day and another and another. The first day I said nothing, this was normal. Day two I mentioned it to my husband. Two days became ten days and ten days became twenty days. All of a sudden I was having more good days than bad days. I asked Helena if there was anything she was doing differently because I'm feeling really great. She mentioned that she had changed the protocol a bit since she was almost done with the, what I call, Alice band part of the brain. She asked me when it started and it was spot on with when she started changing the protocol. I was so excited, for once there was progress but steady progress. Of course, I feared that it might go away, everything was always short lived but this was great, my legs were feeling heavy. Heavy legs were always a good indicator of a good day. You see my legs would normally feel as though they are there but as light as a feather and you have no control over where a feather blows. Heavy legs were good, great, amazing. I had to go to hospital for something, can't remember what and decided to show my neurosurgeon, Dr V what had transpired. Dr V was a kind man – he was definitely living his calling. He was empathetic and compassionate. One day he said to me that if he could fix me his career would be made. I had wished he could. That day I waited for an hour to see him since he was already busy with a patient when I arrived. When he could eventually see me, I told him that I had something to show him. I went on to show him how I could bend without struggling to get up. I could go down on the floor and actually get up not having to crawl until I found somewhere to pull myself up on. I could turn around in a circle which I wouldn't dare do before. I could walk and look up. I could walk and actually look ahead of myself. That was probably the most profound part of it all. I could walk and look up. For all of those years I would walk and had to always be looking down. I had to look down so that I could see potential hazards and try to avoid them. How beautiful life was looking up, if only we look up and really mean it instead of looking up because it's normal. If only we looked up and actually absorbed the beauty around us rather than to rush to the shop to buy that extra pair of jeans because the price is good. Have we just looked up to greet the person passing us or looked up to notice the baby trying to walk or just looked up at the sky at the wonder of the clouds? Those are things I had not been privileged to do unless I was standing stationary and holding on to something or someone. That was liberating. I was walking to work without aid. Every morning and afternoon someone would escort me to and from work to my car just in case I didn't make it all in one piece. Perhaps the one piece was my dignity more than my physical appearance because the great risk for me is that I would trip and fall or that someone would walk past me and knock me off my feet, literally.

Neurotherapy changed my life, but I've said that before haven't I. This time I'm saying it again because it has changed my life twofold. It's given our son the confidence to be who he is, to be him and no-one else. It's given him a calm that he has not had before and has matured him the right way. If you have a conversation with Tristan, you will have to remind yourself that he is only eleven years old. It has restored my liberation. I was once a prisoner in my body but now I'm free. Though I still can't dance the way I used to, I can dance without having to hold on to anybody. Though I still can't walk normally, I can walk looking up. Though I still can't run, I can be wherever you are running. Life is better. I do believe if I had met Helena and her gift at the start of this journey, I would've been far ahead in my healing. God asks us to trust that HE will send the right person, not that we go and find the right person. He did send her, and I am eternally grateful.

The following neurofeedback training protocols have been used thus far:

- Fifteen sessions amplitude training on the sensory motor strip at Cz, C3 and C4

- Five sessions at T3 - T4 (15 minutes at T3 rewarding 15–18 Hz plus 12 minutes

- at T4 rewarding 12–15 Hz)

- Combinations of Cz and T3 - T4

- Seven sessions of 4 Channel live Z-score training at Fz, Cz, T5, T6

- Alternating between T3-T4 and live Z-score training at the above-mentioned placement areas

- Ongoing Live Z-Score training at T3, C3, C4, T4

13.2 The Testimony of a 60-Year-Old Female

This attestation statement is mainly the translation of the testimony by Carmen (pseudonym), the opera singer referred to earlier in this book.

It is weird to be sitting here and writing this, but I can't think of a more appropriate place. (Carmen is referring to the deck of the lodge overlooking the Kavango River where I was on retreat in a tented camp for a month to write this book. It was completely coincidental or probably serendipitous that we crossed paths there, three thousand kilometers away from Cape Town in the wilderness). Where does one even begin to describe and analyse a person's life that has been in existence for sixty years? And in fact, I don't want to. For the first time I am not fragmented. It is as if the puzzle pieces have fallen into place and I don't want to take the puzzle apart and analyse the separate pieces to the puzzle. I don't want to wonder about the protrusions and the cavities, it suffices that the pieces fit and complete one another. I am at peace within my body and my soul and that is very precious. I can't ignore my previous life – or rather, I am not suppressing it. The regrets of choices I have made are no longer intensely haunting me. Things are the way they are, and I can be mindfully present in my life. I am so much happier than so many other people and for that I am grateful to you and your equipment. I would not have been able to enjoy this holiday that I am on now with my husband prior to the training sessions with you. I would not have been able to enjoy the endless traveling for thousands of kilometers on a seemingly endless road with the vast expanse of grass fields. On this journey I could feast my senses on every unfolding scene and treasure it.

I have always said that my life is fragmented, and it was difficult to navigate myself through such a life. My life still exists of many different components but with all the components integrated it is just so much easier and so significantly less stressful.

13.3 The Testimony of Margaret

This attestation statement is a translation of a thirty-eight-year-old female, Margaret (pseudonym).

I always had a sense that everything wasn't a 100% normal. It often felt to me as if I didn't belong in my body.

350

I carried a label since I was very young. I remember what it felt like when I was angry. I would start crying in an attempt to express the emotion or to be able to vent it. When I was angry, I would voice any thought or feeling that came to mind without filtering it. In my opinion I was at least being direct and honest-irrespective of the consequences. Because I did well academically, my parents didn't really regard my fiery temper and overreactions to be a serious problem.

I recall being scared – being terribly scared often. I still don't know what I was so overwhelmingly afraid of. When the feeling started it felt as if I couldn't breathe properly – there was tightness in my chest and it felt as if my heart was beating in my throat.

When I was a grown up, I sought out answers and assistance and went to consult with different general practitioners, psychologists, and psychiatrists. Different diagnoses were thrown at me including borderline depression, bipolar disorder and after the birth of each of my children my discomfort was labelled as postnatal depression. I got various prescriptions for different types of medications and underwent different treatments – none of which made a significant difference. When I became a mother, my mother repeatedly pointed out to me that I had so much suppressed anger   and that I needed to see someone who could assist me. When my youngest son started coming home from school with messages about his temper outbursts and oppositional behavior, I could see my own tendencies reflected in him. Strangely enough, this did not make it easier for me to understand him and be accommodating. It rather caused a rift between us. I found it difficult to bond with him. It was as if I needed to push him away from me – I guess it was too close for comfort. He too was prescribed different types of medications at different stages to calm him down and have him behave more acceptably in social situations.

It really started dawning on me that I needed to get assistance. If it were too late for me, at least my son could possibly still be helped. I started researching all possibilities and when I came across neurofeedback training, it felt to me to be a more acceptable option than experimenting with yet another medication.

Both my son and I embarked on a neurofeedback journey. I could feel a difference right from the word go and also detected an immediate difference in my son's behavior. It was amazing. The aftereffects of some sessions were better than others. Sometimes I had a slight headache or felt slightly down but what I knew for a fact was that things were shifting and changing.

The biggest benefit to me was that I started feeling more calm and grew more accepting of myself. For the first time in my life I could consider my responses to situations. I no longer just reacted, I responded according to a conscious choice. I could actually just keep quiet and not respond at all if I so chose. I could reprimand my children without scolding them and I could just calmly and contently spend quality time with them. I was no longer constantly my own worst enemy!

I could also for the first time decide who I wanted to engage with and allow into my inner circle and who not. I learnt to say "no" in an assertive and liberating way without being aggressive. For the first time in my journey of thirty-seven years, I have found myself. I can actually distinguish between pleasant and unpleasant experiences and make choices that honor me.

I see changes in my son on a daily basis. We can sit down and have a calm and pleasant conversation about almost anything. His gentle nature is now shining forth. I can see emotions other than anger.

It is difficult for me to explain the changes that have occurred inside of me. It can best be described as a shift. There is a song in Afrikaans that when I hear it, I associate it with the shift that neurofeedback brought about in my life. The words translated say more or less the following: "Although the sky has always been blue, it is now bluer. Although I have always been here, I now belong here".

The following neurofeedback training protocols were used for Margaret:

- Sixteen sessions of amplitude training on the sensory motor strip at Cz,
- C4 and combinations of C3 and C4. The training on C3 never exceeded one minute.
- Three sessions amplitude training at T4-P4
- Eleven sessions 4Channel Z-score training at F3, F4, P3, P4

The following neurofeedback training protocols were used for Margaret's son:

- Nine sessions on Cz (12–15 Hz)
- One session on P4
- Two 4Channel Z-score training at C3, C4, P3, P4
- Four sessions 4Channel Z-score at F3, F4, P3, P4

The training was ongoing at the time this book went to the press.

13.4 Katerina's Story

This is the unedited story of Katerina (pseudonym), written by herself.

By the time I arrived at neurotherapy I was profoundly ready for change. I knew and understood much about my trauma history and its long-term effects. I had done great work in psychotherapy (18 years' worth) and was no longer dissociating. I had been meditating for years and intensively practicing mindfulness for four years. Mindfulness has helped me observe my mind getting "stuck" in unrelenting repetitive thinking. My thoughts were mostly self-critical and self- judgmental from the moment I woke in the morning. Yet with all I had learnt and all I could observe I could not change what I was experiencing. This left me feeling both helpless, at the mercy of this "noise" and hopeless, feeling that no one "got" what I was saying. I knew there was something more, something I was struggling to get words for. All the tools and strategies I had learnt in therapy didn't work and I felt I was failing and that I was a failure because I couldn't change or control what was happening in my thoughts.

The intake procedure at the onset of my neurofeedback journey was already profound. The questionnaires indicated that I was severely depressed and also showed significant signs of anxiety. This gave me a physical jolt. I knew that I had been struggling but had no idea it was this bad.

Arriving for my first session I was a shell. I was unable to connect with others or myself. I was hiding and was not managing to sleep through the night. I was unable to think or plan and found it challenging to string a coherent sentence together. I was impatient and irritable with myself and those around me. I was both in deep pain and numbed out and the list goes on.

So started a remarkable journey . . .

Here are some of the most profound moments, experiences, and insights so far: I had made a very conscious decision at the beginning of this course of neurotherapy that I was going to "try". I was not going to continue all those strategies I had been using trying to cope. I was going to stop struggling and see what happened and where it led.

From the initial consult, Helena expressed the belief that neurotherapy could help me. During sessions I learnt that my treatment was a normal protocol. WOW-what this gave me was a sense of hope – something I had not felt in a long time. The feeling I had about the possibility that this agony could end and that I could possibly get my life back is indescribable.

Another hugely important aspect in my process of healing is the validation of my experience which has happened in two important ways. Firstly, Helena "got" my experience after having tried for over a year to explain what I was experiencing. From what I said, she knew what was going on in the brain and could tell me what was happening. It both validated my experience and normalized it. Relief – now I knew I wasn't nuts. This was also the first time that when I said that I was freezing, that I knew that the person I was speaking to, understood. I was not making it up. I was not in conscious control of how the brain was responding and I understood that I was not a failure.

Secondly, she showed me the amplitude of the frequency that a fear circuit was running at and it brought tears to my eyes. This is what I have been living with for as long as I can remember and this is part of what has made my daily life so hard and there it was on a screen – it was real!

I am only one quarter through the process so far and there are already so many changes: By the time I started neurotherapy I was perhaps sleeping through every third or fourth night and would often get only three- or four-hours uninterrupted sleep per night. Now I sleep through most nights. I can think and plan and prioritize. Two months ago, writing this would have been virtually impossible and now I love doing it. Instead of just battling through a day I can make choices and have clarity. I know what works for me and what doesn't, what I have capacity for and what I am not quite ready for yet. And I have energy: the simplest of tasks used to defeat and overwhelm me and now I can achieve several tasks in a day.

I can breathe again. The volume of the "noise" and the sense of agitation are both turned way down. And on some days, they are not there at all and then I am me and I am home.

The following neurofeedback training protocols have been used for Katerina so far:

- Seven sessions at Cz (12–15 Hz)
- Two sessions T4-P4 (10–13 Hz)
- Eight sessions 2Channel training at C3, C4
- Two sessions eyes closed training at Pz (5–8; 8–11 Hz)

13.5 Testimonial from Edward's Mother

This attestation statement was contributed by Edward's (pseudonym) mother.

Edward is the third born of my four boys. He has always been a very friendly, jovial boy who loved people and thoroughly enjoyed being the number one joker at every event. Younger children adored his kind nature and especially his ability to bring more fun into any situation. He was an endless fountain of mischievous ideas and my husband jokingly referred to him as the catalyst – for trouble!

Social interaction with peers of Edward's own age was unfortunately much more difficult, especially when a group of children was present. He had no friends of his own age and his perceptions regarding social situations were extremely skewed. He always seemed to think he was treated in an unfair manner and from his description of situations, I sometimes wondered if we were thinking of the same situation – his story not reflecting what really happened at all.

Edward always felt like the scapegoat, the outcast and the rejected friend in every group. This resulted in him being a very sad and lonely boy who craved friendship but did not have the ability to cultivate one. His behavior obviously influenced how people treated him, but somehow, he could never understand his role in it, he simply thought he was being bullied.

The problems seemed to stem out of group situations, for when I communicated and spent time with Edward one on one I was able to enjoy him immensely. I home schooled my children over a period of six years and for the last of those years, it was only Edward and I – the others were back in school. I remember how much fun we had during the mornings, but as soon as the others arrived back from school, it seemed as if he was a different child. To me it felt as if he was intentionally looking for trouble all through the afternoon – taunting and teasing his brothers.

It felt as if any form of correction or explanation around social situations would float around in his brain but somehow was unable to hook unto something solid and settle. It was as if there was no foundation of emotional intelligence and no matter how hard I tried; I could not make any progress.

He was not very self-aware and seemed not to understand social boundaries. He had very little boundaries of his own in terms of personal space, belongings and "me time". Furthermore, he failed to understand the importance of building trust and having integrity in friendships.

I can very vividly remember a friend of my husband visiting us and playing around with Edward while coffee was being made. Not long after that Edward walked passed the lounge where we were sitting and casually knocked the guy's cap off his head, laughed and walked on – completely unaware of how offending that was to the adults, even though he was theoretically old enough to understand.

Another time a gentleman, old enough to be Edward's grandfather, stretched out his hand to greet Edward. Edward stayed sitting, looked the man in his eyes and completely ignored the outstretched hand. He was taught to greet all people, to shake hands and to treat others with respect and make them feel welcome. Somehow the "theory" was not transferrable to practice and he did not seem to understand and grasp the disrespect he showed.

Edward had many typical ADHD symptoms. He was very impulsive, talked loudly and without end and his mind and world was unorganized and messy. He is a very intelligent boy with a vivid interest in the world around him, but he has serious reading problems and despite several interventions, was two and a half years behind on reading skills. I remember thinking that my son would never be able to attend a school – because of the reading problems, but more so because of his lack of social skills and his prominent ADHD related symptoms.

We were therefore quite desperate when we started with neurotherapy. When I first heard Helena Bester speak about neurotherapy I was very skeptical. Then, within a short time period I read feedback from two moms on a home school Facebook group about the positive changes in their children after neurofeedback. We decided to give it a try and never looked back.

It changed his whole world and because of that our world as well. After a few weeks, his reading started to improve and today his reading is almost on par with his peers, although he still hates reading! The most significant thing for us was that his perceptions of social situations changed. He became more self-aware and he was finally able to understand social clues, cues, and boundaries. Suddenly when I corrected Edward on something, he was able to absorb the information and adjust his behavior. The road was not without bumps and a lot of ups and downs week after week. But within a year after our first neurotherapy session he was in school, making friends and loving every moment of it. Our home is no longer a war zone. His concentration levels improved drastically and his hockey coach could not believe the difference in skill.

I am so grateful for this chance on life that Edward got.

The following neurofeedback training protocols were used with Edward:

- Ten sessions at C4 at 12–15 Hz
- One session at C3 at 15–18 Hz (3 minutes) + C4 at12–15 Hz (24 minutes)
- One session at C3 at 15–18 Hz (6 minutes) + C4 at 12–15 Hz (21 minutes)
- Six sessions at C3 at 15–18 Hz (1 minute) + C4 at 12–15 Hz (25 minutes)
- Twenty-seven sessions at C4 at 10–13 Hz
- Two sessions at C4 at 12–15 Hz (3 minutes) + C4 at 10–13 Hz (24 minutes)
- Eight sessions at C4 at 12–15 Hz (30 sec) + C4 at 10–13 Hz (26,5 minutes)
- One session at Cz at 12–15 Hz

(All specified frequencies are reward frequencies. The same two frequency bands were inhibited throughout, namely 4–7 Hz and 22–36 Hz).

13.6 Veronica's Story

This report is a contribution by Veronica (pseudonym) translated by the author.

Veronica was 31 years old when I met her in June 2017. She shared her story as follows:

Neurotherapy changed my life completely.

I have had to deal with depression during various stages of my life. I was diagnosed with depressive disorder as a child and was prescribed different anti- depressants throughout the years.

I met the love of my life a few years ago and we got married soon after. I have always loved babies and children since I was a little girl. Babies brought me joy and I really looked forward to having my own little bundle of joy. After a miscarriage in 2015 we decided to do fertility treatment which was extremely costly and unfortunately not successful. At that stage I had stopped using anti-depressants in an attempt to increase the possibility of falling pregnant. The process was draining on more level than one. I started feeling the familiar symptoms of depression creeping up on me. We were planning on having another in vitro fertilization later that year so I did not want to start on anti-depressants again and jeopardize my chances of having a viable pregnancy.

My brother recommended that I considered neurotherapy because of the relief he has experienced through the therapy. I was a bit skeptical, but my brother made an appointment with Helena anyway. Soon after the onset of the neurofeedback intervention program, I fell pregnant spontaneously. I was ecstatic! My prayers were answered and my biggest dream fulfilled. I was over the moon and felt so ready to receive our own child into our lives. I continued with neurotherapy throughout the pregnancy which I believe is the main reason why our child is so content and happy. She has slept well since birth, she hardly ever cries and she is almost always happy. Holding her for the first time brought the realization that one is capable of love beyond what one can imagine.

Unfortunately this chapter did not have a fairy tale ending. That which I feared, happened. I wanted to give birth to her as I believe giving birth was intended to be. I wanted natural birth. I was petrified of the idea of a Caesarean Section! But so it unfolded that I had to have the procedure. I was extremely anxious but when I heard Emily's announcement of her arrival into this world the anxiety dissipated.

After we were discharged, Emily contracted yellow jaundice and had to be hospitalized again. I felt so helpless. The repeated probing and poking with needles to conduct different tests caused Emily discomfort and pain. I was supposed to protect my child and I couldn't. For the first time in a long time I felt the characteristic suffocating grip of anxiety – it wasn't the normal fear and anxiety associated with the C-section. I recognized this enemy. It had me in what felt like a potentially fatal grip. When we were discharged and I could finally be home with my child, I realized that I was not okay. I could feel that I needed to go back onto my mood stabilizing medication. I was so terribly afraid that I would get postnatal depression and here it was! Despite the endless love and gratitude that caused my metaphorical cup to overflow, I was now sliding into a deep and dark place. I could not stop crying. I did not manage to take care of the simplest of tasks and I am a very hands- on person–especially when it comes to children. My wonderful husband took care of what was necessary and his only concern was that I would become healthy again. My mother stayed with us for one month and gave everything that I was not able to give Emily at the time. I will remain forever grateful to all the assistance I received from all my family members and friends.

I re-commenced with neurotherapy as soon as I could and was confronted with a difficult reality. I would have to stop the breastfeeding, start with medication again and probably be admitted to a clinic until I felt more stable. I just could not bear the thought of being without my baby for an extended period of time and decided to start on my medication again and pray that it would bring relief soon. With every bout of depression that I have had in my life, it felt that the current one was the worst. The intensity with which the depression blocked out the light this time around was worse than anything I had experienced before. The added feelings of guilt and resentment tightened the grip of despair and although I feel ashamed to admit it, I felt that my child did not deserve to have me as a mother. My mother reminded me on a daily basis that I would feel better again and that my child needed me.

Although it felt like forever at the time, in retrospect the depression subsided relatively quickly and soon I could love and hold my child the way I had dreamed of and yearned for. I could be the mother I wanted to be and wake up every morning with joy in my heart, eager to see Emily's angelic smile. She does that-she smiles every time she sees me and it is gift that I am aware of every single time I see it.

I have never recovered from a bout of depression so quickly ever and I have no doubt in my mind that it is due to the neurotherapy. I will definitely have neurotherapy again if I am blessed to fall pregnant again because I also firmly believe that my child's smooth development and emotional contentment is due to the neurotherapy during pregnancy.

When I look back, I can hardly imagine that darkness I was in. The gratitude I feel for where I am at is almost as abundant as the love I have for our child that colors every day with love and joy.

The following neurofeedback training protocols were used with Veronica:

The sessions were not done in the order mentioned. Protocol decisions were based on the most severe presenting symptoms per session. Symptoms were tracked meticulously.

- 14 Sessions at C3 at 15–18 Hz for between six to nine minutes, plus C4 at 12–15 Hz for between 18 to 21 minutes
- Two sessions at Pz at 8–11 Hz
- 12 Sessions at Cz at between 12.5–15.5 Hz to 15–18 Hz
- 4 Sessions at T4-P4 at 10–13 Hz

(All specified frequency bands are reward frequencies. The inhibit bands were 4–7 Hz and 22–36 Hz and 0–7 Hz for T4-P4).

In Closing

May we – therapists, clients and patients alike – experience a time in which the world will no longer be dominated by fear driven models of intervention- fear of not having authority, fear of rejection by peers, fear of sharing and other fears based on a scarcity mentally that excludes possibilities of growth and the reassessment of the limitations of our perceptions. May we be entering a period in which we will be willing to learn from one another with open minds and join our skills in support of mankind in an attempt to relieve suffering and promote growth to the best of our abilities!

I had to consult with a neurosurgeon in 2019 who asked me what I did for a living. "I love elephants" amongst many other things that I do, was not going to suffice. I replied appropriately with "I am a clinical neurotherapist". He responded with: "so what do you do?" My ego wanted to attack him with jargon that would make his head spin. Instead it left me with sadness. Here I was thinking that nobody could possibly still be ignorant of the field – surely not with all of the research freely available everywhere! But it is true that many mainstream medical specialists in related fields still do not consider neurofeedback a viable option or alternative to invasive therapies.

How does one go about changing judgmental perceptions so that the benefits of a non-invasive option of treatment can become more accessible to all? We do exactly what we are doing – we keep at it: The individuals who have benefited should keep telling their stories; the neuroscientists and scientists with open minds from related fields should continue with their research; the brave neurotherapists who sought out training and pursued certification should continue with their heartfelt work to which their convictions lead them and inspire colleagues to embark in the field.

Thank you to every individual with an open mind that was willing to choose to read this book. Thank you to every therapist that contributed to this book through which many other therapists may possibly be inspired to include the modalities of bio-/neurofeedback to their practices. Thank you to all the individuals that were courageous enough to share their stories – through sharing their experiences, they empower others to seek help.

Thank you to every board member, past and current and yet to serve, of every international association and society of bio-/neurofeedback — the implications of your service are too vast to imagine.

References

Acheson, D. J., & Hagoort, P. (2014). Twisting tongues to test for conflict-monitoring in speech production. *Frontiers in Human Neuroscience, 8,* 206. http://dx.doi.org/10.3389/fnhum.2014.00206

Adrian, E. D., & Matthews, B. C. H. (1934). The Berger rhythm: Potential changes from occipital lobes in man. *Brain, 57,* 355-385.

Aftanas, L. I., & Golocheikine, S. A. (2001). Human anterior and frontal midline theta and lower alpha reflect emotionally positive state and internalized attention: High-resolution EEG investigation of meditation. *Neuroscience Letters, 310*(1), 57-60. ttps://doi.org/10.1016/s0304-3940(01)02094-8

Agnihotri, H., Paul, M., & Sandhu, J. S. (2007). Biofeedback approach in the treatment of generalized anxiety disorder. *Iranian Journal of Psychiatry, 2*(3), 90-95.

Aladjalova, N. A. (1957). Infra-slow rhythmic oscillations of the steady potential of the cerebral cortex. *Nature, 179*(4567), 957-959. https://doi.org/10.1038/179957a0

Allen, J. J., Iacono, W. G., Depue, R. A., & Arbisi, P. (1993). Regional electroencephalographic asymmetries in bipolar seasonal affective disorder before and after exposure to bright light. *Biological Psychiatry, 33*(8-9), 642-646. https://doi.org/10.1016/0006-3223(93)90104-l

Allen, J. J. B., Urry, H. L., Hitt, S. K., & Coan, J. A. (2004). Stability of resting frontal EEG asymmetry across different clinical states of depression. *Psychophysiology, 41*(2), 269-280. https://doi.org/10.1111/j.1469-8986.2003.00149.x

Amen, D. G. (1998). *Change your brain, change your life: The revolutionary, scientifically proven program for mastering your moods, conquering your anxieties and obsessions, and taming your temper.* Times Books.

Amen, D. G. (2001). *Healing ADD: The breakthrough program that allows you to see and heal the six types of attention deficit disorder.* New York, NY: Putnam.

Amen, D. (2012). Daniel Amen, MD: The impact of brain imaging on psychiatry and treatment for improving brain health and function. Interview by Karen Burnett. *Alternative Therapies in Health and Medicine, 18*(2), 52-58.

Amen, D. G. (2018). *Feel better fast and make it last: Unlock your brain's healing potential to overcome negativity, anxiety, anger, stress, and trauma.* Carol Stream, IL: Tyndale Momentum.

American Psychiatric Association. (1994). *Diagnostic and statistical manual of mental disorders* (DSM-IV). Washington, DC: Author.

American Psychiatric Association. (2013). *Diagnostic and statistical manual of mental disorders (DSM-5)* (5th ed.). Arlington, VA: Author.

Andreassi, J. L. (2010). *Psychophysiology: Human behavior and physiological response* (5th ed.). Mahwah, NJ: Lawrence Erlbaum Associates, Inc.

Apkarian, A. V., Sosa,Y., Sonty, S., Levy, R. M., Harden, R. N., Parrish, T. B., & Gitelman, D. R. (2004). Chronic back pain is associated with decreased prefrontal and thalamic gray matter density. *Neuroscience, 24*(46), 10410-104105. https://doi.org/10.1523/JNEUROSCI.2541-04.2004

Arns, M., de Ridder, S., Strehl, U., Breteler, M., & Coenen, A. (2009). Efficacy of neurofeedback treatment in ADHD: The effects on inattention, impulsivity and hyperactivity: A meta-analysis. *Clinical EEG and Neuroscience, 40*(3), 180-189. https://doi.org/10.1177/155005940904000311

Arns, M., Heinrich, H., & Strehl, U. (2014). Evaluation of neurofeedback in ADHD: The long and winding road. *Biological Psychology, 95*, 108-115. https://doi.org/10.1016/j.biopsycho.2013.11.013

Askew, J. (2001). *The diagnosis of depression using psychometric instruments and quantitative measures of electroencephalographic activity.* (Unpublished doctoral dissertation). University of Tennessee, Knoxville, TN.

Ayers, M. E. (1995). Long-term follow-up of EEG neurofeedback with absence seizures. *Biofeedback & Self-Regulation, 20*(3), 309-310.

Baehr, E., Rosenfeld, J. P., & Baehr, R. (1997). Clinical use of an alpha asymmetry protocol in the neurofeedback treatment of depression. *Journal of Neurotherapy, 2*(3), 10-23. https://doi.org/10.1300/J184v02n03_02

Baehr, E., Rosenfeld, J. P., Baehr, R., & Earnest, C. (1999). Clinical use of an alpha asymmetry neurofeedback protocol in the treatment of mood disorders. In J. R. Evans & A. Abarbanel (Eds.), *Introduction to quantitative EEG and neurofeedback* (pp. 181-201). Academic Press.

Baehr, E., Rosenfeld, J. P., & Baehr, R. (2001). Clinical use of an alpha asymmetry neurofeedback protocol in the treatment of mood disorders. *Journal of Neurotherapy, 4*(4), 11-18. https://doi.org/10.1300/J184v04n04_03

Bandura, A. (1977). Self-efficacy: Toward a unifying theory of behavioral change. *Psychological Review, 84*(2), 191-215. https://doi.org/10.1037/0033-295X.84.2.191

Barlow, D. H. (2002). *Anxiety and its disorders* (2nd ed.). New York, NY: Guilford Press.

Basar, E., Schürmann, M., Basar-Eroglu, C., & Karakas, S. (1997). Alpha oscillations in brain functioning: An integrative theory. *International Journal of Psychophysiology, 26*(1-3), 5-29. https://doi.org/10.1016/s0167-8760(97)00753-8

Basmajian, J. V. (1963). Control and training of individual motor units. *Science, 141*(3579), 440-441. https://doi.org/10.1126/science.141.3579.440

Basmajian, J. (1989). *Biofeedback: Principles and practice for clinicians*. Philadelphia, PA: Williams & Wilkens.

Beck, A., Emery, G., & Greenberg, R. (1985). *Anxiety disorders and phobias. A cognitive perspective*. New York, NY: Basic Books.

Berger, H. (1929). Ueber das Elektroenkephalogramm des Menschen. *Archiv für Psychiatrie und Nervenkrankheiten, 87*, 527-570.

Beidel, D. C., Bulik, C. M., & Stanley, M. A. (2014). *Abnormal psychology* (3rd ed.). New York, NY: Pearson.

Bester, H. (2014). *New hope for AD/HD in children and adults: A practical guide*. Cape Town, South Africa.

Bigler, E. D., Mortensen, S., Neeley, E. S., Ozonoff, S., Krasny, L., Johnson, M., ... Lainhart, J. E. (2007). Superior temporal gyrus, language function, and autism. *Developmental Neuropsychology, 31*(2), 217-238. https://doi.org/ 10.1080/87565640701190841

Birbaumer, N., Elbert, T., Canavan, A., & Rockstroh, B. (1990). Slow potentials of the cerebral cortex and behavior. *Physiological Reviews, 70*, 1-41.

Birbaumer, N. (1999). Slow cortical potentials: Plasticity, operant control, and behavioral effects. *The Neuroscientist, 5*, 74-78.

Bird, B. L., Newton, F. A., Sheer, D. E., & Ford, M. (1978a). Behavioral and electroencephalographic correlates of 40-Hz EEG biofeedback training in humans. *Biofeedback and Self-Regulation, 3*(1), 13-28. http://dx.doi.org/10.1007/bf00998560

Bird, B. L., Newton, F. A., Sheer, D. E., & Ford, M. (1978b). Biofeedback training of 40-Hz EEG in humans. *Biofeedback and Self-Regulation, 3*(1), 1-11. http://dx.doi.org/10.1007/bf00998559

Blanco, C., Okuda, M., Wright, C., Hasin, D.S., Grant, B. F., Liu, S. M., & Olfson, M. (2008). Mental health of college students and their non-college-attending peers: Results from the National Epidemiologic Study on Alcohol and Related Conditions. *Archives of General Psychiatry, 65*(12), 1429-1437. https://doi.org/10.1001/ archpsyc.65.12.1429

Bourne, E. J. (2000). *The anxiety and phobia workbook* (3rd ed.). Oakland, CA: New Harbinger Publications.

Brandmeyer, T., & Delorme, A. (2013). Meditation and neurofeedback. *Frontiers in Psychology, 4*, 688. https://doi.org/10.3389/ fpsyg.2013.00688

Brooks, M. (2012, February 16). *Lancet weighs in on DSM-5 bereavement exclusion.* https://www.medscape.com/viewarticle/758788

Brown, B. (1977). *Stress and the art of biofeedback* (1st ed.). Harper & Row. https://www.amazon.com/Stress-Art-Biofeedback-Barbara-Brown/dp/0060105445

Broyd, S. J., Helps, S. K., & Sonuga-Barke, E. J. S. (2011). Attention-induced deactivations in very low frequency EEG oscillations: Differential localisation according to ADHD symptom status. *PloS One, 6*(3), e17325. https://doi.org/10.1371/journal.pone.0017325

Buckner, R. L., Andrews-Hanna, J. R., & Schacter, D. L. (2008). The brain's default network: Anatomy, function, and relevance to disease. *Annals of the New York Academy of Sciences, 1124*, 1-38. https://doi.org/10.1196/annals.1440.011

Cavanna, A., & Trimble, M. R. (2006). The precuneus: A review of its functional anatomy and behavioural correlates. *Brain, 129*(3), 564-583. https://doi.org/10.1093/brain/awl004

Chabot, R. J.,& Serfontein, G. (1996). Quantitative electroencephalographic profiles of children with attention deficit disorder. *Biological Psychiatry, 40*(10), 951-963. https://doi.org/10.1016/0006-3223(95)00576-5

Chabot, R. J., di Michele, F., & Prichep, L. (2005). The role of quantitative electroencephalography in child and adolescent psychiatric disorders. *Child and Adolescent Psychiatric Clinics of North America, 14*(1), 21-53. https://doi.org/10.1016/j.chc.2004.07.005

Chakravarthy, V., Joseph, D., & Bapi, R. S. (2010). What do the basal ganglia do? *Biological Cybernetics, 103*(3), 237-253. https://doi.org/10.1007/s00422-010-0401-y

Chopra, D. (1994). *The seven spiritual laws of success: A practical guide to the fulfillment of your dreams.* Amber-Allen Publishing and New World Library.

Coben, R., Mohammad-Rezazadeh, I., & Cannon, R. L. (2014). Using quantitative and analytic EEG methods in the understanding of connectivity in autism spectrum disorders: A theory of mixed over- and under-connectivity. *Frontiers in Human Neuroscience, 8*, 45. http://dx.doi.org/10.3389/fnhum.2014.00045

Collura, T. F. (2014). *Technical foundations of neurofeedback.* New York and London: Routledge.

Collura, T. F., & Thatcher, R. (2006, April 29). *Real-time EEG Z-score training – Realities and prospects.* https://brainmaster.com/wp-content/themes/brainmasters/kb_file/ZScore_White_Paper.pdf

Collura, T. F. (2008). Whole head normalization using live Z-score for connectivity training. *NeuroConnections, April*, 12-18.

Collura, T. F., & Frederick, J. A. (Eds.). (2017). *Handbook of clinical QEEG and neurotherapy.*New York and London: Routledge.

Conn, P. M. (Ed.). (2003). *Neuroscience in medicine* (2nd ed.). Totowa, NJ: Humana Press.

Crane, A., & Soutar, R. (2000). *MindFitness training: Neurofeedback and the process.* Lincoln, NE: iUniverse.

Craigmyle, N. A. (2013). The beneficial effects of meditation: Contribution of the anterior cingulate and locus coeruleus. *Frontiers in Psychology, 4*, 731. https://doi.org/10.3389/fpsyg.2013.00731

Crottaz-Herbette, S., & Menon V. (2006). Where and when the anterior cingulate cortex modulates attentional response: Combined fMRI and ERP evidence. *Journal of Cognitive Neuroscience, 18*(5), 766-780. https://doi.org/10.1162/jocn.2006.18.5.766

Davidson, R. J. (1994). Asymmetric brain function, affective style, and psychopathology: The role of early experience and plasticity. *Development and Psychopathology, 6*(04), 741-758. https://doi.org/10.1017/S0954579400004764

Davidson, R. J. (1995). Cerebral asymmetry, emotion, and affective style. In R. J. Davidson & K. Hugdahl (Eds.), *Brain asymmetry* (pp. 361-387). The MIT Press.

Dawson, G., Klinger, L., Panagiotides, H., Hill, D., & Spieker, S. (1992). Frontal lobe activity and affective behavior of infants of mothers with depressive symptoms. *Child Development, 63*(3), 725-737.

Demos, J. N. (2005). *Getting started with neurofeedback.* New York and London: W. W. Norton & Company.

Demos, J. N. (2019). *Getting started with neurofeedback* (2nd ed.). New York and London: W. W. Norton & Company.

Denkowski, K. M., & Denkowski, G. C. (1984). Is group progressive relaxation training as effective with hyperactive children as individual EMG biofeedback treatment. *Biofeedback and Self-Regulation, 9*(3), 353-364. https://doi.org/10.1007/bf00998978

Di Michele, F., Prichep, L., John, E. R., & Chabot, R. J. (2005). The neurophysiology of attention-deficit/hyperactivity disorder. *International Journal of Psychophysiology, 58*(1), 81-93. https://doi.org/10.1016/j.ijpsycho.2005.03.011

Diamond, D. M., Campbell, A. M., Park, C. R., Halonen, J., & Zoladz, P. R. (2007). The temporal dynamics model of emotional memory processing: A synthesis on the neurobiological basis of stress-induced amnesia, flashbulb and traumatic memories, and the Yerkes-Dodson law. *Neural Plasticity, 2007*, 60803. https://doi.org/10.1155/2007/60803

Dingledine, R., Borges, K., Bowie, D, & Traynelis, S. F. (1999). The glutamate receptor ion channels. *Pharmacological reviews, 51*(1), 7-61.

Donaldson, S., Donaldson, M., & Moran, D. (2017). Investigating the neuroplasticity of chronic pain utilizing biofeedback procedures. In T. F. Collura & J. A. Frederick (Eds.), *Handbook of clinical QEEG and neurotherapy* (pp. 82-91). New York and London: Routledge.

Dunn, B. R., Hartigan, J. A., & Mikulas, W. L. (1999). Concentration and mindfulness meditations: Unique forms of consciousness? *Applied Psychophysiology and Biofeedback, 24*(3), 147-165. https://doi.org/10.1023/a:1023498629385

Egner, T., & Sterman, M. B. (2006). Neurofeedback treatment of epilepsy: From basic rationale to practical application. *Expert Review of Neurotherapeutics, 6*(2), 247-257. https://doi.org/10.1586/14737175.6.2.247

Ellis, R. (1997). *Second language acquisition.* Oxford: Oxford University Press.

Evans, J., & Abarbanel, A. (1999). *Introduction to quantitative EEG and neurofeedback* (1st ed.). New York: Academic Press.

Faraone, S., & Buitelaar, J. (2009). Comparing the efficacy of stimulants for ADHD in children and adolescents using meta-analysis. *European Child and Adolescent Psychiatry, 19*(4), 353-364. https://doi.org/10.1007/s00787-009-0054-3

Fehmi, L. G. (2008). Multichannel EEG phase synchrony training and verbally guided attention training for disorders of attention. In J. R. Evans (Ed.), *Handbook of neurofeedback* (Haworth Series in Neurotherapy) (pp. 301-311). New York: The Haworth Medical Press/Routledge

Fehmi, L., & Robbins, J. (2008). *The open-focus brain: Harnessing the power of attention to heal mind and body.* Boston & London: Trumpeter.

Fehmi, L., & Robbins, J. (2010). *Dissolving pain: Simple brain-training exercises for overcoming chronic pain.* Boston, MA: Trumpeter.

Ferster, C. B., & Skinner, B. F. (1957). *Schedules of reinforcement.* New York, NY: Appleton-Century-Crofts. http://dx.doi.org/10.1037/10627-000

Field, T. (1995). Infants of depressed mothers. *Infant Behavior and Development, 18*(1), 1-13. https://doi.org/10.1016/0163-6383(95)90003-9

Fisch, B. (1999). *Fisch and Spehlmann's EEG primer: Basic principles of digital and analog EEG* (3rd ed). Elsevier.

Fisher, S. F. (2014). *Neurofeedback in the treatment of developmental trauma: Calming the fear-driven brain.* New York, NY: W.W. Norton & Company.

Fischer, M. H., & Lowenbach, H. (1934). Aktionsstrome des Zentralnervensystems unter der Einwirkung von Krampfgiften. I Mitteilung. Strychnin und Pikrotoxin. *Archiv für Experimentelle Pathologie und Pharmakologie, 174*, 357-382.

Frances, A. J. (2012, February 18). *DSM 5 to the barricades on grief.* Psychology Today. https://www.psychologytoday.com/us/blog/dsm5-in-distress/201202/dsm-5-the-barricades-grief

Fusiform gyrus. (n. d.). In Wikipedia. https://en.wikipedia.org/wiki/Fusiform_gyrus

Gazzaniga, M. S. (2009). *The cognitive neurosciences* (4th ed.). Cambridge: MIT Press.

Gervirtz, R. (2013). The promise of heart rate variability biofeedback: Evidence-based applications. *Biofeedback, 41*(3), 110-120. https://doi.org/10.5298/1081-5937-41.3.01

Geschwind, D. H. (2011). Genetics of autism spectrum disorders. *Trends in Cognitive Sciences, 15*(9), 409-416. https://doi.org/10.1016/j.tics.2011.07.003

Getter, N., Kaplan, Z., & Todder, D. (2017). sLORETA neurofeedback as a treatment for PTSD. In T. F. Collura & J. A. Frederick (Eds.), *Handbook of clinical QEEG and neurotherapy* (pp. 300-311). New York and London: Routledge.

Gevensleben, H., Holl, B., Albrecht, B., Schlamp, D., Kratz, O., Studer, P., ... Heinrich, H. (2010). Neurofeedback training in children with ADHD: 6-month follow-up of a randomized controlled trial. *Journal of Child Psychology and Psychiatry, 19*(9), 715-724. https://doi.org/10.1007/s00787-010-0109-5

Gibbs, F. A., Davis, H., & Lennox, W. G. (1935). The electro-encephalogram in epilepsy and in conditions of impaired consciousness. *Archives of Neurology and Psychiatry, 34*(6), 1133-1148. http://dx.doi.org/10.1001/archneurpsyc.1935.02250240002001

Ginsberg, J. (2018, May). *2018-05 webinar recording: Applied HRV data interpretation for the clinician.* https://certify.bcia.org/store/2018-05-webinar-recording/21104/

Gotlib, I. H., Ranganath, C., & Rosenfeld, J. P. (1998). Frontal EEG alpha asymmetry, depression, and cognitive functioning. *Cognition and Emotion, 12*(3), 449-478. https://doi.org/10.1080/026999398379673

Gracefire, P. (2017). Introduction to the concepts and clinical applications of multivariate live Z-score training, PZOK and sLORETA feedback. In T. F. Collura & J. A. Frederick (Eds.), *Handbook of clinical QEEG and neurotherapy* (pp. 326-383). New York and London: Routledge.

Green, E. (1993). Alpha theta brainwave training: Instrumental Vipassana? *Subtle Energies and Energy Medicine, 10*(1), 221-230.

Gruzelier, J. H., & Egner, T. (2004). Physiological self-regulation:

Biofeedback and neurofeedback. In A. Williamon (Ed.), *Musical excellence: Strategies and techniques to enhance performance* (pp. 197-219). Oxford: Oxford University Press.

Guan, J. (2017). The efficacy of Z-score neurofeedback training. In T. F. Collura & J. A. Frederick (Eds.), *Handbook of clinical QEEG and neurotherapy* (pp. 312-325). New York and London: Routledge.

Haldane, M., Cunningham, G., Androutsos, C., & Frangou, S. (2008). Structural brain correlates of response inhibition in bipolar disorder. *Journal of Psychopharmacology, 22*(2), 138-143. https://doi.org/10.1177/0269881107082955

Hammond, D. C. (2000). Neurofeedback treatment of depression with the Roshi. *Journal of Neurotherapy, 4*(2), 45-56. https://doi.org/10.1300/J184v04n02_06

Hammond, D. C. (2005). Neurofeedback treatment of depression and anxiety. *Journal of Adult Development 12*(2), 131-137. https://doi.org/10.1007/s10804-005-7029-5

Hardt, J. V. (1993, March 25). *Alpha EEG feedback: Closer parallel with zen than yoga.* Applied Psychophysiology and Biofeedback 24th Annual Meeting, Los Angeles, CA.

Haxby, J. V., Hoffman, E. A., & Gobbini, M. I. (2000). The distributed human neural system for face perception. *Trends in Cognitive Sciences, 4*(6), 223-233. https://doi.org/10.1016/s1364-6613(00)01482-0

Henriques, J. B., & Davidson, R. J. (1991). Left frontal hypoactivation in depression. *Journal of Abnormal Psychology, 100*(4), 535-545. https://doi.org/10.1037//0021-843x.100.4.535

Hodgson, K., Hutchinson, A. D., & Denson, L. (2014). Nonpharmacological treatments for ADHD: A meta-analytic review. *Journal of Attention Disorders, 18*(4), 275-282 (Epub 2012). https://doi.org/10.1177/1087054712444732

Horvat, J. J. (2009). Coherence and the quirks of coherence/phase training: A clinical perspective. In J. R. Evans (Ed.), *Handbook of Neurofeedback* (Haworth Series in Neurotherapy) (pp. 213-230). New York: The Haworth Medical Press.

Horwitz, A. V. (2010). How an age of anxiety became an age of depression. *The Milbank Quarterly, 88*(1), 112-138. https://doi.org/10.1111/j.1468-0009.2010.00591.x

Horwitz, A. V. (2014). *DSM - I and DSM - II.* In The Encyclopedia of Clinical Psychology. https://doi.org/10.1002/9781118625392

Horwitz, A. V., & Wakefield, J. C. (2007). *The loss of sadness: How psychiatry transformed normal sorrow into depressive disorder.* New York: Oxford University Press.

Horwitz, A. V., Wakefield, J. C., & Lorenzo-Luaces, L. (2017). History of depression. In R. J. DeRubeis & D. R. Strunk (Eds.), *The Oxford handbook of mood disorders* (Oxford Library of Psychology) (pp. 11-23). Oxford University Press.

Hölzel, B. K., Carmody, J., Vangel, M., Congleton, C., Yerramsetti, S. M., Gard, T., & Lazar, S. W. (2011). Mindfulness practice leads to increases in regional brain gray matter density. *Psychiatry Research, 191*(1), 36-43. https://doi.org/10.1016/j.pscychresns.2010.08.006

Hughes, J. R., & John, E. R. (1999). Conventional and quantitative electroencephalography in psychaitry. *Journal of Neuropsychiatry and Clinical Neurosciences, 11*(2), 190-208. https://doi.org/10.1176/jnp.11.2.190

IMAIOS (n. d.). *Anatomy, medical imaging and e-learning for healtcare professionals.* https://www.imaios.com/en

Inanaga, K. (1998). Frontal midline theta rhythm and mental activity. *Psychiatry and Clinical Neurosciences, 52*(6), 555-566. https://doi.org/10.1046/j.1440-1819.1998.00452.x

Insula (n. d.). *Neuroscientifically challenged.* https://www.neuroscientificallychallenged.com/blog/2013/05/what-is-insula

Isaacs, J. (n. d.). *Neurofeedback, QEEG brain mapping, EFT.* http://julianisaacs.com

Jacobson, E. (1938). *Progressive relaxation.* Chicago: University of Chicago Press.

Jacofsky, M. D., Santos, M. T., Khemklani-Patel, S., & Neziroglu, F.

(2013, August 9). *Normal and abnormal anxiety: What's the difference.* https://www.mentalhelp.net/contributors/biobehavioral/

Jones, R., & Bhattacharya, J. (2014). A role for the precuneus in thought-action fusion: Evidence from participants with significant obsessive-compulsive symptoms. *NeuroImage. Clinical, 4,* 112-121. https://doi.org/10.1016/j.nicl.2013.11.008

Joo, M. S., Park, D. S., Moon, C. T., Chun, Y., Song, S. W., & Roh, H. G. (2016). Relationship between gyrus rectus resection and cognitive impairment after surgery for ruptured anterior communicating artery aneurysms. *Journal of Cerebrovascular and Endovascular Neurosurgery, 18*(3), 223-228. https://doi.org/10.7461/jcen.2016.18.3.223

Kaas, J. H. (1993). The functional organization of somatosensory cortex in primates. *Annals of Anatomy, 175*(6), 509-518. http://dx.doi.org/10.1016/s0940-9602(11)80212-8

Kabat-Zinn, J., & Chapman-Waldrop, A. (1988). Compliance with an outpatient stress reduction program: Rates and predictors of program completion. *Journal of Behavioral Medicine, 11*(4), 333-352. https://doi.org/10.1007/bf00844934

Kamiya, J. (1962). *Conditioned discrimination of the EEG alpha rhythm in humans.* Proceedings of the Western Psychological Association. San Francisco, California.

Kamiya, J. (1969). Operant control of the EEG alpha rhythm. In C. Tart (Ed.), *Altered states of consciousness.* NY: Wiley.

Kerasidis, H. (2017). Concussionology: Sport concussion management. In T. F. Collura & J. A. Frederick (Eds.), *Handbook of clinical QEEG and neurotherapy* (pp. 184-209). New York and London: Routledge.

Kerson, C. (2017). Neurofeedback as a treatment for anxiety in adolescents and young adults. In T. F. Collura & J. A. Frederick (Eds.), *Handbook of clinical EEG and neurotherapy* (pp. 455-463). New York and London: Routledge.

Kessler, R. C., Chiu, W. T., Demler, O., & Walters, E. E. (2005). Prevalence, severity, and comorbidity of twelve-month DSM-IV disorders in the national comorbidity survey replication (NCS-R). *Archives of General Psychiatry, 62*(6), 617-627. https://doi. org/10.1001/archpsyc.62.6.617

Kirk, I. J., & Mackay, J. C. (2003). The role of theta-range oscillations in synchronising and integrating activity in distributed mnemonic networks. *Cortex, 39*(4-5), 993-1008. https://doi.org/10.1016/ s0010-9452(08)70874-8

Kleitman, N. (1987). *Sleep and wakefulness* (Midway Reprint). Chicago IL: University of Chicago Press.

Koenigs, M., Barbey, A. K., Postle, B. R., & Grafman, J. (2009). Superior parietal cortex is critical for the manipulation of information in working memory. *The Journal of Neuroscience, 29*(47), 14980- 14986. http://dx.doi.org/10.1523/JNEUROSCI.3706-09.2009

Kwon, J. S., Youn, T., & Jung, H. Y. (1996). Right hemisphere abnormalities in major depression: Quantitative electroencephalographic findings before and after treatment. *Journal of Affective Disorders, 40*(3), 169-173. https://doi.org/10.1016/0165- 0327(96)00057-2

Laird, A. R., Eickhoff, S. B., Fox, P. M., Uecker, A. M., Ray, K. L., Saenz J. J., ... Fox, P. T. (2011). The Brain Map strategy for standardization, sharing, and meta-analysis of neuroimaging data. *BMC Research Notes, 4*, 349. https://doi.org/10.1186/1756-0500- 4-349

Laird, A. R., Eickhoff, S. B., Rottschy, C., Bzdok, D., Ray, K. L., & Fox, P. T. (2013). Networks of task co-activations. *Neuroimage, 80*, 505-514. https://doi.org/10.1016/j.neuroimage.2013.04.073

Lateral inhibition. (n. d.). In Wikipedia. https://en.wikipedia.org/wiki/ Lateral_inhibition

Lazarus, R. S., & Folkman, S. (1984). *Stress, appraisal and coping.* New York, NY: Springer Publishing Company.

Ledoux, J. E. (1998). Cognitive-emotional interactions in the brain. *Cognition and Emotion, 3*(4), 267-289. https://doi. org/10.1080/02699938908412709

Legg, T. J. (n. d.). *Articles.* Muck Rack. https://muckrack.com/timothy-j-legg/articles

Lehmann, D., Faber, P. L., Achermann, P., Jeanmonod, D., Gianotti, L. R., & Pizzagalli, D. (2001). Brain sources of EEG gamma frequency during volitionally meditation-induced, altered states of consciousness, and experience of the self. *Psychiatry Research, 108*(2), 111-121. https://doi.org/10.1016/s0925-4927(01)00116-0

Lehrer, P., & Eddie, D. (2013). Dynamic processes in regulation and some implications for biofeedback. *Applied Psychophysiology and Biofeedback, 38*(2), 143-155. https://doi.org/10.1007/s10484-013-9217-6

Li, W., Qin, W., Liu, H., Fan, L., Wang, J., Jiang, T., & Yu, C. (2013). Subregions of the human superior frontal gyrus and their connections. *NeuroImage, 78*, 46-58. http://dx.doi.org/10.1016/j.neuroimage.2013.04.011

Lingual gyrus. (n. d.). In Wikepedia. https://en.wikipedia.org/wiki/Lingual_gyrus

Litchfield, P. (n. d.). *Webinar lectures*. Better Physiology, Ltd. https://betterphysiology.com/webinar-lectures/

Loukas, M., Pennell, C., Groat, C., Tubbs, R. S., & Cohen-Gadol, A. A. (2011). Korbinian Brodmann (1868-1918) and his contributions to mapping the cerebral cortex. *Neurosurgery, 68*(1), 6-11. https://doi.org/10.1227/NEU.0b013e3181fc5cac

Lubar, J. F. (1991). Discourse on the development of EEG diagnostics and biofeedback treatment for attention deficit/hyperactivity disorders. *Biofeedback and Self-Regulation, 16*(3), 201-225. http://dx.doi.org/10.1007/bf01000016

Lubar, J. O., & Lubar, J. F. (1984). Electroencephalographic biofeedback of SMR and beta for treatment of attention deficit disorders in a clinical setting. *Biofeedback and Self-Regulation, 9*(1), 1-23. http://dx.doi.org/10.1007/bf00998842

Lubar, J. F., & Shouse, M. N. (1976). EEG and behavioral changes in a hyperkinetic child concurrent with training of the sensorimotor rhythm (SMR): A preliminary report. *Biofeedback and Self-Regulation, 1*(3), 293-306. https://doi.org/10.1007/bf01001170

Lubar, J. F., Swartwood, M. O., Swartwood, J. N., & O'Donnell, P. H. (1995a). Evaluation of the effectiveness of EEG neurofeedback training for ADHD in a clinical setting as measured by changes in T.O.V.A. scores, behavioral ratings, and WISC-R performance. *Biofeedback and Self-Regulation,* *20*(1), 83-99. https://doi. org/10.1007/bf01712768

Lubar, J. F., Swartwood, M. O., Swartwood, J. N., & Timmermann, D. L. (1995b). Quantitative EEG and auditory event-related potentials in the evaluation of attention-deficit disorder: Effects of methylphenidate and implications for neurofeedback training. *Journal of Psychoeducational Assessment Monographs*, (Special ADHD Issue), 143-160.

Mikosch, P., Hadrawa, T., Laubreiter, K., Brandl,J., Pilz, J., Stettner, H., & Grimm, G. (2010). Effectiveness of respiratory-sinus-arrhythmia biofeedback on state-anxiety in patients undergoing coronary angiography. *Journal of Advanced Nursing, 66*(5), 1101-1110. https://doi.org/10.1111/j.1365-2648.2010.05277.x

Miller, N. E. (1969). Learning of visceral and glandular responses. *Science, 163*(3866), 434-445. http://dx.doi.org/10.1126/science.163.3866.434

Monto, S., Palva, S., Voipio, J., & Palva, J. M. (2008). Very slow EEG fluctuations predict the dynamics of stimulus detection and oscillation amplitudes in humans. *Journal of Neuroscience, 28*(33) 8268-8272. https://doi.org/10.1523/JNEUROSCI.1910-08.2008

Moss, D., & Shaffer, F. (2016). *Foundations of heart rate variability biofeedback: A book of readings.* Wheat Ridge, CO: Association for Applied Psychophysiology and Biofeedback.

Nakagawa, T. T., Jirsa, V. K., Spiegler, A., McIntosh, A. R., & Deco, G. (2013). Bottom up modeling of the connectome: Linking structure and function in the resting brain and their changes in aging. *NeuroImage, 80*, 318-329. https://doi.org/10.1016/j.neuroimage.2013.04.055

Nakasone, A., Prendinger, H., & Ishizuka, M. (2013). *Emotion recognition from electromyography and skin conductance.* Fifth International Workshop on Biosignal Interpretation (BSI-05), Tokyo, Japan.

Niedermeyer, E., & Da Silva, F. (1999). *Electroencephalography: Basic principles, clinical applications and related fields* (4th ed.). Philadelphia, PA: Williams & Wilkins.

Niedermeyer, E., & Da Silva, F. H. (Eds). (2005). *Electroencephalography: Basic principles, clinical applications and related fields* (5th ed.). Philadelphia, PA: Lippincott Williams & Wilkins.

Nolan, R. P., Floras, J. S., Ahmed, L., Harvey, P. J., Hiscock, N., Hendrickx, H., & Talbot, D. (2012). Behavioural modification of the cholinergic anti-inflammatory response to C-reactive protein in patients with hypertension. *Journal of Internal Medicine, 272*(2), 161-169. https://doi.org/10.1111/j.1365-2796.2012.02523.x

Nolte, J. (2008). *The human brain: An introduction to its functional anatomy* (6th ed.). Philadelphia, PA: Mosby.

Olshansky, S. J., & Carnes, B. A. (2008). The future of human longevity. In P. Uhlenberg (Ed.), *International handbook of population aging* (pp. 731-745). New York, NY: Springer.

Othmer, S., & Othmer, S. F. (2017). *Development history of the Othmer method: 1987 to 2016.* http://www.eeginfo.com/research/research-papers/Research-w-Othmer-Method-2017.pdf

Othmer, S., Othmer, S. F., & Kaiser, D. A. (1999). EEG biofeedback: Training for AD/HD and related disruptive behavior disorders. In J. A. Incorvaia, B. F. Mark-Goldstein, & D. Tessmer (Eds.), *Understanding, diagnosing, and treating AD/HD in children and adolescents: An integrative approach* (Vol. 3) (pp. 235-296). New York: Jason Aronson Inc.

Pacak, K., Palkovits, M., Kopin, I. J., & Goldstein, D. S. (1995). Stress-induced norepinephrine release in the hypothalamic paraventricular nucleus and pituitary-adrenocortical and sympathoadrenal activity: In vivo microdialysis studies. *Frontiers in Neuroendocrinology, 16*(2), 89-150. https://doi.org/10.1006/frne.1995.1004

Pascual-Leone, A., Freitas, C., Oberman, L., Horvath, J. C., Halko, M., Eldaief, M., … Rotenberg, A. (2011). Characterizing brain cortical plasticity and network dynamics across the age-span in health and disease with TMS-EEG and TMS-fMRI. *Brain Topography,*

24(3-4), 302-315. https://doi.org/10.1007/s10548-011-0196-8

PascualMarqui, R. D., Michel, C. M., & Lehmann, D. (1994). Low resolution electromagnetic tomography: A new method for localizing electrical activity in the brain. *International Journal of Psychophysiology, 18*(1), 4965. https://doi.org/10.1016/0167-8760(84)90014-x

Peniston, E. G., & Kulkosky, P. J. (1989). Alpha-theta brainwave training and beta endorphin levels in alcoholics. *Alcoholism: Clinical and Experimental Results, 13*(2), 271-279. http://dx.doi.org/10.1111/j.1530-0277.1989.tb00325.x

Peniston, E. G., & Kulkosky, P. J. (1990). Alcoholic personality and alpha-theta brainwave training. *Medical Psychotherapy: An International Journal, 3*, 37-55.

Peniston, E. G., & Kulkosky, P. J. (1991). Alpha-theta brainwave neurofeedback therapy for Vietnam veterans with combat-related posttraumatic stress disorder. *Medical Psychotherapy: An International Journal, 4*, 47-60.

Peeters, F., Oehlen, M., Ronner, J., van Os, J., & Lousberg, R. (2014). Neurofeedback as a treatment for major depressive disorder – A pilot study. *PloS One, 9*(3), e91837. https://doi.org/10.1371/journal.pone.0091837

Petersen, S. E., & Posner, M. I. (2012). The attention system of the human brain: 20 years after. *Annual Review of Neuroscience, 35*, 73-89. https://doi.org/10.1146/annurev-neuro-062111-150525

Pigott, H. E., De Biase, L., Bodenhamer-Davis, E., & Davis, R. E. (2013, April 17). *The evidence-base for neurofeedback as a reimbursable healthcare service to treat attention deficit/hyperactivity disorder.* White Paper, International Society of Neurofeedback and Research. https://isnr.org/wp-content/uploads/2019/07/NFB-as-an-Evidence-Based-Treatment-for-ADHD.pdf

Porges, S. W. (1995). Cardiac vagal tone: A physiological index of stress. *Neuroscience and Biobehavioral Reviews, 19*(2), 225-233. https://doi.org/10.1016/0149-7634(94)00066-a

Porges, S. W. (2007). The polyvagal perspective. *Biological Psychology,*

74(2), 116-143. https://doi.org/10.1016/j.biopsycho.2006.06.009

PracticeWise (n. d.). *What works in children's mental health.* https://www.practicewise.com/

Prinsloo, G. E., Rauch, H. G. L., Lambert, M. I., Muench, F., Noakes, T. D., & Derman, W. E. (2011). The effect of short duration heart rate variability (HRV) biofeedback on cognitive performance during laboratory induced cognitive stress. *Applied Cognitive Psychology, 25*(5), 792-801. https://doi.org/10.1002/acp.1750

Reuter, P. (2005). *Der Große Reuter. Springer Universalwörterbuch Medizin, Pharmakologie und Zahnmedizin.* Berlin: Springer.

Ricard, M., Lutz, A., & Davidson, R. J. (2014). Mind of the meditator. *Scientific American, 311*(5), 38-45. https://doi.org/10.1038/scientificamerican1114-38

Rice, K., Blanchard, E., & Purcell, M. (1993). Biofeedback treatments of generalized anxiety disorder: Preliminary results. *Biofeedback & Self-Regulation, 18*(2), 93-105. https://doi.org/10.1007/BF01848110

Rojas, A., & Dingledine, R. (2013). Ionotropic glutamate receptors: Regulation by G-protein-coupled receptors. *Molecular Pharmacology, 83*(4), 746-752. https://doi.org/10.1124/mol.112.083352

Rosenfeld, J. P. (1977). Conditioning changes in the evoked response. In G. E. Schwartz & J. Beatty (Eds.), *Biofeedback: Theory and research* (pp. 377-388). New York: Academic Press.

Rosenfeld, J. P. (1997). EEG biofeedback of frontal alpha asymmetry in affective disorders. *Biofeedback, 25*(1), 8-25.

Rosenfeld, J. P. (2000). An EEG biofeedback protocol for affective disorders. *Clinical EEG and Neuroscience, 31*(1), 7-12. http://dx.doi.org/10.1177/155005940003100106

Rosenfeld, J. P., Baehr, E., Baehr, R., Gotlib, I. H., & Ranganath, C. (1996). Preliminary evidence that daily changes in frontal alpha asymmetry correlate with changes in affect in therapy sessions. *International Journal of Psychophysiology, 23*(1-2), 137-141. http://dx.doi.org/10.1016/0167-8760(96)00037-2

Schmidt, S., Schneider, R., Utts, J., & Walach, H. (2004). Distant intentionality and the feeling of being stared at: Two meta-analyses. *British Journal of Psychology, 95*(2), 235-247.

Seifert, F., & Maihöfner, C. (2011). Functional and structural imaging of pain-induced neuroplasticity. *Current Opinion in Anaesthesiology, 24*(5), 515-523. https://doi.org/10.1097/ACO.0b013e32834a1079

Sherlin, L., Arns, M., Lubar, J., & Sokhadze, E. (2010). A position paper on neurofeedback for the treatment of ADHD. *Journal of Neurotherapy, 14*(2), 66-78. https://doi.org/10.1080/10874201003773880

Skinner, B. F. (1938). *The behaviour of organisms: An experimental analysis* (Century Psychology Series). New York: Appleton-Century-Crofts, Inc.

Skinner, B. F. (1958). Reinforcement today. *American Psychologist, 13*, 94.

Smith, M. L. (n. d.). *Infra-low frequency: A proposed mechanism.* Brain Enhancement Centre. https://www.bec-eeg.com/resources/infra-low-frequency-a-proposed-mechanism/

Smith, M. L., Leiderman, L. M., & de Vries, J. (2017). Infra-slow fluctuation (ISF) training for autism spectrum disorders. In T. F. Collura & J. A. Frederick (Eds.), *Handbook of clinical QEEG and neurotherapy* (pp. 488-499). New York and London: Routledge.

Smith, M. (2018, March 2). *Infra-slow fluctuation (ISF) training workshop, Orlando, Fl.* http://stresstherapysolutions.com/2018/01/infra-slow-fluctuation-isf-training-workshop/

Sonuga-Barke, E. J., Brandeis, D., Cortese, S., Daley, D., Ferrin, M., Holtmann, M., Stevenson, J., Danckaerts, M., van der Oord, S., Döpfner, M., Dittmann, R. W., Simonoff, E., Zuddas, A., Banaschewski, T., Buitelaar, J., Coghill, D., Hollis, C., Konofal, E., Lecendreux, M., … Sergeant, J.; European ADHD Guidelines Group. (2013). Nonpharmacological interventions for ADHD: Systematic review and meta-analyses of randomized controlled trials of dietary and psychological treatments. *American Journal of Psychiatry, 170*(3), 275-289. https://doi.org/10.1176/appi.ajp.2012.12070991

Soutar, R. (2017). Perspective and method for a QEEG based two channel bi-hemispheric compensatory model of neurofeedback training. In T. F. Collura & J. A. Frederick (Eds.), *Handbook of clinical QEEG and neurotherapy* (pp. 387-403). New York and London: Routledge.

SparkNotes (n. d.). *Neurons, hormones and the brain.* https://www.sparknotes.com/psychology/psych101/thebrain/

Sterman, M. B. (1996). Physiological origins and functional correlates of EEG rhythmic activities: Implications for self-regulation. *Biofeedback & Self-Regulation, 21*(1), 3-33. https://doi.org/10.1007/BF02214147

Sterman, M. B. (2000). Basic concepts and clinical findings in the treatment of seizure disorders with EEG operant conditioning. *Clinical Electroencephalography, 31*(1), 45-55.

Sterman, M. B., & Wyrwicka, W. (1967). EEG correlates of sleep: Evidence for separate forebrain substrates. *Brain Research, 6*(1), 143-163. http://dx.doi.org/10.1016/0006-8993(67)90186-2

Sterman, M. B., & Egner, T. (2006). Foundation and practice of neurofeedback for the treatment of epilepsy. *Applied Psychophysiology and Biofeedback, 31*(1), 21-35. http://dx.doi.org/10.1007/s10484-006-9002-x

Sterman, M. B., Wyrwicka, W., & Roth, S. R. (1969a). Electrophysiological correlates and neural substrates of alimentary behavior in the cat. *Annals of the New York Academy of Sciences, 157*(2), 723-739. http://dx.doi.org/10.1111/j.1749-6632.1969.tb12916.x

Sterman, M. B., Wyrwicka, W., & Howe, R. (1969b). Behavioral and neurophysiological studies of the sensorimotor rhythm in the cat. *Electroencephalography and Clinical Neurophysiology, 27*(7), 678-679. https://doi.org/10.1016/0013-4694(69)91281-4.

Sterman, M. B., Howe, R. C., & Macdonald, L. R. (1970). Facilitation of spindle-burst sleep by conditioning of electroencephalographic activity while awake. *Science, 167*(3921), 1146-1148. http://dx.doi.org/10.1126/science.167.3921.1146

Stoyva, J. (1986). Wolfgang Luthe: In memoriam. *Biofeedback and*

Self-Regulation, 11, 91-93. https://doi.org/10.1007/BF00999976

Subcallosal gyrus - An overview. (n. d.). *ScienceDirect Topics.* https://www.sciencedirect.com/topics/medicine-and-dentistry/subcallosal-gyrus

Sutton, S., Braren, M., Zubin, J., & John, E. R. (1965). Evoked-potential correlates of stimulus uncertainty. *Science, 150*(3700), 1187-1188. http://dx.doi.org/10.1126/science.150.3700.1187

Szentágothai, J., & Hamori, J. (1969). Growth and differentiation of synaptic structures under circumstances of deprivation of function and of distant connections. In S. H. Barondes (Ed.), *Cellular dynamics of the neuron* (Vol. 8) (pp. 301-320). London, UK: Academic Press, Inc. https://doi.org/10.1016/B978-0-12-611908-4.50021-6

Talati, A., & Hirsch, J. (2005). Functional specialization within the medial frontal gyrus for perceptual go/no-go decisions based on "what", "when", and "where" related information: An fMRI study. *Journal of Cognitive Neuroscience, 17*(7), 981-993. https://doi.org/10.1162/0898929054475226

Tamraz, J. C., & Comair, Y. G. (2000). *Atlas of regional anatomy of the brain using MRI: With functional correlations.* New York: Springer.

Tan, G., Shaffer, F., Teo, I., & Lyle, R. R. (2016). *Evidence-based practice in biofeedback and neurofeedback* (3rd ed.). Wheat Ridge, CO: The Association for Applied Psychophysiology and Biofeedback.

Tarrant, J. M. (2017). Neuromeditation: An introduction an overview. In T. F. Collura & J. A. Frederick (Eds.), *Handbook of clinical QEEG and neurotherapy* (pp. 64-81). New York and London: Routledge.

Teipel, S. J., Pogarell, O., Meindl, T., Dietrich, O., Sydykova, D., Hunklinger, U., … Hampel, H. (2009). Regional networks underlying interhemispheric connectivity: An EEG and DTI study in healthy ageing and amnestic mild cognitive impairment. *Human Brain Mapping, 30*(7), 2098-2119. 10.1002/hbm.20652

Thatcher, R. W. (2008). Z-score EEG biofeedback: Conceptual foundations. *NeuroConnections, April*, 22-25.

Thayer, J. F., Hansen, A. L., Saus-Rose, E., & Johnsen, B. H. (2009). Heart rate variability, prefrontal neural function, and cognitive performance: The neurovisceral integration perspective on self-regulation, adaptation, and health. *Annals of Behavioral Medicine, 37*(2), 141-153. https://doi.org/10.1007/s12160-009-9101-z

Thompson, M. (Ed.). (1979). *A resident's guide to psychiatric education.* New York: Plenum Publishing.

Thompson, M., & Thompson, L. (2003). *The neurofeedback book: An introduction to basic concepts in applied psychophysiology* (1st ed.). Wheat Ridge, CO : Association for Applied Psychophysiology and Biofeedback.

Thompson, M., & Thompson, L. (2015). *The neurofeedback book: An introduction to basic concepts in applied psychophysiology* (2nd ed.). Wheat Ridge, CO: The Association for Applied Psychophysiology and Biofeedback.

Thorndike, E. L. (1911). *Animal intelligence: Experimental studies* (Animal Behavior Series). New York: Macmillan Company.

Travis, F., & Shear, J. (2010). Focused attention, open monitoring and automatic self-transcending: Categories to organize meditations from Vedic, Buddhist and Chinese traditions. *Consciousness and Cognition, 19*(4), 1110-1118. https://doi.org/10.1016/j.concog.2010.01.007

Van der Kolk, B. A. (2014). *The body keeps the score: Brain, mind, and body in the healing of trauma.* New York, NY: Viking Books.

Van Doren, J., Arns, M., Heinrich, H., Vollebregt, M., Strehl, U., & K Loo, S. (2019). Sustained effects of neurofeedback in ADHD: A systematic review and meta-analysis. *European Child & Adolescent Psychiatry, 28*(3), 293-305. https://doi.org/10.1007/s00787-018-1121-41121–4

Vossel, S., Thiel, C. M., & Fink, G. R. (2006). Cue validity modulates the neural correlates of covert endogenous orienting of attention in parietal and frontal cortex. *NeuroImage, 32*(3), 1257-1264. https://doi.org/10.1016/j.neuroimage.2006.05.019

Walker J. E., Lawson, R., & Kozlowski, G. (2007). Current status of QEEG and neurofeedback in the treatment of clinical depression. In J. R. Evans (Ed.), *Handbook of neurofeedback* (Haworth Series in Neurotherapy) (pp. 341-351). New York: The Haworth Medical Press/Routledge.

Walter, W. G., Cooper, R., Aldridge, V. J., McCallum, W. C., & Winter, A. L. (1964). Contingent negative variation: An electric sign of sensori-motor association and expectancy in the human brain. *Nature, 203*, 380-384. http://dx.doi.org/10.1038/203380a0

Warner, S. (2013, January). *Cheat sheet for neurofeedback.* http://www.stresstherapysolutions.com/uploads/STSCheatSheetoftheBrain.pdf

Warrier, C., Wong, P., Penhune, V., Zatorre, R., Parrish, T., Abrams, D., & Kraus, N. (2009). Relating structure to function: Heschl's gyrus and acoustic processing. *Journal of Neuroscience, 29*(1), 61-69. http://dx.doi.org/10.1523/JNEUROSCI.3489-08.2009

Watson, J. B., & Rayner, R. (1920). Conditioned emotional reactions. *Journal of Experimental Psychology, 3*(1), 1-14.

WebMD. (n. d.). *Dystonia: Causes, types, symptoms, and treatments.* https://www.webmd.com/brain/dystonia-causes-types-symp-toms-and-treatments#1

White, N. E. (1999). Theories of the effectiveness of alpha-theta training for multiple disorders. In J. Evans & A. Abarbanel (Eds.), *Intro-duction to quantitative EEG and neurofeedback* (pp. 341-367). San Diego, CA: Academic Press.

Yerkes, R. M., & Dodson, J. D. (1908). The relation of strength of stimulus to rapidity of habit formation. *Journal of Comparative Neurology & Psychology, 18*, 459-482. https://doi.org/10.1002/cne.920180503

Yucha, C. B., & Montgomery, D. (2008). *Evidence-based practice in biofeedback and neurofeedback* (2nd ed.). Association for Applied Psychophysiology and Biofeedback.

Additional Reading

Abbott, K. (2017). The use of surface 19-channel Z-score training to ameliorate symptoms remaining or apparently caused after withdrawal of those medications. In T. F. Collura & J. A. Frederick (Eds.), *Handbook of clinical QEEG and neurotherapy* (pp. 421-430). New York and London: Routledge.

Acheson, D. T., Twamley, E. W., & Young, J. W. (2013). Reward learning as a potential target for pharmacological augmentation of cognitive remediation for schizophrenia: A roadmap for preclinical development. *Frontiers in Neuroscience, 7*, 103. https://doi.org/10.3389/fnins.2013.00103

Allen, A. J., Leonard, H., & Swedo, S. E. (1995). Current knowledge of medications for the treatment of childhood anxiety disorders. *Journal of the American Academy of Child and Adolescent Psychiatry, 34*(8), 976-986. https://doi.org/10.1097/00004583-199508000-00007

Allen, M. D., Bigler, E. D., Larsen, J., Goodrich-Hunsaker, N. J., & Hopkins, R. O. (2007). Functional neuroimaging evidence for high cognitive effort on the Word Memory Test in the absence of external incentives. *Brain Injury, 21*(13-14), 1425-1428. https://doi.org/10.1080/02699050701769819

Arns, M., & Kenemans, J. L. (2014). Neurofeedback in ADHD and insomnia: Vigilance stabilization through sleep spindles and circadian networks. *Neuroscience and Biobehavioral Reviews, 44*, 183-194. https://doi.org/10.1016/j.neubiorev.2012.10.006

Beck, E. C., Doty, R. W., & Kooi, K. A. (1958). Electrocortical reactions associated with conditioned flexion reflexes. *Electroencephalography and Clinical Neurophysiology, 10*(2), 279-289. https://doi.org/10.1016/0013-4694(58)90035-x

Bennett, C., Gupta, R., Prabhaka, P., Christopher, R., Sampath, S., Thennarasu, K., & Rajeswaran, J. (2018). Clinical and biochemical outcomes following EEG neurofeedback training in traumatic brain injury in the context of spontaneous recovery. *Clinical EEG and Neuroscience, 49*(6), 433-440. https://doi.

org/10.1177/1550059417744899

Biggs, A., Brough, P., & Drummond, S. (2017). Lazarus and Folkman's psychological stress and coping theory. In C. L. Cooper & J. C. Quick (Eds.), *The handbook of stress and health: A guide to research and practice* (1st ed.) (pp. 351-364). John Wiley & Sons. https://doi.org/10.1002/9781118993811.ch21

Gapen, M.,Van der Kolk, B., Hamlin ,E., Hirshberg, L., Suvak, M., & Spinazzola, J. (2016). A pilot study of neurofeedback for chronic PTSD. *Applied Psychophysiology and Biofeedback, 41*(3), 251-261. https://doi.org/10.1007/s10484-015-9326-5

Gessel, A. H. (1989). Edmund Jacobson, M.D., Ph.D: The founder of scientific relaxation. *International Journal of Psychosomatics, 36*(1-4), 5-14.

Ghaziri, J., Tucholka, A., Larue, V., Blanchette-Sylvestre, M., Rey-burn, G., Gilbert, G., … Beauregard, M. (2013). Neuro-feedback training induces changes in white and grey matter. *Clinical EEG and Neuroscience, 4*(4), 265-272. https://doi.org/10.1177/1550059413476031

Hamilton, J. P., Glover, G. H., Bagarinao, E., Chang, C., Mackey, S., Sacchet, M. D., & Gotlib, I. H. (2016). Effects of salience- net-work-node neurofeedback training on affective biases in major depressive disorder. *Psychiatry Research. Neuroimaging, 249*, 91-96. https://doi.org/10.1016/j.pscychresns.2016.01.016

Hammond, D. C. (2005). Neurofeedback with anxiety and affective dis-orders. *Child and Adolescent Psychiatric Clinics of North Ameri-ca, 14*(1), 105-123. https://doi.org/10.1016/j.chc.2004.07.008

Hammond, D. C. (2011). Placebos and neurofeedback: A case for facil-itating and maximizing placebo response in neurofeedback treat-ments. *Journal of Neurotherapy, 15*(2), 94-114. https://doi.org/10.1080/10874208.2011.570694

Hammond, D. C., & Baehr, E. (2009). Neurofeedback for the treatment of depression: Current status of theoretical issues and clinical research. In T. H. Budzynski, J. R. Evans, H. Kogan Budzynski, & A. Abarbanel (Eds.), *Inroduction to quantitative EEG and neuro-feedback: Advanced theory and applications* (2nd ed.) (pp. 295-

313). New York, NY: Academic Press.

Hardt, J. V., & Kamiya, J. (1978). Anxiety change through electroencephalographic alpha feedback seen only in high anxiety subjects. *Science, 201*(4350), 79-81. https://doi.org/10.1126/science.663641

Johnson, R. (1986). A triarchic model of P300 amplitude. *Psychophysiology, 23*(4), 367-384. https://doi.org/10.1111/j.1469-8986.1986.tb00649.x

Koberda, J. L. (2017). QEEG (brain mapping) and LORETA Z-score neurofeedback in neuropsychiatric practice. In T. F. Collura & J. A. Frederick (Eds.), *Handbook of clinical QEEG and neurotherapy* (pp. 158-183). New York and London: Routledge.

Larson, S. (2006). *The healing power of neurofeedback: The revolutionary LENS technique for restoring optimal brain function.* Rochester, VT: Healing Arts Press.

Longo, R. E. (2018). *A consumer's guide to understanding QEEG brain mapping and neurofeedback training.* Bloomington, IN: iUniverse.

Longo, R. E., & Russo, G. M. (2017). Working with forensic populations: Incorporating peripheral biofeedback and brainwave biofeedback into your organisation or practice. In T. F. Collura & J. A. Frederick (Eds.), *Handbook of clinical QEEG and neurotherapy* (pp. 92-105). New York and London: Routledge.

Lubar, J. F., & Bahler, W. W. (1976). Behavioral management of epileptic seizuresfollowing EEG biofeedback training of the sensorimotor rhythm. *Biofeedback and Self-Regulation, 7,* 77-104.

MacKay, D. J. C. (2003). *Information theory, inference and learning algorithms* (1st ed.). Cambridge, UK: Cambridge University Press.

Pascual-Marqui, R. D. (2002). Standardized low-resolution brain electromagnetic tomography (sLORETA): Technical details. *Methods and Findings in Experimental and Clinical Pharmacology, 24*(D), 5-12.

Pineda, J. A., Friedrich, E. V. C., & LaMarca, K. (2014). Neurorehabilitation of social dysfunctions: A model-based neurofeedback approach for low and high-functioning autism. *Frontiers in Neu-*

roengineering, 7, 29. https://doi.org/10.3389/fneng.2014.00029

Porges, S. W. (2009). The polyvagal theory: New insights into adaptive reactions of the autonomic nervous system. *Cleveland Clinic Journal of Medicine, 76*(S2), 86-90. https://doi.org/10.3949/ccjm.76.s2.17

Rossiter, T. R., & La Vaque, T. J. (1995). A comparison of EEG biofeed-back and psychostimulants in treating attention deficit/hyperac-tivity disorders. *Journal of Neurotherapy, 1*(1), 48-59. https://doi.org/10.1300/J184v01n01_07

Rutter, M. (2011). Research review: Child psychiatric diagnosis and classification: concepts, findings, challenges and potential. *Journal of child psychology and psychiatry, and allied disciplines, 52*(6), 647-660. https://doi.org/10.1111/j.1469-7610.2011.02367.x

Schabus, M., Heib, D. P., Lechinger, J., Griessenberger, H., Klimesch, W., Pawlizki, A., ... Hoedlmoser, K. (2014). Enhancing sleep quality and memory in insomnia using instrumental sensorimotor rhythm conditioning. *Biological Psychology, 95*, 126-134. https://doi.org/10.1016/j.biopsycho.2013.02.020

Sherrington, C. E. (1975). Charles Scott Sherrington (1857-1952). *Notes and Records of the Royal Society of London, 30*(1), 45-63. https://doi.org/10.1098/rsnr.1975.0005

Smith, M. L. (2017). sLORETA in clinical practice. In T. F. Collura & J. A. Frederick (Eds.), *Handbook of clinical QEEG and neurothera-py* (pp. 283-299). New York and London: Routledge.

Steffert, T., & Steffert B. (2017). Rhythms of dyslexia: EEG, ERP and neurofeedback. In T. F. Collura & J. A. Frederick (Eds.), *Handbook of clinical QEEG and neurotherapy* (pp. 213-234). NewYork and London: Routledge.

Steiner, N. J., Frenette. E. C., Rene, K. M., Brennan, R. T., & Perrin, E. C. (2014). In-school neurofeedback training for ADHD: Sustained improvements from a randomized control trial. *Pediatrics, 133*(3), 483-492. https://doi.org/10.1542/peds.2013-2059

Stoller, L. (2017). Alpha-theta-based clinical outreach. In T. F. Collura & J. A. Frederick (Eds.), *Handbook of clinical QEEG and neu-*

rotherapy (pp. 464-473). New York and London: Routledge.

Sudre, G., Szekely, E., Sharp, W., Kasparek, S., & Shaw, P. (2017). Multimodal mapping of the brain's functional connectivity and the adult outcome of attention deficit hyperactivity disorder. *Proceedings of the National Academy of Sciences of the United States of America, 114*(44), 11787-11792. https://doi.org/10.1073/pnas.1705229114

Swingle, P. (2017). Neurotherapy for clinicians in the trenches: The clinical and braindriving. In T. F. Collura & J. A. Frederick (Eds.), *Handbook of clinical QEEG and neurotherapy* (pp. 404-419). New York and London: Routledge.

Tan, G., Wang, P., & Ginsberg, J. (2013). Heart rate variability and post-traumatic stress disorder. *Biofeedback, 41*(3), 131-135. https://doi.org/10.5298/1081-5937-41.3.05

Thapar, A., Cooper, M., & Rutter, M. (2017). Neurodevelopmental disorders. *The Lancet. Psychiatry, 4*(4), 339-346. https://doi.org/10.1016/S2215-0366(16)30376-5

Thornton, K. E. (2016). Neurotherapy and connectivity. *Biofeedback, 4,* 218-224. https://doi.org/10.5298/1081-5937-44.4.03

Toyama, K., & Matsunami, K. (1976). Convergence of specific visual and commissural impulses upon inhibitory interneurones in cats visual cortex. *Neuroscience, 1*(2), 107- https://doi.org/12.10.1016/0306-4522(76)90004-x

Trans Cranial Technologies Ltd. (2012*). Cortical functions. Manual.* https://thebrainstimulator.net/docs/external/Trans_Cranial_Technologies-cortical_functions_ref_v1_0.pdf

Walker, J. E. (2017). QEEG-guided neurofeedback to normalize brain function in various disorders. In T. F. Collura & J. A. Frederick (Eds.), *Handbook of clinical EEG and neurotherapy* (pp. 149-157). New York and London: Routledge.

Walton, R. G. (n. d.). *Survey of Aspartame studies: Correlation of outcome and funding sources.* https://www.lightenyourtoxicload.com/wp-content/uploads/2014/07/Dr-Walton-survey-of-aspartame-studies.pdf

Index

19Channel PZOK 159

Firing In Unison 56, 57
Fissure 82, 95, 108
Flat EEG 72
Focal Epileptiform Activity 67
Focused Attention 66, 134, 199, 201, 204
Forebrain 78, 79, 87, 114, 176
Four Channel Assessment 10, 155
Freeze Mechanism 227

Freeze Response 252, 254, 256, 268
Frontal Alpha Asymmetry 235, 236, 237, 239, 242
Frontal Lobe 42, 52, 62, 84, 85, 91, 92, 94, 95, 212, 237, 288, 306, 339
Front Temporal 85
Functional Groups 57, 112

G

GABA 113, 115, 176, 177, 226
Gamma 56, 64, 65, 66, 115, 118, 124, 198, 199, 200
Generalized Asynchronous Slow Waves 72
George Ohm 116
Glia 78
Glial Cells 49, 78, 83
Globus Pallidius 87
Glutamate 108, 115, 148

Glycine 115
Grey Matter 82, 94, 188, 319
Ground 25, 49, 51, 117, 129, 144, 154, 166, 171, 172, 196, 212, 300, 309, 334
Gyri 78, 92, 93, 94, 95
Gyrus 82, 90, 91, 92, 93, 94, 95, 97, 98, 101, 103, 104, 105, 152, 202

H

Handbook of Clinical EEG and Neurotherapy 148, 230, 231
Headache 46, 53, 54, 136, 138, 288, 304, 327, 333, 352
Heart Rate (HR) 53, 133, 162, 173, 174, 175, 178, 180, 181, 182, 183, 194, 226, 229, 234, 256, 284, 287, 297, 309
Heart Rate Variability (HRV) 162, 182, 183, 229, 284, 287, 297, 309
Heightened Activity 53
Heroine 115
High Beta 64, 65, 66, 122
Higher Cortical Regions 265
High Pass Filter 118

Hindbrain 78
Hippocampal Formation 259
Hippocampus 58, 60, 89, 94, 114, 176, 192, 223, 231
Horizontal 150
Horizontal Axis 132
Hyperalgesia 188
Hyper- Arousal 63, 180
Hyperarousal 270
Hyper-Aroused 63, 256
Hyper- Aroused Nervous System 265
Hyper- Coherence Of Beta 65
Hypervigilance 64, 143, 259
Hypo- Aroused 63
Hypothalamus 89

I

Imagery 11, 102, 184

Immersed Attention 193

Immune Response 177
Impedance 116, 117
Impulsiveness 53
Impulsivity 136, 137, 141, 142, 145, 267
Inferior 80, 81, 86, 91, 92, 93, 94, 95, 259
Inferior Frontal Gyrus 91, 105
Inferior Parietal Lobule 86, 259
Inferior Parietal Lobule 152
Inferior Temporal Gyrus 92, 101
Infinite Impulse Response (IIR) 10, 119
Inhibition 68, 89, 91, 112, 113, 134, 182, 212, 216, 251, 262, 263, 264, 266

Inhibitory 88, 107, 108, 109, 111, 113, 114, 115, 173, 174, 243
Inion 51, 52, 253, 254, 270, 273
Inion Ridge 253, 254, 270, 273
Insomnia 12, 47, 75, 309
Instability Of The Cns 272
Insula 95, 152
Intake Procedure 40, 48, 353
Inter-Ictal 67
International 10/20 Placement System 39
Intrinsic Rhythm 58
Intuitive Approaches 40
Irritability 53, 137, 179, 189, 234
Isf 10, 120, 126, 161, 162, 163, 210, 231, 275, 297, 301, 304

J

Joint Time Frequency Analysis 10, 120

Joint Time Frequency Analysis (JTFA) 10, 120

K

K Complexes 70

L

Laminar Nuclei 113
Lamina Terminalis 95
Laplacian Montage 121
Lateral 81, 90, 91, 92, 93, 94, 95, 105, 112, 113, 254, 339
Learned Normalization 41
Learning Paradigms 34, 37, 51, 128
Left Frontal Lobe 42, 62, 237
Left Hemisphere 16, 79, 80, 83, 86, 93, 130, 134, 149, 150, 210, 235, 257
Levels Of Efficacy 45, 48, 128
Limbic Oscillatory Activity 131
Limbic System 60, 79, 84, 85, 89, 90, 94, 116, 223
Linear Analysis 111

Lithium 124
Live Z-Score 34, 50, 126, 141, 153, 154, 210, 291, 297, 350
Localized Slow Waves 71
Locus Coeruleus 175, 176, 238
Longitudinal Cerebral Fissure 82
Long Term Potentiation (LTP) 115
Loving Kindness 192, 200
Low Arousal 59, 123, 134, 140, 210, 315, 322
Low Beta 64, 65, 66, 70, 111, 112, 119, 123
Low Blood Sugar Symptoms 54
Low Pass Filter 118, 120

M

Macrocolumn 109
Marijuana 124
Medial 80, 81, 86, 89, 92, 94, 95, 251, 259, 263
Medial Frontal Gyrus 92
Medial Pre-Frontal Cortex 251
Medial Surface 86, 92, 95
Medial Temporal Lobe 89
Meditation 16, 26, 28, 30, 33, 62, 163, 165, 169, 178, 184, 185, 186, 190, 191, 192, 193, 196, 197, 198, 199, 200, 201, 202, 203, 204, 205, 251, 285, 327
Melatonin 114
Memory Network 76
Mental Disorder 209
Metacognition 85
Metacognitive Skills 38
Methylphenidate 124, 212, 215, 216
Micro Voltages 56
Midbrain 78, 88, 253, 254, 255

Middle Frontal Gyrus 92
Middle Temporal Gyrus 92, 101
Midrange Beta 65
Mindfulness 192, 200, 203, 204, 251, 285, 353
Mini-Q 155
Mini QEEG Recording 49
Minnesota Multiphasic Personality Inventory (MMPI) 236
Modulation 57, 155, 250, 304, 370
Modulation Of Stress 250
Montage 109, 121, 122, 301, 369
Morphine 115, 124, 253
Morphology 56, 58, 59, 60, 61, 64, 65
Motor Homunculus 84
Mu Rhythm 8, 69
Muscle Artefact 66, 122
Myelinated 83, 227, 285
Myelinated Axons 83
Myofascial Pain 47, 188

N

Narrow Focus 191, 193, 194, 196, 197
Nasion 51, 52
National Institute Of Mental Health 15, 26, 207, 220
Negative Reinforcement 35
Neglect 246, 248, 249, 250, 252, 254, 261, 262, 265, 266, 267, 269, 271, 275
Neuroanatomy 77, 128, 275
Neuroception 256
Neurofeedback 4, 15, 16, 17, 18, 19, 20, 21, 22, 23, 24, 25, 26, 27, 28, 29, 30, 31, 32, 33, 34, 36, 37, 38, 39, 40, 41, 42, 43, 44, 45, 48, 49, 50, 54, 55, 56, 61, 66, 67, 68,

69, 74, 76, 79, 96, 106, 107, 111, 113, 115, 116, 120, 122, 123, 126, 127, 128, 129, 130, 131, 132, 134, 135, 139, 140, 143, 144, 147, 148, 149, 152, 153, 154, 155, 158, 161, 163, 166, 167, 168, 169, 170, 173, 176, 177, 184, 190, 191, 192, 193, 198, 199, 201, 202, 203, 205, 206, 210, 212, 213, 214, 215, 216, 217, 218, 219, 222, 225, 229, 230, 231, 232, 233, 235, 236, 237, 238, 242, 243, 244, 245, 246, 248, 252, 253, 254, 256, 257, 259, 261, 265, 266, 269, 270, 271, 273, 274, 275,

R

Raphe Nuclei 237
RAS 58, 134
Ratio 29, 36, 60, 72, 73, 210, 213, 214
Ratios 9, 72
Rauwolfia 124
Reactive Attachment Disorder 138, 146
Receptive Aphasia 95
Receptor Site 114
Reference 45, 48, 49, 51, 64, 117, 118, 121, 129, 144, 153, 159, 160, 171, 172, 181, 191, 212, 236, 314
Reflex Response 36
Refractory Period 110
Regulation 16, 22, 23, 28, 33, 37, 43, 44, 53, 54, 55, 57, 80, 89, 90, 113, 114, 123, 139, 145, 148, 156, 159, 161, 162, 168, 176, 177, 181, 182, 199, 212, 245, 248, 249, 250, 251, 256, 257, 259, 265, 266, 267, 270, 271, 274, 275, 276, 288, 291, 294, 315, 364, 366, 370
Reinforcers 36, 170
Relaxing State 28, 56, 260
REM Sleep 124
Research Information 45, 106, 235
Resistance 24, 116, 158, 230, 335
Respiratory Rate 133, 173
Respiratory Sinus Arrhythmia (RSA) 178, 182, 287
Resting Rhythm 65, 215
Reticular Activating System 58, 114, 134
Rhinencephalon 95
Right Hemisphere 65, 79, 80, 83, 93, 131, 134, 149, 150, 189, 211, 235, 284
Rostral 80, 98

S

Sadness 54, 181, 233, 234, 239, 241, 242, 245, 269, 345, 361
Sagittal 81, 150
Salience Network 258
Sampling 9, 118
Schizophrenia 31, 59, 63, 88, 94, 209
Scientific Foundation 39
Scientific Principles 40, 41
SCP 161, 213, 214, 215, 217
Secondary Reinforcement 36
Seizure 29, 31, 56, 67, 68, 69, 70, 124, 126, 127, 128, 180, 272, 274, 317, 318, 319, 335, 362
Seizure Activity 29, 56, 67, 69, 70, 124, 126, 127, 180, 318, 319
Self-Harm 267
Self-Regulation 22, 181, 199, 212, 245, 276
SEMG 29, 187, 188
Sensorimotor System 131
Sensory-Motor Cortex 76
Sensory Motor Strip 211, 271, 296, 322, 350, 353
Sensory Overload 268
Septal Area 60
Septal Nucleus 89
Sequential Montage 121
Serotonin 114, 124, 176, 226
Serotonin (5-Hydroxy-Trypamine, 5-Ht) 114
Sexual Abuse 247, 248, 267, 320
Sharp Transients 8, 70
Sharp Waves 67, 70

List of Illustrations